Ethical Foundations of Palliative Care for Alzheimer Disease

Ethical Foundations of Palliative Care for Alzheimer Disease

Edited by

Ruth B. Purtilo, Ph.D.

James Marsh Presidential Professor-at-Large, University of Vermont, Burlington, Vermont
Professor Emerita, MGH Institute of Health Professions, Boston, Massachusetts

and

Henk A.M.J. ten Have, M.D., Ph.D.

Professor of Medical Ethics
University Medical Centre Nijmegen, The Netherlands
Director, Division of Ethics of Science and Technology
UNESCO, Paris, France

Foreword by

Christine K. Cassel, M.D.

The Johns Hopkins University Press
Baltimore

© 2004 The Johns Hopkins University Press
All rights reserved. Published 2004
Printed in the United States of America on acid-free paper

Johns Hopkins Paperback edition, 2010

9 8 7 6 5 4 3 2 1

The Johns Hopkins University Press
2715 North Charles Street
Baltimore, Maryland 21218-4363
www.press.jhu.edu

*The Library of Congress has catalogued the hardcover edition of this book
as follows:*

Ethical foundations of palliative care for Alzheimer disease / edited by
Ruth B. Purtilo and Henk A.M.J. ten Have.
    p.   ; cm.
Includes bibliographical references and index.
ISBN 0-8018-7870-5 (hardcover : alk. paper)
1. Alzheimer's disease—Patients—Palliative treatment—Moral and ethical
aspects. 2. Palliative treatment—Moral and ethical aspects.
3. Alzheimer's disease—Patients—Hospice care—Moral and ethical
aspects.
[DNLM: 1. Alzheimer Disease—nursing. 2. Ethics, Professional.
3. Palliative Care. WT 155 E84 2004] I. Purtilo, Ruth B. II. Have, H. ten.
RC522.E86 2004
362.196′831—dc22   2003017424

A catalog record for this book is available from the British Library.

ISBN 13: 978-0-8018-9839-6
ISBN 10: 0-8018-9839-0

Contents

Foreword

Alzheimer disease has been a classic paradigm in medical ethics. The progressive and inexorable loss of cognitive function challenges every principle on which Western medical ethics is based. These include the fundamental respect for the autonomy of the individual on which the principles of informed consent are based, premised on an individual's capacity and inalienable right to decide what should be done with his or her own body. As one loses one's memory, one's personality, and indeed one's identity to the dementing illness of Alzheimer disease, all of those principles are called into question. The tidy nostrum of advance directives does not really provide psychological, spiritual, or personal reassurance that one is doing the right thing for a patient who seems to be a different person from the one who executed the directive. Of course, directives themselves have not been used as widely as ethicists had hoped, leaving many people facing decisions throughout the course of their medical care where quality of life must be balanced by surrogate decision makers. Health care professionals who value intelligence—perhaps above all else—struggle to make sense of quality-of-life determinations for a person who does not recognize even the closest family members and must be assisted in every aspect of basic daily living functions.

Alzheimer disease has also challenged the deeper philosophies of mind and of identity. The very nature of personhood and the meaning of memory are challenged by this disorder. In the United States, our focus is almost entirely on the rights and values of the individual patient and yet the experience of dementing illness—as much as any other human experience—is one that is shared with family, friends, caregivers, and those who happen to share one's room in the nursing home. What has been the meaning of the phenomenon of dementia not only in the person who suffers the illness but also in the person who suffers the experience of watching it happen? Or in the broader community of aging societies around the world? Does it give rise to a collective empathy that transcends individualism? Does it vary from society to society, even within Western nations?

Dementing illness has a major role in our understanding of societal attitudes about aging—an issue of enormous importance as the success story of the aging of advanced civilizations worldwide challenges our concepts of family, of priorities, and of the productivity and role of older people in our society. I believe that dementing illness is the single most powerful factor in the negative attitudes about aging that occur in our society and throughout the world. If modern biomedical science can find an effective treatment or preventive measure for this disease, it would do more to improve attitudes toward aging than would anything else. This, of course, is vitally important because the vast majority of older people do not have dementia; and as we move into a time in the next few decades when one out of five individuals in this country and in developed European nations that participated in this conference will be over the age of 65, it is essential that this population not be marginalized but rather find an integral and meaningful role in every aspect of society. The stereotype of the elderly person as inevitably "losing it" is an enormous barrier to progress in productive aging.

And yet, frailty is an inevitable concomitant of our increased longevity. How we treat our most vulnerable citizens is as much a marker of progress as the advance of biomedical science. Moral dimensions of this challenge are identified and clarified by the authors of the essays in this volume. They treat the issues with the full complexity they deserve, in a spectrum from early diagnosis to end-of-life care.

The palliative care movement in the United States has reminded modern medicine of human mortality and has shown us that even though we cannot cure many illnesses, it is not true that "there is nothing left to do." The leaders in palliative care have dramatically shifted our understanding of the role of medicine, health care, and indeed communities and families in enhancing the quality of life to relieve suffering and give meaning to each day. This movement has progressed beyond the pharmacological treatment of pain and the model of an individual with widely metastatic cancer in rapid decline to the less predictable, more prolonged, and more clinically challenging question of the palliative care of a person with Alzheimer disease. These authors remind us that a neat division between life-prolonging treatment and palliative treatment is not always so clear and that important subtle and sophisticated distinctions rest on a much broader understanding of the nature of suffering and the inclusion of family and caregivers in that experience of suffering.

The chapters in this book were developed from a conference that brought together all these different directions at a perfect time for health care and for bioethics. The worlds of policy and practice are hungry for such a thoughtful set of discussions. Its unique advantage is the interaction of clinicians and philosophers in an international context where idiosyncrasies of each individual country quickly become less important as one realizes that the universal challenges of identity, compassion, and personhood affect all of us. Anthropologists have pointed out that some populations in India do not know the concept of dementia in old age. In their research, they discovered not that there is a unique genetic phenomenon in which those populations escape the ravages of dementia in old age, but rather that they have ways of understanding it not as an illness but as a characteristic of the person. This allows an approach to caring for those older people within the family and community in ways that do not exclude them or make them "other." Modern science has called the phenomenon of dementia in old age a disease, leading to major commitments to important research and giving families a way to understand what is happening to their loved one. The challenge for the medical model is not to let that disease designation create a stigma that isolates and distances us from the basic humanity at the core of the caring professions. This remarkable collection of essays reminds us of the importance of looking cross-culturally in our approach to illness, disability, and mortality as we understand the universality of the moral claim that Alzheimer disease represents.

Christine K. Cassel, M.D.
President, American Board of Internal Medicine and ABIM Foundation

Preface

The editors and chapter contributors invite you, the reader, into a dialogue focused on a set of engaging and important issues emerging around Alzheimer disease (AD). As a group, we are exploring the ethical foundations of a palliative care approach to AD, drawing on the perspectives of scholars and clinicians in Europe and the United States.

Today's student may assume that AD "has always been with us," but—as the introduction to this book highlights—it is a relative newcomer to the world of identified diseases. Not surprisingly, new information continues to be released about how to diagnose and treat the condition as well as the toll that AD is taking on individuals, families, caregivers in the health professions, and society. Not surprisingly, either, debate about this information flourishes.

The personal, clinical, and social burdens of AD slowly are reaching a level of global consciousness. The growing concern is not only that a sufficient level of care be provided but also that care services meet high moral standards. To articulate and implement such standards, we need ethical research and reflection. Moreover, with the recognition that prevention and cure are ultimate goals but may be many years into the future, that AD as an incurable condition calls for palliative measures, and that the scope and utility of palliative interventions are still being assessed, we identified the need to focus on ethical foundations of palliative care that will serve at least U.S. and European societies well in their attempts to deal humanely with the challenge AD poses.

The purpose of this book is to provide a resource for:

- health professionals, policymakers, and ethicists on both sides of the Atlantic who are becoming aware of and beginning to address challenges imposed on individuals, family members, and society by the presence of AD;

- philosophers and theologians who are prompted to rethink such basic notions as dignity, personal identity, autonomy, authenticity, solidarity, and community in face of the presence of AD; and
- other scholars and policymakers who are focused on creating a just allocation of resources but who are finding themselves pressed to accommodate the financial and other burdens of the condition.

All of these groups must make decisions in, add to the scholarship about, provide thoughtful input into, or prepare others for situations involving palliative care for persons with AD. Today these activities must be carried out within a largely unexplored ethical terrain, since in the main the ethical issues, with rare exceptions, remain at the margins of consideration in mainstream U.S. and European bioethics. This book adds relevant expertise while redressing an increasingly serious gap in the literature.

Claiming what we saw as an important opportunity to provide leadership in this emerging area, the editors of this volume contacted thirty scholars whom we believed were not only qualified but would be willing to contribute to a joint European—U.S. exploration into the ethical foundations of palliative care for AD. Each was to participate in the dialogue over a period of at least three years. The twenty-two who responded favorably included health professionals (physicians, nurses, a physical therapist, a dentist) and scholars in the fields of bioethics, philosophy, and law. Everyone contributed a draft manuscript to be critiqued in a working conference sponsored by the Greenwall Foundation, New York. The conference was held in Berg en Dal, Netherlands, in November 2001. Participants returned home to further develop their articles as well as engage in continuing online discussion with each other and other scholars in the fields represented. During the next two years, the articles were updated and further refined, then peer reviewed in preparation for publication in this volume.

Several practical challenges have arisen in this multidisciplinary, international exploration. One was the term to use in referring to persons who have AD. Authors varied in their terminology, some using "demented patient" or "patients with dementia" as well as "patients with Alzheimer disease." Through discussion, we learned that the term "demented" is more acceptable in Europe than in the United States. In any case, we were aware that any terminology is a reflection of moral viewpoints. For example, a quandary arose over use of the term "Alzheimer patient." The U.S. Alzheimer's Association and several other U.S. groups are trying to get away from that designation, substituting, instead, "patient [or, preferably, *person*] with Alzheimer disease" to try to decrease the potential for discrimination that the label "Alzheimer patient" might promote. At the same time, a few members of the dialogue point out that this position may neglect the perspective that the disease brings about deep identity changes in the human person, making the expression "Alzheimer patient" more appropriate. Some chapters in this book continue to probe this issue. In the overall project, we allowed for a variation in the terminology to help readers appreciate ambiguities we discovered and to highlight the importance of the rich diversity of language and ideas in international explorations such as ours.

The book is divided into six parts. In part I, three contributions combine to provide a brief overview of health care and larger societal challenges related to the diagnosis and prognosis of AD in the United States and Europe. Brumback's chapter provides the reader with a rare, accessible look into the incessant march of the brain pathology of AD, noting key behavioral and other manifestations commonly observed in persons with the condition at each stage.

In part II the focus shifts to a critique of palliative care as it is administered worldwide. The contributors are all Europeans who have spent significant time assessing the concepts and practices of palliative care and palliative medicine on both sides of the Atlantic. We chose these chapters to enhance the current U.S. discussions of palliative care with insights not often gleaned from U.S. approaches, as well as to bring European colleagues up to date on current international themes.

Part III addresses several key philosophical and theological concerns central to understanding AD (e.g., personal embodiment, autonomy, dependence, dignity) and engages the reader in current discussion around the positions raised in each of the chapters. Janssens, for instance, holds that the traditional approaches of medical ethics must be recast in order to deal with some of the moral issues AD raises. This section of the book is not designed to be completely comprehensive; indeed, in keeping with the tone of the book throughout, the goal is to provoke further debate and reflection on vital topics.

Part IV is composed of five chapters that take up familiar clinical ethics issues in palliative care decision making, turning the kaleidoscope to focus on how each issue fares in the situations presented by AD. The formats range from a narrative, in the form of a family caregiver's letter with the author's reflections, to rigorous ethical analyses of advance directive decision making in situations of AD and of euthanasia as an intervention for patients with AD, to a powerful ethics case study on pain by a Swedish dentist who treats such patients. In part IV the reader will be especially struck by how inseparable the well-being of family caregivers and that of the patient are.

Part V concentrates on the larger organizational ethics issues involved in changing societal patterns of care and institutional and societal policies. One theme is how best to prepare patients and families for the intense institutional and social interactions they will be required to broker in the interest of survival during the months and years following diagnosis, their choice of site for that care, and the education of health professionals for the challenges presented by AD. These chapters offer valuable practical information, but their primary purpose is to highlight the serious ethical concerns embodied in current institutional and social arrangements, on both sides of the Atlantic. The contributors invite discussion about their suggestions for laws, policies, and institutional initiatives that will help sustain the strong moral and social fabric that will be needed for the projected explosion of AD in the next decades, as described in part I. The other theme is the urgent need to base allocation decisions for AD on sound ethical principles and practical realities, thereby assuring sustainable policies and practices that meet with the demands of justice. Understandably, this part includes two authors from Central and East Europe, where the overall resources of health care fall far below those available in West Europe and the United States.

Part VI ends the book appropriately with several ethical aspects of biomedical research regarding AD. The urgent need for responsible research in this area is balanced by several caveats about the direction U.S. and European societies might take in their zeal for preventive and curative successes. The authors share the commitment to such applaudable outcomes, but also provide the reader with guidance on how and when to temper research initiatives so as to sustain family and other relationships as well as the well-being of the purported end point of the entire research enterprise; namely, the person living with AD.

We also call your attention to the two appendixes at the end of this volume—the Declaration of Berg en Dal, which lists ethical principles for palliative care for Alzheimer disease, and a framework for a course on the same topic.

Acknowledgments

The editors acknowledge with gratitude:

The Greenwall Foundation, New York, for a grant to support the development of this book, including the funds for an international working group of scholars to convene at Berg en Dal, Netherlands. This Greenwall Foundation support made it feasible for this book to emerge as one outcome of the ongoing European and U.S. dialogue;

The administration of Creighton University, Omaha, Nebraska, and the University Medical Centre Nijmegen, in Nijmegen, Netherlands, for their commitment to an international dialogue on Alzheimer disease, expressed through their financial and other substantive support for expenses incurred by the coeditors, authors, and support staff in their preparation of this volume.

We also are grateful to:

Ms. Helen Shew, Creighton University Center for Health Policy and Ethics—for her skill, commitment, and patience with us during several phases of the project. We thank her for her key role in coordinating and staffing the Berg en Dal conference and, even more critical, for the hours upon hours she devoted to two years of follow-up, correcting, editing, retyping, and proofing the draft manuscripts while coordinating the efforts of the twenty-two contributors. Without her assistance, this book simply would not have seen the light of day;

Ms. Valesca Hulsman, Department of Ethics, Philosophy, and History of Medicine, University Medical Centre Nijmegen, in Nijmegen, Netherlands, for her leadership, with Helen Shew, in coordinating and staffing the Berg en Dal conference. Her contribution in taking care of the on-site logistics was invaluable;

Ms. Rita Nutty and Ms. Marybeth Goddard, Creighton University Center for

Health Policy and Ethics, for their able assistance as support staff to Helen Shew and the coeditors on this project.

Ruth Purtilo also expresses her gratitude to Ann Caldwell, president, and the faculty and staff of the MGH Institute of Health Professions, Boston, Massachusetts, for their support while she completed the final editing during her nine-month tenure as the Henry Knox Sherrill Visiting Scholar in Ethics (October 2002–July 2003).

We have deeply appreciated the gentle but expert guiding hand of Ms. Wendy Harris, medical editor, and the staff at the Johns Hopkins University Press, throughout the process of producing this book.

Finally, we would be amiss if we failed to thank the families of the participants who bravely supported the attendance of their loved ones at the Berg en Dal conference, held shortly after September 11, 2001. We had an opportunity while there to acknowledge that many of them were reticent to allow their loved ones to travel, some of them far from home, at such an uncertain time. We thank them once again for overcoming their fears—and helping us overcome ours—so that we could proceed with the important work of finding humane solutions to the challenges posed by Alzheimer disease.

Contributors

David A. Bennahum, M.D., Professor of Medicine, Family and Community Medicine and Law, Gerontology Division, and Senior Bioethicist, Ethics Institute, University of New Mexico, Albuquerque, New Mexico

Pierre Boitte, Ph.D., Associate Professor, Faculté Libre de Médecine, and Director, Centre d'éthique médicale, Catholic University of Lille, Lille, France

Roger A. Brumback, M.D., Professor and Chairman, Department of Pathology, Creighton University Medical Center, and Chief, Pathology and Laboratory Medicine Department, Omaha Veterans Affairs Medical Center, Omaha, Nebraska

Wim J. M. Dekkers, M.D., Ph.D., Senior Researcher, Department of Ethics, Philosophy and History of Medicine, University Medical Centre Nijmegen, Nijmegen, The Netherlands

Elizabeth Furlong, R.N., Ph.D., J.D., Associate Professor, School of Nursing, and Faculty Associate, Center for Health Policy and Ethics, Creighton University Medical Center, Omaha, Nebraska

Eugenijus Gefenas, M.D., Ph.D., Associate Professor and Chairman, Department of Medical History and Ethics, Medical Faculty of Vilnius University, and Senior Researcher, Institute of Culture, Philosophy and Art, Vilnius, Lithuania

Bert Gordijn, Ph.D., Senior Researcher, Department of Ethics, Philosophy and History of Medicine, University Medical Centre Nijmegen, Nijmegen, The Netherlands

Amy M. Haddad, R.N., Ph.D., Professor, Department of Pharmacy Sciences, School of Pharmacy and Health Professions, and Professor and Associate Director, Center for Health Policy and Ethics, Creighton University Medical Center, Omaha, Nebraska

Søren Holm, M.D., Ph.D., Dr.Med.Sci., Professor of Clinical Bioethics, Institute of Medicine, Law and Bioethics, University of Manchester, Manchester, United Kingdom, and Centre for Medical Ethics, University of Oslo, Oslo, Norway

Franz J. Illhardt, D.D., Ph.D., Professor of Medical Ethics, Center for Ethics and Law in Medicine, Freiburg University, Freiburg, Germany

Rien Janssens, Ph.D., Senior Researcher, Department of Ethics, Philosophy and History of Medicine, University Medical Centre Nijmegen, Nijmegen, The Netherlands

Givi Javashvili, M.D., Ph.D., Head of the Chair of Family Medicine, State Medical Academy of Georgia, and Vice-chairman, National Council on Bioethics, Tbilisi, Republic of Georgia

Judith Lee Kissell, Ph.D., Assistant Professor, Center for Health Policy and Ethics, Creighton University Medical Center, Omaha, Nebraska

Gunilla Nordenram, D.D.S., Ph.D., Associate Professor, Institute of Odontology, Karolinska Institute, Stockholm, Sweden

Richard L. O'Brien, M.D., University Professor, Center for Health Policy and Ethics, Creighton University Medical Center, Omaha, Nebraska

Marcel G. M. Olde Rikkert, M.D., Ph.D., Associate Professor, Chairman, Department of Geriatric Medicine, University Medical Centre Nijmegen, Nijmegen, The Netherlands

Winifred J. Ellenchild Pinch, R.N., Ed.D., Professor, School of Nursing, and Center for Health Policy and Ethics, Creighton University Medical Center, Omaha, Nebraska

Patricio F. Reyes, M.D., Professor of Neurology, Pathology, and Psychiatry, and Director, Center for the Study of Aging, Alzheimer's Disease, and Neurodegenerative Disorders, Creighton University Medical Center, Omaha, Nebraska

Anne-Sophie Rigaud, M.D., Ph.D., Professor, Chair of Department of Geriatric Medicine, Hôpital Broca, Paris, France

Linda S. Scheirton, Ph.D., Associate Professor, Department of Occupational Therapy, and Faculty Associate, Center for Health Policy and Ethics, Creighton University Medical Center, Omaha, Nebraska

Jos V. M. Welie, M.Med.S., J.D., Ph.D., Associate Professor, Center for Health Policy and Ethics, Creighton University Medical Center, Omaha, Nebraska

Ethical Foundations of Palliative Care
for Alzheimer Disease

Introduction

Historical Overview of a Current Global Challenge

Henk A.M.J. ten Have, M.D., Ph.D., and
Ruth B. Purtilo, Ph.D.

Alzheimer disease (AD) was identified as a particular disease in 1910. The construct was rooted in the concepts and methods of psychiatry and neuropathology in nineteenth-century Germany. However, its existence was disputed from the time of its identification; in particular, it was controversial whether it was distinct from senile dementia and the normal processes of aging (Dillmann, 1990).

The first case was reported by Alois Alzheimer (1864–1915) at a scientific meeting in 1906 in Tübingen, a famous university town in southern Germany. A fifty-one-year-old woman had unusual clinical symptoms that could not be classified within the existing nosological system. Starting with memory failures and an intense jealousy toward her husband, she soon became helpless and disoriented to time and place, with perception disorders and deliria. Her mental state deteriorated rapidly until she was fully bedridden, apathetic, and severely demented. Furthermore, the anatomical patterns found during autopsy were different from those of the usual disease processes. Specific changes in the brain cells were discovered, with tangled bundles of fibrils subsequently replacing the normal neurons, and multiple foci of deposits of a peculiar substance in the cerebral cortex were noted (later known as plaques).

These typical clinical and anatomical observations were possible because of the particular conditions in which Alzheimer worked. He was director of the research laboratories of the newly built psychiatric clinic in Munich. This clinic was established (in 1904) and headed by Emil Kraepelin (1856–1926), one of the leaders of German psychiatry and a professor of psychiatry at the University of Munich. Alzheimer, after working with Kraepelin in Heidelberg, in 1902 moved with his teacher to Munich. Under the direction of Alzheimer, the laboratories developed into the leading research facilities for the neuropathological study of mental disorders. A school of psychiatric researchers was trained there, with Fritz Lewy, Alfons Jakob, and Hans Creutzfeld as disciples of Alzheimer. The focus of the laboratories was on neuropathology, using innovative techniques and instruments such as chemical staining and powerful microscopes to investigate the brains of deceased patients. At the same time, due to the efforts of Kraepelin, psychiatric patients were hospitalized in academic centers for diagnosis and research. This growth of institutional psychiatric care not only was a reaction against the dehumanizing conditions of *Irrenanstalten* ("lunatic asylums"), where patients were merely boarded, but it also was motivated by the need for care and possible cures. For Kraepelin, psychiatry as a medical discipline could emerge only when patients were observed and examined, in order to delineate particular diseases, combining clinical data (Kraepelin introduced a system of patient records) with autopsy findings (van Bakel, 2000).

The interconnection of psychiatric care and neuropathological research was characteristic of German psychiatry for a long time (until 1930). Alzheimer was the first (in 1904) to describe the histopathological changes in the brains of patients with dementia paralytica. In 1907, Alzheimer published his case of the unusual brain disease. Three years later, G. Perusini, an assistant to Alzheimer, published a more extensive report, with four cases (including Alzheimer's earlier one). Perusini did extensive pathological investigations of the brain. He concluded that the findings indicated a disease picture of a characteristic type: the clinical symptoms as well as neuropathology were similar to the changes in senile dementia, but progressed further and at an earlier stage, which he termed "the presenile age period." Both publications motivated Kraepelin to proclaim the existence of a new disease named after Alzheimer. There was a particular set of clinical symptoms that could not be classified under a known clinical pattern. There was also a particular anatomical pattern, made visible with the latest staining techniques and microscopes, indicating particular chemical transformations. For Kraepelin, the clinical symptoms were distinctive and, therefore, determinative in delineating this new disease. However, in Alzheimer's point of view, specific neuropathological changes were considered basic and primary, the clinical symptoms secondary. This scientific view made it rather problematic to demarcate the clinical picture; since the disease basically could exist only when a particular neuropathology (especially neurofibrillary tangles and plaques) had been confirmed, the clinical diagnosis could be made only retrospectively.

Finally, in the eighth edition of his widely read textbook, Kraepelin introduced the concept of "Alzheimer disease," based on the four published cases. Kraepelin assumed a parallel manifestation of clinical symptoms and brain pathology; he therefore concluded that this disease was different from "senile dementia." He gave priority to the peculiar symptoms and the course of the disease (starting at a "presenile" age). Alzheimer himself did not agree: since the neuropathological changes could not always be demonstrated, he dismissed the idea that there was a separate disease. This controversy about the existence of a specific disease was in fact a debate between clinical medicine (giving priority to symptoms and the patient perspective) and medical science (giving priority to pathological changes and the brain-research perspective)—a controversy that has continued for decades in disputes about the nosological status of Alzheimer disease.

It took a long time before it was generally acknowledged that it was unfruitful to discuss whether AD was different from senile dementia and that it was a disease entity not identical with the processes and changes associated with regular aging. Only in the 1970s did a pragmatic consensus emerge that Alzheimer disease was to be regarded as a special category of the clinical syndrome of dementia, a constellation of psychological and behavioral phenomena. The search for related biological phenomena and possible explanations still continues.

In more recent times, the larger social implications have become as compelling as the scientific and medical. Alzheimer disease exacts a heavy toll from afflicted persons, families, and society. Whether it be the gradual, conscious loss of memory and intellectual function, the shame or embarrassment, or the substantial loss of roles and relationships it is a situation that is dreaded by any potential patient. As this book strikingly highlights, Alzheimer caregivers carry heavy personal and social burdens in both economically developed and developing countries. O'Brien and other contributors to this volume show that societal costs of AD are large, and growing larger. Aging populations and slow growth or decline in nations' workforces will increase the societal burden, with fewer productive workers to support the large increase in numbers of AD and related dementia patients. This demographic time bomb affects all nations. It is particularly serious for Europe. These facts present major challenges of distributive justice, of our benevolence to fellow humans, and our respect for those who have contributed to human society but who have become dependent.

In response to these challenges, families, religious groups, grassroots organizations, the health care system, the pharmaceutical industry, governments, and others have begun to search in earnest for answers. Many attempts to discover preventive strategies and curative interventions are being sought. Although hopefully such strategies and interventions will be effective in the future, they do not yet exist. At present, the best we can do is to develop and maintain a high level of care. Persons with AD need interventions that are directed to relief of suffering, pain control, and comfort, often associated with "palliative" rather than preventive or curative measures. However, the symptoms of AD often fail to place such persons in a situation where traditional palliative care resources are available to them. Indeed, more often than not clinicians and others may be unsure about what constitutes effective "palliation" in this case.

In short, the range of ethical and social issues is not new, but societal trends and more knowledge about Alzheimer disease and how to meet the challenges of compassionate, competent, affordable care create an urgent call for attention.

REFERENCES

van Bakel, T. (2000). *Kraepelin over zichzelf* [Kraepelin about himself]. Nijmegen: Sylvius/Candide.
Dillmann, R. (1990). *Alzheimer's disease: The concept of disease and the construction of medical knowledge.* Amsterdam: Thesis Publishers.

Part I / The Health Care Challenge of Alzheimer Disease

Basic Societal, Pathological, and Clinical Issues

CHAPTER ONE

Darkness Cometh

Personal, Social, and Economic Burdens
of Alzheimer Disease

Richard L. O'Brien, M.D.

Alzheimer disease (AD) and related dementias impose immensely heavy burdens on individuals, families, and society. Those with AD suffer terribly, caregivers are robbed of familial and social relationships, families and society pay exorbitant costs for care and lost productivity.

Persons with Alzheimer Disease

Dementia is unfathomable to one who has never experienced it. It can be described, but it can be known only to those who have it. The onset and progress of dementia is insidious and progressive. Those afflicted become slowly aware of memory loss and diminution of their ability to concentrate and sustain higher intellectual functions. At first there is worry over failing memory, then fear that disastrous changes are occurring. When they and their families learn the diagnosis and that the outcome is inevitable, that they will continue to deteriorate, lose cherished human relationships, and become increasingly, and ultimately completely, dependent on others, the sense of loss and impending doom is devastating. Once diagnosed, those with AD are frequently depersonalized by others who position them as incompetent, unable to comprehend or to function, having lost personal attributes, having lost their "self" (Sabat, 2001).

Persons in early stages of dementia experience frustration, embarrassment, and shame from increasing forgetfulness, inability to find words to express themselves, episodes of not knowing where they are, where they have been, or what they have done, and not knowing for certain to whom they are speaking.

> You so often feel that you are stupid for not remembering things or for not knowing things. . . . Just the knowledge that I've goofed again or I said something wrong or I feel like I did something wrong or that I didn't know what I was saying or I forgot. (Henderson, Henderson, & Main, 1998)

> I feel so stupid. . . . I don't remember what I did from minute to minute. (Hoffman, 1994)

> One of the problems of having such a bad memory is the unbelievable waste of time spent looking for things. (Shelia, 2000, p. 3)

Those in the early stages of AD experience fear, guilt, depression, and despair—

> I have pushed myself into depression, and feelings of failure, and guilt for the destruction this disease has wrought. . . . I'm tortured with guilt, and yet I'm helpless to change what has happened to me. (Jan/Mina, 2001)

especially when they are aware that failing memory and their behavior endangers or hurts their loved ones.

> My poor dear husband didn't stop me very much unless it was too outrageous and then I'd get very angry. (Tennis, 1992)

> The worst feeling is that of not being able to trust yourself. (Shelia, 2000, p. 3)

> I can still cook and yet without a doubt can be distracted . . . and completely forget that I have anything on the stove. (Jan/Mina, 2001)

> I never cook when alone . . . but I still can microwave. (Tennis, 1992)

Uncertainty plagues them.

> There's no such thing as having a day which is like another day. Every day is separate. . . . It's as if every day you have never seen anything before like what you're seeing right now. (Henderson, 1998)

> Time seems to run a little differently. (Hoffman, 1994)

The shame and the insecurity of never knowing whether they are or have been functioning well or not, of appearing demented to others, frequently leads persons in these early stages to cover their uncertainty by expressions of anger, confabulation, excuses for lapses, and deceit.

> I'm not sure why I cannot be honest with those around me. (Jan/Mina, 2001)

> I knew something was wrong with me, but I didn't want this to be seen by anyone else. I wanted to stay normal. I was always terrified my wife would find out. (Marshall, 1997)

Increasing uncertainty of how they function and knowledge of growing more dependent on others renders them much more susceptible to depression than others of similar age who are not in these early stages of dementia. As they continue the spiral into the disease, persons with AD reach a point when they are never certain where they are, whom they are with, what time, day, month, or year it is. Uncertainty, disorientation of time, place, and person gives rise to anxiety and fear that manifest themselves in agitation, pacing, sleeplessness, anger, hostility, and combativeness.

> It's a feeling like no other—like your engine is racing 100 mph and you can't go anywhere.... I'm getting cross at people and I hate that. When my psychologist kept asking me questions—the same ones over and over, I got so impatient inside that I had a strange impulse to throw my purse on the floor or better yet to bite him and say, NO MORE! (Tennis, 1992)

Even when the descent into madness has reached a stage of deep dementia, when a person appears to be completely "out of it," the suffering continues and is intense. They are still conscious and still retain substantial selves (Sabat, 2001), though they may perceive confused, frequently delusional and threatening, circumstances. They are surrounded by the unknown and unknowable, misunderstood by those around them, with little control of their environment and their person, plagued with confusing and shifting conceptions of their world and their place. Around them is incomprehensible turmoil over which they have no influence. Sometimes they react with apathy, other times by lashing out. Everyone in their world is a stranger with unknown intentions, frequently imposing their will. Under these circumstances, they understandably react defensively, fearfully, angrily, sometimes violently. It is world of fearful and threatening unknowns against which one is powerless.

And finally, AD destroys all their intellectual power and their ability to formulate and express coherent thought.

> The power of concentration has gone, along with the ability to form coherent sentences and to remember where she is, or has been. She does not know she has written 26 remarkable novels, as well as her books on philosophy; received honorary doctorates from the major universities; become a *Dame of the British Empire.* (Bayley, 2000)

❧ Caregivers

The overwhelming burdens of AD are shared by family, friends, and colleagues of those afflicted. Caregivers commonly experience denial, anger, hostility, depersonalization, despair, guilt, loss of control, and social isolation (Lindgren, Connelly, & Gaspar, 1999). Early symptoms of dementia in loved ones or colleagues cause worry and sometimes fear.

> I notice a change in our lives, but don't know what to do about it. Sam is confused a lot and is often restless and irritable. I cannot shake the eerie feeling that something is very wrong. (Wilhoite & Buschmann, 1991, p. 18)

Return to normal behavior, or denial, frequently alleviates concern.

> Sam was in a good mood and I was happy. I felt as though things were back on track. (Wilhoite & Buschmann, 1991, p. 18)

But increasing frequency of episodes of forgetfulness or apparently irresponsible behavior magnify concern. When a diagnosis of AD is pronounced, the bottom drops out for both the patient and those who care for her or him.

> An incredible blow. (Hoffman, 1994)

Caregivers usually manifest denial and anger, sometimes feel guilt and shame because they have not acted soon enough on behalf of their loved one or have reacted with resentment or anger to their loved one's efforts to cover his or her loss of intellectual function.

> The doctor still cannot be sure that it is Alzheimer's Disease. Great! Just great! I am in shock! (Wilhoite & Buschmann, 1991, p. 20)

The children could not accept the changes they saw in Sam. (Wilhoite & Buschmann, 1991, p. 21)

As the patient's condition deteriorates, the burden on the caregiver grows.

The carer must be prepared to be verbally abused, disbelieved and to be seen as an enemy by the patient. (Wood, 1990, p. 30)

I have to readjust my whole way of relating to my husband. (Wilhoite & Buschmann, 1991, p. 20)

She would turn on me. It was really painful. (Hoffman, 1994)

More time and attention is required to monitor the AD sufferer to protect her or him against the consequences of forgetfulness and confusion, to attend daily needs of dressing, eating, and toilet. There is need to curtail their freedom of movement and association in order to protect them. One of the most difficult issues is to prohibit driving or find subterfuges to make it impossible to drive. The person with AD almost always reacts with anger and hostility, resulting in guilt in the caregiver.

Friends, and frequently family, begin to distance themselves to avoid the pain and uncertainty of being around one who is becoming unknown to them.

We no longer meet with our friends. Entertaining became a disaster. Our social life is gone. (Wilhoite & Buschmann, 1991, p. 21)

The sense of social isolation can become overwhelming, leading to resentment and anger at the patient and, subsequently, feelings of guilt for anger at someone utterly undeserving of it.

The sleeplessness and wandering that characterize AD seem almost to be infectious; caregivers become sleepless worrying about their charges and fearing that they may wander away or do something that may endanger themselves or others around them.

I developed a guilt complex about falling asleep. (Wood, 1990, p. 30)

I slept no more than three hours last night. Tonight I slept only an hour, but I don't dare go to sleep now, at 2:00 A.M. . . . I'm so tired. But I have to stay awake. . . . And so I began another day, more tired than I was the night before. (Sibley, 1994)

Sleeplessness, social isolation, the sense of helplessness to influence the course of a loved one's deterioration lead to despair.

> I felt like a zombie or robot. I thought to myself: "Will this ever end? How long can I take this abuse and this struggle?" (Wood, 1990, p. 32)

Dementia caregivers are at substantially higher risk of clinical depression. Nearly half of caregivers are diagnosed as depressed, which compares with approximately 15 to 20 percent of age-matched controls, and caregivers consume twice the psychotropic pharmaceuticals as matched controls (Gallagher et al., 1989; Baumgarten et al., 1994; Baumgarten et al., 1997; Schulz et al., 1995; Ballard et al., 1996).

As persons with AD become more severely demented—aggressive, combative, less able to meet daily living needs, incontinent—the caregiver burden grows and usually ends with the institutionalization of the patient. This is an agonizing decision for caregivers and is commonly accompanied by feelings of intense guilt and a sense of having "failed" the loved one.

> Today I visited nursing homes. . . . I hate doing this, but . . . I have to do something. (Wilhoite & Buschmann, 1991, p. 22)

> The hardest thing I've ever done was walking out there. I had just done the most horrible thing to a person I could ever do. I just felt horrible. (Hoffman, 1994)

> We put my mother in the nursing home last Tuesday . . . today she has pneumonia. I can't help but feel that this is my fault. She may die tonight, and if she does, it will be my fault. (Sibley, 1996)

The burden of caring is not restricted to those who provide care in the home. Institutional caregivers also experience frequent and early burnout dealing with patients with whom they cannot communicate well, who are unappreciative, who resist the caregivers' efforts to help. They lose respect for their patients as persons and, in turn, suffer frustration and guilt about their lost or faded caring. The turnover rate of employed caregivers in long-term care facilities approaches 100 percent per year in the United States.

The burden on patients and caregivers is much more than personal suffering and social isolation. Individuals, their families, and caregivers bear a substantial share of the financial costs of AD and related dementias. Out-of-pocket expenses for the care of AD patients vary greatly, but approximate 45 to 50 percent of direct care costs, or about $12,000 per year in year 2000. In addition, there is great cost to individuals (and to employers) for lost time at work. Individuals often are forced to leave the workforce entirely. Some have estimated total costs to families to be much higher when foregone income is included in the estimates.

❧ The Societal Burden

The burdens of AD extend well beyond the personal, social, and economic costs to patients and caregivers. Society also bears a large financial burden of costs of care and lost productivity. It is estimated that in the United States AD costs businesses $61 billion per year in lost productivity, clinical care, and other costs (Koppel, 2002).

The financial burden on patients and caregivers frequently drives them to marginal economic levels, into poverty, forcing their dependence on public support for the costs of care. U.S. Medicaid costs of dementia are estimated to have been more than $18 billion in 2000 (Lewin Group, 2001). In large part, these costs are in support of patients who have been impoverished by the costs of AD.

In fact, the cost of AD represents one of the most challenging aspects of this disease in an aging society. In the year 2000, direct paid care and total care costs for an AD patient in the United States averaged $25,048 and $31,371, respectively (Leon, Chang, & Neumann, 1998, updated to 2000 using U.S. Bureau of Labor Statistics medical care index). The total societal cost in the United States is estimated to have been nearly $68 billion to care for slightly more than 2 million AD patients (table 1.1). Of the $68 billion, more than $54 billion are paid costs of clinical care; the remainder is the value of unpaid services of caregivers. Of the direct care costs, $36 billion are estimated to have been supported by public funds. This conservative estimate translates to a public cost of AD care of $256 (in taxes) per year for each productive worker in the society. It is also 2.1 percent of the U.S. federal budget. These estimates do not include lost productivity of patients or caregivers. If those are included, the total societal cost is in excess of $100 billion per year.

These costs are apparently manageable at present, but they are large enough to cause concern among policymakers, who struggle to find ways to contain

TABLE 1.1.   Alzheimer Disease, United States, 2000–2050 (selected years)

	2000	2010	2025	2050
Prevalence (000)	2,167	2,929	3,868	7,975
Total annual cost of care (000)	$67,981,000	$105,955,000	$139,923,000	$288,492,000
Annual paid care costs (000)	$54,279,000	$ 87,435,000	$115,466,000	$238,067,000
% GDP	0.55	0.88	1.2	2.4
Total annual Medicare cost (000)	$17,876,000	$ 29,814,000	$ 39,372,000	$ 81,178,000
Total excess Medicare cost (000)	$ 8,722,000	$ 14, 583,000	$ 19,259,000	$ 39,708,000
Total annual Medicaid cost of AD (000)	$18,200,000	$ 33,018,000	$ 43,604,000	$ 89,902,000
Total government cost of AD (000)	$36,076,000	$ 62,832,000	$ 82,976,000	$171,080,000
% federal budget	2.1	3.6	4.8	9.9
Workers per AD patient	65	52	41	23
Government cost per worker	$ 256	$ 413	$ 523	$ 933

NOTE: Estimates of the prevalence and costs of AD are quite variable owing to differences in sampling and diagnostic criteria. The figures in this table are conservative best estimates based on comprehensive analyses. Figures are estimated using U.S. General Accounting Office (1998) estimated prevalence rates, U.S. Census Bureau demographic projections, and cost data and estimates from Leon, Chang, & Neumann (1998), the Lewin Group (2001), and U.S. Bureau of Labor Statistics price indexes. Estimated prevalence rates are similar to those of Brookmeyer and Gray (2000). All monetary values are expressed in constant 2000 dollars. GDP 2000 is from U.S. Department of Commerce Bureau of Economic Analysis. It is assumed that GDP increases will parallel health care price increases. Future costs are computed assuming that per patient costs will not increase above 2000 and 2010 estimated costs. Excess Medicare cost is the difference in Medicare payments for AD patients and age-matched controls without dementia. The Lewin Group projects much higher total costs. See table 1.2. The number of workers was estimated by assuming that the fraction of the population in each age group working in 1996 will remain constant (U.S. Bureau of Census).

them. Though costs are managed today, there remain unmet needs of care by patients, of respite for family caregivers, of training and compensation for institutional caregivers. And what current high costs portend for the future is ominous. According to U.S. Census Bureau demographic projections (fig. 1.1), aging baby boomers and increased longevity will result in a disproportionate increase of the elderly population that will rely on support of a workforce that is a declining fraction of the whole. If there is no change in prevalence or effective treatments are not found, the societal burden will grow exponentially.

Demographic projections and conservative estimates of prevalence predict nearly 8 million AD sufferers in the United States in the year 2050, with an annual total cost of care approaching $300 billion (constant year 2000 dollars). If there are no changes in public benefits, the Medicare and Medicaid costs will rise to more than $170 billion, representing 2.4 percent of the GDP and 9.9 percent of the federal budget. Each AD patient in this dependent elderly population will be supported by twenty-three workers—a tax cost of $933 per worker.

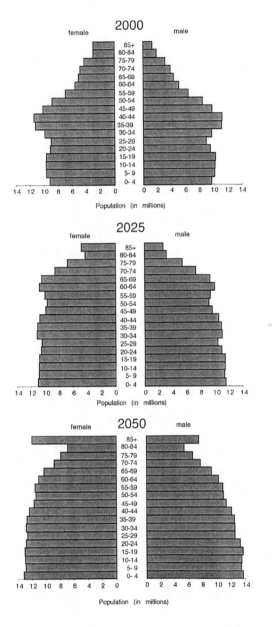

Fig. 1.1. Projected population age distribution in the United States from 2000 to 2050.
Data from U.S. Bureau of Census, International Data Base, table 094.

TABLE 1.2.   Alzheimer Disease Costs, United States, 2000–2050 (selected years)

	2000	2010	2025	2050
Total annual Medicare cost of AD (000)	$31,879,000	$49,283,000	$ 70,160,000	$130,052,000
Total annual Medicaid cost (000)	$18,200,000	$33,018,000	$ 47,005,000	$ 87,131,000
Total annual government cost of AD (000)	$50,079,000	$82,301,000	$117,165,000	$217,183,000
Total government cost of AD per worker (Lewin)	$ 355	$ 540	$ 733	$ 1,175

SOURCE: The Lewin Group Estimates

NOTE: These estimates are based on Evans et al. (1989), who estimated prevalence rates much higher than other studies. The Evans prevalence rates give total prevalence of AD as 4.9 million in 2000, 5.76 million in 2010, 8.2 million in 2025, and 15.2 million in 2050. The figures are expressed in constant 2000 dollars. It is assumed that the per patient costs of Medicare and Medicaid in 2010 remain constant in 2025 and 2050. Lewin adjusts its estimate of Medicare costs per AD patient by assuming that younger patients have milder disease and thus are less costly. Costs per worker are based on workforce projections computed from U.S. Bureau of Census data.

TABLE 1.3.   Alzheimer Disease in Europe, 2000–2050 (selected years)

	2000	2010	2025	2050
Prevalence (000)				
Western Europe	4,300	5,310	7,178	10,966
Eastern Europe, including Baltics	803	1,132	1,630	2,653
Workforce (000)				
Western Europe	180,960	179,945	165,617	137,557
Eastern Europe, including Baltics	60,503	61,974	56,541	41,050
Workers per AD patient				
Western Europe	42 (33–54)	34 (24–44)	23 (17–30)	13 (8–16)
Eastern Europe	75 (49–78)	55 (40–64)	35 (27–45)	15 (12–23)
Direct paid care costs per patient UK	£ 14,465			
Total annual costs UK (000)	£9,341,000	£10,907,000	£14,248,000	£22,580,000
NHS and local health authority per patient	12,959			
Total annual health system cost (000)	8,449,000	9,771,000	12,765,000	20,229,000
Government health costs per worker	266	320	436	785
Annual costs of care Netherlands (000)	€3,309,000	€4,113,000	€6,193,000	€10,519,000
Direct costs per worker	437	543	864	1,600

NOTE: Prevalence was estimated using U.S. General Accounting Office (1998). This meta-analysis was used because it draws on several European studies and American studies populated predominantly by European Americans. It results in prevalence quite similar to EURODEM figures (Launer et al., 1999). In the row "Workers per AD patient," the numbers in parentheses are the range in the nations analyzed. Workforce estimates were computed using U.S. Census Bureau demographic projections and workforce data from 1996 (except those of Bulgaria and Czech Republic, 1991; Slovakia, 1993; Estonia, 1995). The number of workers was estimated by assuming that the fraction of the population in each age group working in 1996 (or other base year) remained constant (France, Germany, Italy, Netherlands, Spain, and United Kingdom used as representative of Western Europe; those six nations constitute >80% of Western European population. Bulgaria, Czech Republic, Hungary, Poland, Romania, and Slovakia used as representative of Eastern Europe and Estonia, Latvia, and Lithuania; those nations are >80% of Eastern European and Baltic populations). Estimates of costs for 2010, 2025, and 2050 assume no major change in per patient costs and are expressed in constant 2000 currency units. Price data from National Statistics (UK) and Statistics Netherlands.

Other estimates (Lewin Group, 2001) have put public support (Medicare and Medicaid) as high as $50 billion in 2000, rising to more that $217 billion in 2050 (table 1.2), representing 12.6 percent of the federal budget. Using similar prevalence rates, one can estimate that the portion of GDP consumed by paid services

for AD and related dementias will reach 3.5 percent. Using the prevalence estimates used by Lewin, each worker contributed $355 per year in 2000 and will
contribute $1,175 in 2050.

But the United States is relatively favored. The U.S. population is projected
to include continued growth of its productive workforce because of immigration and relatively high birth rates among immigrant groups. In fact, some
project that for the reasonably foreseeable future, funding of the Medicare trust
fund in the United States is sound enough to avoid crisis or hard decisions
(Vladek, 2001). It is projected that the Medicare trust fund reserve will remain
intact until 2029 (Board of Trustees of the Federal Hospital Insurance Trust
Fund, 2001).

Europe may not be so fortunate. Low birth rates and low immigration are
projected to result in declining populations and workforce and a striking increase in dependent elderly persons (figs. 1.2 and 1.3), including major increases
in the numbers suffering from AD. Using conservative prevalence estimates,
there were 4.8 million persons with AD in East and West Europe in 2000, and the
number will rise to 6.4 million by 2010, 8.8 million by 2025, and 13.6 million by
2050. Between 2000 and 2050, the number of workers funding each AD patient
will decline from forty-two to thirteen in West Europe and from seventy-five to
fifteen in East Europe (table 1.3).

Estimates of the costs of AD in Europe are comparable with U.S. estimates.
Two of the European estimates—one from the United Kingdom (Souêtre,
Thwaites, & Yeardly, 1999) and one from the Netherlands (McDonnell et al.,
2001)—put paid costs of £14,465 (US$23,400) and €22,638 (US$26,000) per pa-
tient-year, respectively. Assuming no change in per patient cost and no change in
prevalence rates, these allow estimates of total national costs of £9.3 billion in the
United Kingdom and €3.3 billion in the Netherlands in 2000, increasing to £22.6
billion and €10.5 billion in 2050. The increasing numbers of aged persons and
AD patients and the declining workforces in these nations result in cost estimates
that were £266 and €437 per worker in 2000, rising to £785 and €1600 by 2050.

These burdens will affect every region and nation of the world as the fraction
of elderly persons in their populations grows. The 1066 research group of
Alzheimer's Disease International projects sharply growing worldwide prevalence of AD and estimates that, by 2025, 71 percent of all dementia cases will be
in developing countries (www.alz.co.uk/alz/wp.htm).

These projections are of course fraught with risk. They assume no changes in

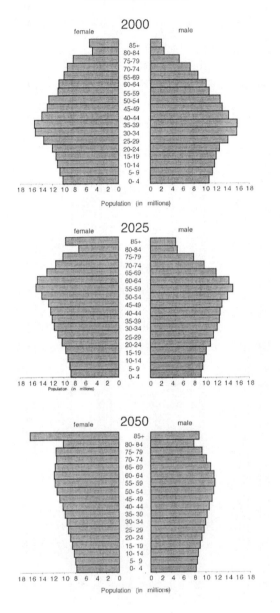

Fig. 1.2. Projected population age distribution in Western Europe from 2000 to 2050. Data from U.S. Bureau of Census, International Data Base, table 094.

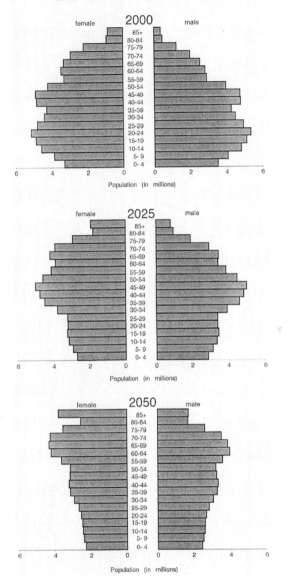

Fig. 1.3. Projected population age distribution in Eastern Europe and the Baltic states from 2000 to 2050. Data from U.S. Bureau of Census, International Data Base, table 094.

scientific knowledge, no changes in economies, no changes in the relationships between the costs of health care and other prices or economic productivity. One hopes that research will produce effective means of preventing or treating AD and thus alleviating the burdens. One hopes for continued robust economic growth in developed and developing nations. But there is a near certain likelihood of cyclic swings in economies that will bring crises (or perceived crises) of health care funding. Though the future is uncertain, prudence demands that we attempt to predict and anticipate it as best we can in order to plan effective policies with what is certain to be a human population increasingly at risk of AD and related dementias.

❧ Societal Responses

The increasing societal burden of AD seriously challenges policymakers in all nations and regions. Callahan (1995) addressed the demographic challenges to health care resulting from an increasingly aged population. He has proposed age as a criterion for limiting life-extending treatment for elderly persons. He did not, however, suggest limits or curtailment of palliative care, the only available therapy for persons with AD and the subject of this volume. The escalating costs of care for AD and the fact that the costs will be borne by fewer productive workers is certain to lead to societal consideration of means to increase resources and to constrain costs. Measures likely to be considered include

- raising the retirement age to increase the workforce
- increasing taxes to pay the escalating costs of greater numbers of dependent elderly and AD patients
- decreasing benefits, thus shifting a greater portion of the burden to patients and their caregivers
- increasing research on prevention or treatment to delay or control manifestations of dementia in the hope of controlling costs and their rise
- diminishing the quality of care to reduce per patient costs (e.g., herd patients with dementia into large holding facilities where bare survival needs are met, as was done in the past with mental patients)

These societal and individual burdens raise important ethical questions, many of which are addressed by other authors in this book:

- What is the societal responsibility to alleviate personal and economic burdens on patients, families, and caregivers?
- Are there limits of the responsibilities of society to care for its frail and elderly persons with dementia?
- What sacrifices can be reasonably expected of productive workers to support the care of those suffering from dementia?
- Is it just to shift large resources from younger generations, for education and quality of life, to support care for masses of dying older people?
- What are the limits of acceptable burdens for caregivers and families? What are the remedies for those burdens?
- Do elderly persons have a "duty to die"? (Lamm, 1984; Hardwig, 1997). Will this "duty" be interpreted to justify that elderly persons should not expect or receive extensive medical services? Will it perhaps be extended to acceptance of more active interventions to cause death rather than simply not preventing it?

It seems obvious that in seeking means of prevention and treatment, large investments in research funding should be made. But that will likely mean the redeployment of resources from other priorities—either from other biomedical research or from other societal priorities.

REFERENCES

Ballard, C. G., Eastwood, C., Gahir, M., & Wilcock, G. (1996). A follow up study of depression in the carers of dementia sufferers. *British Medical Journal, 312,* 947.

Baumgarten, M., Battista, R. N., Infante-Rivard, C., Hanley, J. A., Becker, R., Bilker, W. B., & Gauthier, S. (1997). Use of physician services among family caregivers of elderly persons with dementia. *Journal of Clinical Epidemiology, 50* (11), 1265–1272.

Baumgarten, M., Hanley, J. A., Infante-Rivard, C., Battista, R. N., Becker, R., & Gauthier, S. (1994). Health of family members caring for elderly persons with dementia. *Annals of Internal Medicine, 120,* 126–132.

Bayley, J. (2000). *Iris and her friends: A memoir of memory and desire.* New York: W. W. Norton. Quote found at the Eurohealth web site, www.eurohealth.ie/remind//intro.htm (accessed August 2001).

Board of Trustees, Federal Hospital Insurance Trust Fund. (2001). *Annual Report.* Washington, DC: Government Printing Office. Also available at www.hcfa.gov/pubforms/tr (accessed August 2001).

Brookmeyer, R., & Gray, S. (2000). Methods for projecting the incidence and prevalence of chronic diseases in aging populations, application to Alzheimer's disease. *Statistics in Medicine, 19* (11–12), 1481–1493.

Callahan, D. (1995). *Setting limits: Medical goals in an aging society.* Washington, DC: Georgetown University Press.

Evans, D. A., Funkenstein H. H., Albert, M. S., Scherr, P. A., Cook, N. R., Chown, M. J., et al. (1989). Prevalence of Alzheimer's disease in a community population of older persons. Higher than previously reported. *Journal of the American Medical Society, 262,* 2551–1556.

Gallagher, D., Rose, J., Rivera, P., Lovett, S., & Thompson, L. W. (1989). Prevalence of depression in family caregivers. *Gerontologist, 29* (4), 449–456.

Hardwig, J. (1997). Is there a duty to die? *Hastings Center Report, 27* (2): 34–42.

Henderson, C. S., Henderson, R. D., & Main, J. H. (Eds.) and Andrews, N. (Photog.). (1998). *Partial view: An Alzheimer's journal.* Dallas, TX: Southern Methodist University Press. Quotes found at www.alzheimers.org/unravel.html (accessed July 2001).

Hoffman, Deborah. (1994). *Complaints of a dutiful daughter* (video recording). New York: Women Make Movies.

Jan/Mina. (2001). My journal (of an Alzheimer's disease patient) www.google.com (accessed July 2003).

Koppel, R. (2002). Alzheimer's disease: The cost to U.S. business in 2002. Study prepared for the Alzheimer's Association. Available at www.alz.org/Media/newsreleases/current/062602ADCosts.pdf (accessed January 2003).

Lamm, R. (1984). Quoted in *New York Times,* March 29, section A. p. 16.

Launer, L. J., Andersen, K., Dewey, M. E., Letenneur, L., Ott, A., Amaducci, L. A., et al. and the EURODEM Incidence Research Group and Work Groups. (1999). Rates and risk factors for dementia and Alzheimer's disease. Results from EURODEM pooled analyses. *Neurology, 52* (1), 78–84.

Leon, J., Chang, C-K., & Neumann, P. J. (1998). Alzheimer's disease care, costs, and potential savings. *Health Affairs, 6* (17), 206–216.

Lewin Group. (2001). *Medicare and Medicaid costs for people with Alzheimer's disease.* Report prepared for the Alzheimer's Association. Available at www.alz.org/whatsnew/alzreport.pdf (accessed August 2001)

Lindgren, C. L., Connelly, C. T., & Gaspar, H. L. (1999). Grief in spouse and children caregivers of dementia patients. *Western Journal of Nursing Research, 21* (4), 521–537.

Marshall, M. (Ed.). (1997). *State of the art in dementia care.* Center for Policy on Ageing. Quote of a sixty-seven-year-old man man with AD found at Dementia Care: Challenges for an Ageing Europe. www.eurohealth.ie/remind/alzheimer.htm (accessed June 2001).

McDonnell, J., Redekop, W. K., van-der-Roer, N., Goes, E., Ruitenberg, A., Busschbach, J. J., et al. (2001). The cost of treatment of Alzheimer's disease in the Netherlands: A regression-based simulation model. *Pharmacoeconomics, 19* (4), 379–90.

National Statistics. The official UK statistics site, www.statistics.gov.uk (accessed July 2001).

Sabat, S. R. (2001). *The experience of Alzheimer's disease: Life through a tangled veil.* Malden, MA: Blackwell.

Schulz, R., O'Brien, A. T., Bookwala, J., & Fleissner, K. (1995). Psychiatric and physical morbidity effects of dementia caregiving: Prevalence, correlates, and causes. *Gerontologist, 35* (6), 771–791.

Shelia, a woman with early-stage Alzheimer's disease. (2000). What it's like to live with Alzheimer's. *Alzheimer's Disease International Global Perspective, 10,* 3.

Sibley, B. P. (1994–96). *A year to remember . . . with my mother and Alzheimer's Disease.* www.zarcrom.com/users/yeartorem (accessed August 2001).

Souêtre, E., Thwaites, R. M. A., & Yeardley, H. L. (1999). Economic impact of Alzheimer's disease in the United Kingdom. *British Journal of Psychology, 174,* 51–55.

Statistics Netherlands. www.cbs.nl/en (accessed August 2001).

Tennis, L. (1992). "Alzheimer's diary: I have what!" *Caregiver: Newsletter of the Duke Family Support Program 12* (1), 6–13; and "More from Letty's diary," *Caregiver: Newsletter of the Duke Family Support Program 12* (3), 8–10. Quotes found at www.alzheimers.org/unravel.html (accessed May 2001).

U.S. Bureau of Census, International Data Base, Table 069. Economically active population, 1996. Available at www.census.gov/ipc/www/idbnew.html (accessed August 2001).

U.S. Bureau of Census population projections. Available at www.census.gov/population/www/projections/natsum-T3.html (accessed August 2001).

U.S. Bureau of Labor Statistics. Consumer Price Index (incl. Medical Care Index). Available at stats.bls.gov/cpihome.htm (accessed August 2001).

U.S. Department of Commerce Bureau of Economic Analysis. Available at www.bea.doc.gov (accessed August 2001).

U.S. General Accounting Office. (1998). *Alzheimer's disease: Estimates of prevalence in the United States,* GAO/HEHS-98-16. Washington, DC.

Vladek, B. (2001). Learn nothing, forget nothing—the Medicare Commission redux. *New England Journal of Medicine, 345* (6), 456–458.

Wilhoite, C., & Buschmann, M. T. (1991). Alzheimer's disease, diary of a caregiver. *Nursing Forum, 26* (2), 17–22.

Wood, C. (June 1990). A living death. *Nursing Times Community Outlook,* 30–31.

CHAPTER TWO

Neuropathology and Symptomatology in Alzheimer Disease

Implications for Caregiving and Competence

Roger A. Brumback, M.D.

Alzheimer disease (AD) is one of many conditions that produce the clinical syndrome of dementia, which is the insidiously progressive loss of intellectual, cognitive, and social abilities (Brumback & Leech, 1994). Dementia can occur at any age (e.g., adrenoleukodystrophy causing *dementia* in late childhood) (Riva, Boca, & Bruzzone, 2000). However, the term dementia is most often used to describe conditions affecting adults past the fourth decade of life, of which Alzheimer disease is the most common dementing disorder (Fratiglioni et al., 1991; Evans et al., 1989; Evans et al., 1991; Bachman et al., 1993; Brumback & Leech, 1994; Kukull & Ganguli, 2000). *Dementia* must also be distinguished from *senility,* a term used in the late eighteenth century to imply age-related mental infirmity (*Oxford English Dictionary,* 1971). During the nineteenth and twentieth centuries that term developed the connotation of cognitive incompetency occurring in all older people at a specific age, in particular at age sixty-five years (Brumback & Leech, 1994). This chapter describes the current understanding of the progression of the symptoms in AD, correlating them with the progression of the neuropathologic process.

❧ Dementia as a Clinical Syndrome

Dementia is the result of the progressive loss of brain functioning due to reduced functional connectivity of the billions of synapses linking neurons in the brain. This loss of neuronal interconnectivity can be the result of either or both physiologic impairment of neuronal and synaptic activity or pathologic destruction of neurons, axons, dendrites, and synapses.

Behavioral assessment of dementia has involved the use of a wide variety of rating scales (Gottfries et al., 1982; Shader, Harmatz, & Salzman, 1974; Spiegel et al., 1991; Rosen, Mohs, & Davis, 1984; Overall & Schaltenbrand, 1992; Blessed, Tomlinson, & Roth, 1968; Schmitt et al., 1997; Morris, 1993; Reisberg et al., 1982; Reisberg et al., 1987; Cole & Dastoor, 1983; Schneider et al., 1996; Knopman et al., 1994; Tariot et al., 1995; Cummings et al., 1994; Cohen-Mansfield, 1986; Reisberg, 1988; Lucas et al., 1998). These scales have been used to quantify cognitive function and, by implication of a change in value from normal, the severity and the rate of progression of dementia (Milberg, 1996; Malloy et al., 1997). The Mini-Mental State Examination (MMSE), originally developed by Folstein and colleagues (1975), is the scale most often used (Malloy et al., 1997) (table 2.1). It consists of a series of thirty tasks to be performed by the patient, scored from 0 (lowest) to 30 (highest). Normal individuals usually achieve a score of 25 or higher (although some normal individuals can score as low as 21). Scores of 20 or lower indicate varying degrees of severity of dementia (scores of 10 to 20 for moderate dementia and 9 or lower for severe dementia). In chapter 16, Scheirton refers to this examination as a useful tool for distinguishing the kinds of educational interventions that can assist the patient and family caregivers during early, middle, and late stages of the disease.

Individuals with neurodegenerative dementias such as Alzheimer disease progressively experience a linear decrease of 2 to 4 points per year in score on the MMSE. Similar linear deterioration of function over time has been identified with most of the other rating scales developed to assess dementia. The fallacy in using such linear scales (which assign a single overall number to brain function) is the implication that the brain is a homogenous organ. In contrast to the brain, the kidney (like most other organ systems in the body) is a homogeneous organ composed of millions of units (nephrons) that all perform the same functions.

TABLE 2.1. Mini-Mental State Examination (MMSE) Items Correlated with Cognitive Function and Brain Areas

Basic Instructions	Item for Scoring	Major Cognitive Function Tested	Associated Brain Area
Ask a series of questions about time and place	1. What year is it? 2. What season are we in? 3. What month are we in? 4. What is today's date? 5. What day of the week is it? 6. What state are we in? 7. What county are we in? 8. What city (town) are we in? 9. What hospital (building; street) are we in (on)? 10. What is the floor (street number)?	Orientation (memory)	Limbic lobe
Name three common objects (examples include "ball," "apple," "table" "penny," "cigarette," "car," "door"); pronounce each word carefully; have patient immediately repeat all three and record success; then repeat each until patient learns all three; tell patient to remember these words for the future	11. First object? 12. Second object? 13. Third object?	Registration, learning, immediate recall, language	Limbic lobe, temporal lobe
Serial 7's (starting at 100 serially subtract 7); stop after 5 answers	14. "93" 15. "86" 16. "79" 17. "72" 18. "65"	Attention, concentration, calculation, language	Temporal lobe, parietal lobe
Spell the word *world* backwards	14. "D" 15. "L" 16. "R" 17. "O" 18. "W"		
Ask the patient to recall the three object words memorized earlier	19. First object? 20. Second object? 21. Third object?	Delayed (short-term) recall memory, language	Limbic lobe, temporal lobe

Instruction	Item	Ability	Lobe
Show the patient two objects (examples include "pen," "wristwatch," "pencil," "clock," "cup") and ask the name of each	22. First object? 23. Second object?	Naming	Temporal lobe
Ask the patient to repeat a specific nonsense phrase	24. "No, ifs, ands, or buts"	Spoken language reception and expression	Temporal lobe
Ask the patient to follow a three-stage command. Place a piece of paper on a table and instruct the patient to follow directions	25. "Take the paper in your right hand" 26. "Fold it in half" 27. "Put it on the floor"	Spoken language comprehension and praxis	Temporal lobe, parietal lobe, paracentral lobe
Show the patient a written command and instruct the patient to follow it	28. "CLOSE YOUR EYES"	Written language comprehension (reading ability) and praxis	Temporal lobe, parietal lobe, occipital lobe
Give the patient a blank sheet of paper and a pen and instruct the patient to write	29. "Write a complete sentence, whatever you want to write"	Writing ability	Parietal lobe
Give the patient a blank sheet of paper and a pen and show the patient a picture of a complex design (interlocking pentagons) and instruct the patient to copy the figure	30. "Copy this drawing"	Visuospatial and graphic abilities	Parietal lobe

SOURCE: The table is adapted from "A practical method for grading the cognitive state of patients for the clinician," by M. F. Folstein, S. E. Folstein, and P. R. McHugh, *Journal of Psychiatric Research*, 12 (1975): 189–198.

SCORING: Normal individuals 25 or higher. Mild dementia 21 to 24 (although some normal individuals with limited education can score as low as 21). Moderate dementia 10 to 20. Severe dementia 0 to 9.

Thus, renal function is simply proportional to the number of viable nephrons, and a linear measurement scale (for example, recording changes in serum creatinine, blood urea nitrogen, or creatinine clearance) can be used to determine the progress of degenerative renal disease and the number of remaining nephrons, regardless of the etiology of the underlying kidney problem. However, the brain is an extremely heterogenous organ, with millions of unique functional units performing different tasks. Thus, a single numerical value from a dementia scale cannot possibly distinguish the progressive changes in each of the different functional areas of the brain. Instead, to understand the progression of dementia in a disorder such as Alzheimer disease, it is necessary to identify the pathologic features of the disease, the areas of the brain involved, and the deficits of function that occur when particular brain areas are damaged.

❧ Functional Architecture of the Brain

The brain has multiple different functional systems that normally interact in a precise and well-coordinated manner. Dementia is the result of damage to various functional systems in the cerebral hemispheres that subserve cognition. A general classification of dementia divides the forms into cortical dementias (including Alzheimer disease, Pick disease, and frontotemporal dementia) and subcortical dementias (including Huntington disease, Wilson disease, and progressive supranuclear palsy) (Cummings & Benson, 1984; Savage, 1997). The pathologic changes of the cortical dementias principally involve the cerebral cortex resulting in specific cortical cognitive deficits, while the pathologic changes of subcortical dementias involve structures in the interior of the cerebral hemispheres resulting in slowness of thinking and behavior, apathy, depression, and motoric difficulties.

Characterization of specific cortical cognitive deficits began with the pioneering observation of the French physician-anthropologist Paul Broca that the left inferior frontal gyrus of the cerebral cortex subserved language expression (Broca, 1861, 1865). Many subsequent neuropathologic, neuropsychologic, and neurophysiologic studies have identified the unique functions of the various lobes of the cerebral cortex (Stringer, 1996; Lezak, 1995; Heilman & Valenstein, 1993) (fig. 2.1).

On the lateral surface of the cerebral hemisphere, the central sulcus (Rolandic fissure) divides the anterior frontal lobe from the more posterior parietal lobe, and the Sylvian fissure separates the more inferior temporal lobe from the frontal and parietal lobes. The separation between the posterior occipital lobe and the parietal and temporal lobes is most obvious on the medial surface of the cerebral hemisphere as the occipito-parietal sulcus. A general localization of specific cognitive functions to the lobes has been identified, but the exact arrangement of areas subserving specific functions within each lobe varies from individual to individual (much the same as fingerprints vary from individual to individual).

The cerebral cortical tissue that surrounds the central sulcus directs voluntary movements of the body and interprets sensation (such as touch, vibration, temperature, pain) from the body (termed somatic sensation). The gyrus anterior to the central sulcus (termed the precentral gyrus) subserves voluntary movement, and the gyrus posterior to the central sulcus (postcentral gyrus) subserves somatic sensation. The intimate structural and functional relationship between the precentral and postcentral gyri has resulted in their being grouped together as sensorimotor cortex and designated as a distinct lobe—the paracentral lobe.

The two other major sensory inputs to the brain are vision and hearing. The occipital lobe is the terminus of the optic pathways and subserves visual function. The temporal lobe subserves hearing, as well as language functions. The left temporal lobe contains the circuitry for understanding and using the linguistic, syntactic, and grammatical aspects of language, while the right temporal lobe subserves both the nonverbal aspects of language, such as the lilt and melody of language (termed prosody) and the appreciation of nonlanguage sounds (such as music). The importance of prosody in communication was highlighted in the 1951 hit recording by Stan Freberg entitled *John & Marsha* in which only the names John and Marsha are spoken, but with a variety of melody and inflection resulting in different perceived meanings.

The parietal lobe is strategically situated between the cortical sensory reception areas (temporal auditory, occipital visual, and paracentral somatic sensory areas) and as such serves an associative and integrative function. By integrating perception of the environment, the parietal lobe subserves the ability to understand orientation in space, the manipulation of objects (termed praxis), self-awareness and awareness of the environment (termed gnosis), spatial relationships, and sequencing and ordering. The frontal lobe subserves the executive functions that are key to judgment, logic, and the appropriate interactions (rules of behavior) that allow for civilized intercourse between people.

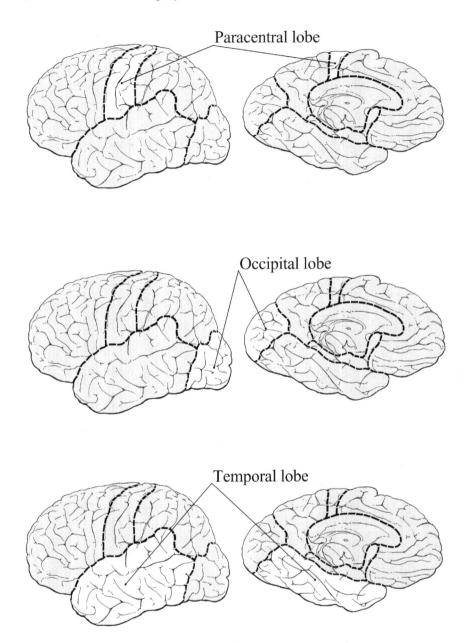

Fig. 2.1. Left cerebral hemisphere, lateral surface (*left*) and inferior/medial surfaces (*right*). *Paracentral lobe* subserving somatic sensation (postcentral gyrus) and voluntary motor control (precentral gyrus). *Occipital lobe* subserving vision. *Temporal lobe* subserving audition, including language, prosody, and nonlanguage sounds.

(*continued*)

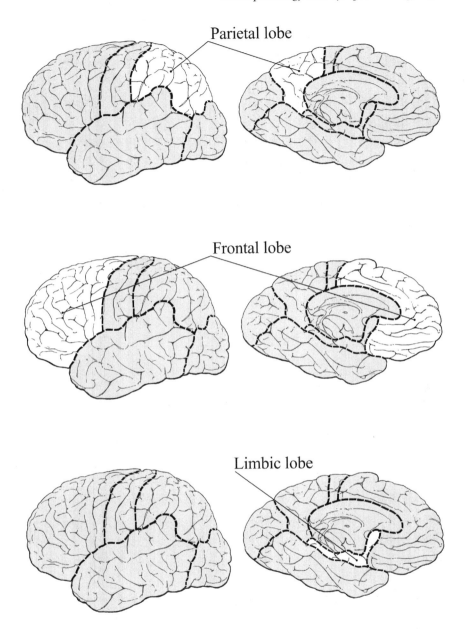

Fig. 2.1. (continued) *Parietal lobe* subserving the integration of visual, auditory, and somatic sensory information, allowing orientation in space, praxis, awareness of self and the environment, and understanding spatial relationships, sequencing, and ordering. *Frontal lobe* subserving personality and executive functions of judgment, logic, and appropriate interactions with others. *Limbic lobe* subserving memory and emotion and acting as a bridge to hypothalamic systems controlling the internal body milieu.

On the medial surface of the cerebral hemisphere is a somewhat dispersed area of cerebral cortex that is phylogenetically ancient (and thus termed corticoid, allocortical, archicortex, and paleocortex) and is equivalent to the olfactory lobe and associated structures in lower animals. This area is known as the limbic lobe (or limbic system) and encompasses the hippocampus, amygdala, septal nuclei, and substantia innominata (including the nucleus basalis of Meynert). The limbic system subserves memory and emotion, as well as acting as a bridge between the other cortical lobes and the hypothalamus that control the body's internal milieu (Mesulam, 2000).

❧ Behavior Associated with Damage to Specific Cerebral Areas

For the first half of the twentieth century, most of the structural-behavioral correlations were made by exhaustive study of individual patients with discrete damage to specific cerebral areas from trauma, stroke, or other injury (Heilman & Valenstein, 1993). Subsequent studies have confirmed these observations using newer techniques for electrical and magnetic stimulation of the brain and imaging with radioactive tracers and magnetic resonance and spectroscopy in larger numbers of individuals.

Damage to the voluntary motor cortex of the paracentral lobe results in paralysis of specific parts of the body. Lesions to the left motor cortex paralyze the right side of the body, but only specific parts depending on the exact location along the precentral gyrus. The inferior areas of the motor cortex nearest the Sylvian fissure subserve the face and hand, while the superior areas near the vertex subserve the leg. Across the central sulcus in the postcentral gyrus, somatic sensation is distributed in the same manner, with facial sensation nearest the Sylvian fissure and leg sensation near the vertex. Damage to the somatosensory cortex results in a loss of ability to discriminate between sensations and to precisely localize the area of the body affected by the sensation.

Occipital lobe damage produces discrete blank spots (visual field defects) in vision or difficulties perceiving color or motion. For example, since the right occipital lobe receives all the information on the left side of the visual space from each eye, lesions to the right occipital lobe generally produce blind areas in the left visual field.

Most of the sound signals from the left ear go to the right temporal lobe, although some information also goes to the left temporal lobe. Thus, damage to one temporal lobe does not produce deafness. However, damage to the left temporal lobe, which subserves linguistics, syntax, and grammar, produces a variety of language disorders. Extensive damage to the left temporal lobe results in an inability to understand any language (termed Wernicke aphasia), but damage more frequently produces varying types of problems with word use (including syntax and grammar) and word finding (termed anomia or dysnomia). In contrast, damage to the right temporal lobe produces problems in interpreting nonlanguage sounds and understanding the melodic and nonlinguistic aspects of language (termed aprosodia) (Ross, 1996).

Damage to the parietal lobe produces difficulty in integrating the input of visual, auditory, and somatosensory information from the occipital, temporal, and paracentral lobes. Parietal lobe damage results in a wide variety of peculiar behaviors involving problems of orientation in space, difficulties with proper manipulation and use of objects (apraxia), problems with recognition of self and/or the environment (agnosia), inattention, and unawareness. These problems can range from poor handwriting to difficulties with manipulating keys or dressing or getting lost to the complete inability to recognize the presence of the left side of the body.

The role of the frontal lobes is to exert "executive control" over the rest of the brain by guiding behavior appropriately and planning for the future through selection of the most advantageous responses for survival in a complex social environment. Thus, frontal lobe damage can produce a myriad of behavioral abnormalities, including deficits in judgment, insight, reasoning, abstraction, planning, and comportment. The behavioral variation possible with frontal lobe lesions is increased by the diversity of experience that molded development of the prelesion function of the frontal lobes. The nebulous term *personality change* is often used to describe the behavior associated with frontal lobe damage, but this requires a knowledge of the prelesion "personality," unless the observed behavior is obviously abnormal, such as rages, profound apathy, or antisocial activity.

Injury to the limbic lobe results in difficulty with memory since the hippocampus serves as a nodal point (gatekeeper function) for the formation of memory (Stringer, 1996; Ross, Homan, & Buck, 1994). Thus, damage to the hippocampus (or its connections in the limbic system) results in a variety of memory problems, varying from discrete memory "holes" to loss of more recent and preservation of older memories or to the loss of all memory.

❧ Symptoms in Dementia

The *Diagnostic and Statistical Manual of Mental Disorders (DSM-IV)* (1994) defines the progressive loss of intellectual and cognitive functioning of dementia as involving memory impairment (impaired ability to learn new information or to recall previously learned information), aphasia (language disturbance), apraxia (impaired ability to carry out motor activities despite intact motor function), agnosia (failure to recognize or identify objects despite intact sensory function), disturbance in executive functioning (i.e., planning, organizing, sequencing, abstracting), and personality changes sufficient to produce social or occupational impairments. The various rating scales used to assess the functional deficits in dementia test a mixture of these functions and then assign a numerical value that presumably describes the extent and severity of the dementia. Even though the deficits encompass dysfunction of widely spaced areas of the cerebral cortex, the implication of the definition of dementia and the rating scales for dementia is that all of the dimensions of cognitive function are equally affected and that any decline occurs equally in all functions. However, the reality of the neuropathologic changes of the underlying diseases causing dementia is that the cerebral cortex is not uniformly damaged and detailed neuropsychological evaluation of affected individuals confirms the nonuniformity of functional deterioration (Gauthier, 1996; Terry et al., 1999).

❧ Behavior-Neuropathology Correlation in Alzheimer Disease

For unknown reasons, the earliest and most severe neuropathologic changes (atrophy, neuronal loss, and deposition of neurofibrillary tangles and β-amyloid-containing neuritic plaques) occur in the limbic lobe (hippocampus and associated limbic structures such as the amygdala, septal nuclei, and substantia innominata basal nucleus of Meynert), which subserves memory (Braak & Braak, 1991, 1997; Terry et al., 1999). Based upon measurements of serial brain magnetic resonance imaging (MRI) scans, reduced volume of the hippocampus is evident years before (and possibly decades before) clinical evidence of dementia appears in those apparently healthy individuals destined to develop AD (Kaye et al., 1997). These imaging changes correlate with the finding that elderly individuals with isolated minimal memory problems (termed mild cognitive impairment) and preservation of all other cognitive functions will develop additional signs of AD over the course of a decade (Morris et al., 2001). The early stage of Alzheimer disease associated with minimal memory loss is usually only clinically identifiable in retrospect, when the individual presents with more obvious symptoms of AD.

After destroying the limbic lobe, the AD process marches from functional area to functional area over the cerebral cortex, involving next the temporal lobe, followed by the parietal lobe and then the frontal lobe, with the paracentral lobe and the occipital lobe affected last (Kaye et al., 1997; Brumback & Leech, 1994; Braak et al., 1998; Braak et al., 1999; Nagy et al., 1999a, 1999b) (fig. 2.2). Symptoms correlating with the destructive march into the temporal lobe (beginning medially and progressing over the inferior, middle, and then superior temporal lobe) consist of language problems, particularly difficulties with word finding and language usage. Initially, the person with Alzheimer disease uses more high-frequency words and fewer low-frequency words, but as the damage proceeds over the temporal lobe, problems become evident in naming, use of fewer nouns and more verbs, substituting words, circumlocutions, and the inability to find the proper word or even any word. Both speaking and the understanding of spoken language are similarly impaired, and writing and reading also deteriorate. Sometimes, however, even this stage of AD is not clinically obvious to observers, but in retrospect families can generally report the appearance of these symptoms many years before the clinical diagnosis of Alzheimer disease.

As the pathologic damage proceeds into the parietal lobes, individuals with AD experience the perceptual problems characteristic of parietal lobe dysfunction (Lezak, 1995; Gauthier, 1996; Heilman & Valenstein, 1993; Stringer, 1996). Getting lost (as a result of the spatial disorientation of parietal lobe dysfunction) is one of the most characteristic symptoms reported by families of individuals with AD, along with problems in the proper manipulation of objects (keys or utensils for eating) and in dressing. When the pathologic process next involves the frontal lobes, the affected individual develops personality changes, difficulties with social interactions (loss of normal comportment), and a lack of proper judgment. It is not until the end stages of the disease process that involvement of the sensorimotor cortex of the paracentral lobe and the visual cortex of the occipital lobe occur and result in the individual becoming immobile and relatively unresponsive.

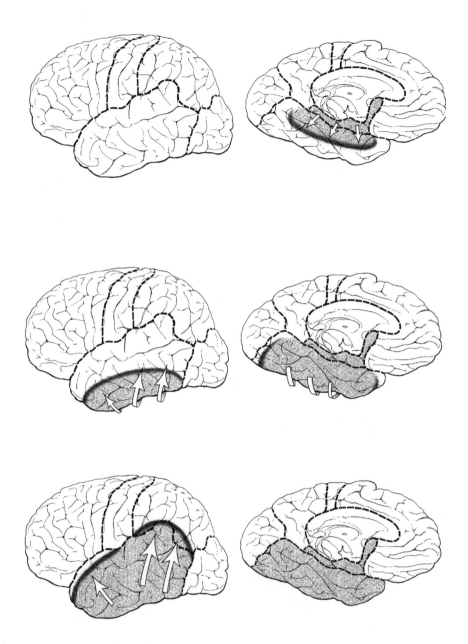

Fig. 2.2. Left cerebral hemisphere, lateral surface (*left*) and inferior/medial surfaces (*right*), demonstrating the progressive march of the destructive process of Alzheimer disease beginning in the limbic lobes and then sequentially involving the temporal lobes, parietal lobes, and frontal lobes.

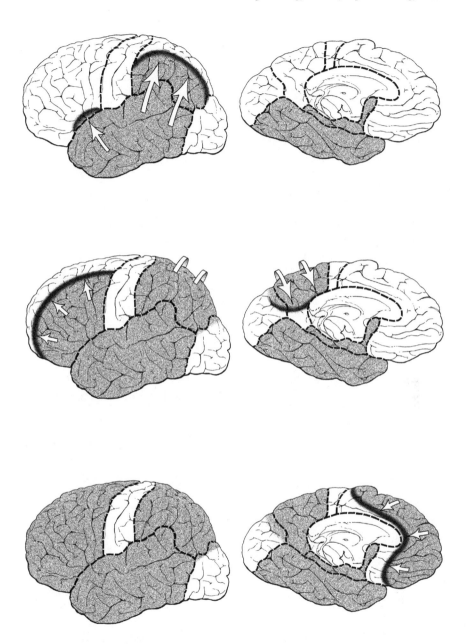

✿ Preserved versus Lost Functioning

Despite the progressive loss of cerebral functions in Alzheimer disease, many cognitive abilities are still preserved during various stages in the illness (Gauthier, 1996; Sabat, 2001). The earliest symptom of AD is the memory loss (from limbic lobe damage); however, only rarely do individuals with mild memory loss present for medical or psychological evaluation (Brumback & Leech, 1994; Breslaw, 1999). Since other brain functions are still intact (particularly the frontal lobe functions of executive control that select the appropriate survival responses), the individual with AD experiencing mild memory loss learns compensatory strategies; for example, relying on someone else such as a spouse, to remember things; and maintaining lists (both of these are well-accepted strategies even among the neurologically healthy population). Additionally, overlap with the syndrome of benign forgetfulness of aging (which appears to be a normal aging phenomenon) means that only in retrospect can those individuals with memory problems who are destined to develop AD years later be identified (Morris et al., 2001). Even after progression of the disease process into the language areas of the temporal lobes, compensatory strategies (by the intact frontal lobe-directed executive functions) can allow the person with AD to adjust to these deficits and continue to function in occupational or other settings that do not require significant language skills. The pathophysiologic basis of such compensation is not completely clear, but there appears to be only a limited amount of individual neuronal plasticity in damaged areas (Buell & Coleman, 1981).

The progression of the disease process to produce parietal lobe dysfunction almost always results in medical evaluation, because the problem of getting lost is frightening to family members, as well as to the affected individual. Nonetheless, even with severe parietal lobe deficits, individuals with AD can often still function in social settings because of intact frontal lobe functions.

Once Alzheimer disease progresses to involve the frontal lobes, personality changes, lack of judgment, and the inability to understand social cues become evident. Activities such as disrobing in public because it is too hot or reacting violently to minor setbacks make it difficult for caregivers to cope with the individual with AD. Often, it is at the stage of frontal lobe dysfunction that caregivers can no longer maintain the affected individual at home, and nursing home placement occurs. Involvement of the paracentral lobe sensorimotor cortex over the vertex of the brain occurs so late in the disease process that even severely affected individuals often still can walk (pacing).

Individual variations in this pattern of the progressive march of the Alzheimer disease destructive process over the cerebral cortex can produce a variety of seemingly unique behavioral syndromes. Most notable have been the reports of remarkably preserved talents in otherwise severely compromised persons with AD (Beatty, 1999). For example, nursing home patients with Alzheimer disease and little remaining self-care abilities have been described as being able to play winning dominos, contract bridge, or checkers when placed at an already set-up game table (Tröster, 1998). Another report described a former professional jazz musician who near the end-stage of Alzheimer disease could still play remarkable jazz performances when his assembled trombone was positioned in his hand and the mouthpiece put up to his lips (Beatty et al., 1994; Beatty et al., 1997).

❧ Implications of Nonuniform, Nonglobal Pathologic Involvement

The progressive march of the pathologic process in Alzheimer disease and its associated neuropsychological course has important implications for caregiving and medical therapy, as well as ramifications for legal and ethical concerns. For example, when should currently available treatment be initiated? The earliest symptom is memory loss, but differentiating Alzheimer disease-associated memory loss from the benign forgetfulness can generally only be done in retrospect. However, even if the Alzheimer disease–associated memory loss could be identified at its onset, should treatment with the currently available medications (that only work on the hippocampal memory system and have significant side effects) be initiated? It is possible that the compensatory strategies of the intact frontal lobe executive functions can be just as efficacious in social and occupational settings with fewer potential side effects.

The only currently available medications for AD act to augment the cholinergic neurotransmission on remaining hippocampal neurons (Grundman & Thal, 2000). Early in the disease process, when only the hippocampal limbic lobe structures are involved and memory problems are the main symptom, such treatment could potentially improve function (Breslaw, 1999). However, by the time the disease has spread over the temporal lobe, language problems are added to the memory difficulties and the temporal lobe language system does not involve cholinergic neurotransmission. In addition, once language problems are prominent, there are fewer viable neurons remaining in the hippocampus to respond to cholinergic augmentation. (Brumback & Leech, 1994). By the time parietal lobe symptoms appear (the stage at which most patients present for medical evaluation), the extent of neuronal loss in the limbic system makes augmentation of its cholinergic neurotransmission almost impossible. Thus, current medication treatment options in stages of AD beyond the period of the discrete memory loss are either ineffective or produce mainly a placebo effect.

Education of the affected individual and caregivers regarding both the lost and the preserved cortical cognitive functions is important in any treatment plan (Sabat, 2001). Instead of focusing on deficits, the focus should be on the preserved abilities and the development of compensatory strategies. This approach is similar to that used for stroke rehabilitation (Good & Couch, 1994). However, in stroke, the deficits from destruction of cerebral cortical areas are stable and compensatory strategies can remain unchanged over many years. In contrast, persons with AD progressively develop new and greater deficits, rendering ineffective compensatory strategies that worked previously and necessitating the identification and substitution of new compensatory strategies.

Competency of individuals with AD in decision making is another important issue. Implications from the dementia rating scales that provide a number value for the severity of the condition obscure the perspective of preserved functions. In the case of stroke patients with discrete cognitive deficits, incompetency is not generally a consideration, and every attempt is made through rehabilitation programs to establish communication and determine the wishes of the affected individual (Good & Couch, 1994). Even in some of the most severe stroke cases (such as the locked-in syndrome, which is not a cortical lesion but involves a brain stem lesion that disconnects the cerebral cortex from all possible motor output except eye blinks), complicated technological systems have been devised to permit the individual to participate in decision making (Allain et al., 1998). In contrast, individuals with Alzheimer disease (particularly those with low scores on dementia rating scales such as the MMSE) are often considered incompetent without regard for the cognitive functioning that is still preserved. For example, memory loss in AD does not preclude meaningful social interactions and the joy derived therefrom (Breslaw, 1999). A number of compensatory strategies have already been developed for the cognitive and language problems experienced by learning-disabled individuals, many of whom can therefore lead productive lives (Weinberg et al., 1995), and some of these strategies could be adapted for use with AD patients.

Driving is a contentious issue for families of individuals with AD (Foley et al., 2001). This becomes more problematic when the destructive march compromises parietal lobe function. Not only do the spatial disorientation and inattention make driving dangerous, but the agnosia and lack of awareness can prevent the individual with AD from recognizing the problem. Meanwhile, intact frontal lobe executive function can cause such an individual to view the removal of driving privileges as unreasonable and socially unacceptable.

Another issue is how long in the course of the AD process is the individual legally competent, and when does incompetence begin (Miner et al., 1989). Damage to the temporal, parietal, paracentral, or occipital lobes from strokes can compromise interactions necessary to participate in decision-making, but affected individuals provided with appropriate compensatory strategies are generally still competent in decision making. It is less clear whether the lack of judgment and insight characteristic of damage to the frontal lobes is compatible with competency in decision making.

Before the stage of frontal lobe involvement and regardless of the degree of compromise of other cognitive functions (or the scores on dementia rating scales), it is possible that persons with AD retain decision-making competency. However, it is not clear whether executive functions of intact frontal lobes can synthesize garbled information input from other lobes of the brain damaged by the AD process and still render appropriate decision making. Nonetheless, preserved frontal lobe functions (particularly preserved social functioning) can make the person with AD appear "normal," prompting casual witnesses to testify that the individual seemed "competent" when signing contracts, wills, or other documents. Legal distinctions are not necessarily helpful in this matter, since the U.S. Code of Federal Regulations provides only a vague definition of mental incompetency: "A mentally incompetent person is one who because of injury or disease lacks the mental capacity to contract or to manage his or her own affairs, including disbursement of funds without limitation" (Determination of Incompetency and Competency, 38 C.F.R., Book B, § 3.353). Thus, it is not clear what cerebral functions are necessary to satisfy the requirements for competency and when, in the course of the illness, individuals with AD become incompetent for decision making (including care decisions).

To summarize, AD is a common cause of the symptom complex of dementia, which is the progressive loss of intellectual and cognitive abilities sufficient to interfere with social or occupational functioning. The neuropathologic changes in AD involve the progressive loss of neurons and deposition of neuritic plaques and neurofibrillary tangles in the cerebral cortex. Involvement of the cerebral cortex is neither global nor uniform, but the process begins in medial structures of the limbic system and then spreads from the inferior temporal lobes over the remainder of the temporal lobes to the parietal lobe and then to the frontal lobe. Symptoms occur in a progressive fashion, with certain cortical functions compromised before others, paralleling the neuropathologic process. The initial symptoms involve memory disturbance, followed by language problems, then difficulties with spatial orientation, dressing, attention, and awareness, finally progressing to personality changes and loss of reasoning and judgment. It is important to recognize that the disease process results in profound deficits in some areas of cortical function, while other functions can remain relatively intact. Thus, the individual with Alzheimer disease should not be categorized solely on a severity rating scale measurement of a few cognitive tasks; nor should it be assumed that such a person is incompetent merely on the basis of certain cognitive deficits. Instead, every effort must be made to identify the specific cortical functional deficits along with the specific preserved cortical functions. The individual with AD (and the caregivers) should be assisted in developing compensatory strategies and, with appropriate accommodations, should be allowed to participate in decision-making processes.

REFERENCES

Allain, P., Joseph, P. A., Isambert, J. L., Le Gall, D., & Emile, J. (1998). Cognitive functions in chronic locked-in syndrome: A report of two cases. *Cortex, 34,* 629–634.

Bachman, D. L., Wolf, P. A., Linn, R. T., Knoefel, J. E., Cobb, J. L., Belanger, A. J., et al. (1993). Incidence of dementia and probable Alzheimer's disease in a general population: The Framingham Study. *Neurology, 43,* 515–519.

Beatty, W. W. (1999). Preserved cognitive skills in dementia: Implications for geriatric medicine. *Journal of the Oklahoma State Medical Association, 92,* 10–12.

Beatty, W. W., Brumback, R. A., & Vonsattel, J. P. (1997). Autopsy-proven Alzheimer disease in a patient with dementia who retained musical skill in life. *Archives of Neurology, 54,* 1448.

Beatty, W. W., Winn, P., Adams, R. L., Allen, E. W., Wilson, D. A., Prince, J. R., et al. (1994). Preserved cognitive skills in dementia of the Alzheimer type. *Archives of Neurology, 51,* 1040–1046.

Blessed, G., Tomlinson, B. E., & Roth, M. (1968). The association between quantitative measures of dementia and of senile change in the cerebral grey matter of elderly subjects. *British Journal of Psychiatry, 114,* 797–811.

Braak, E., Griffing, K., Arai, K., Bohl, J., Bratzke, H., & Braak, H. (1999). Neuropathology of Alzheimer's disease: What is new since A. Alzheimer? *European Archives of Psychiatry and Clinical Neurosciences, 249* (Suppl. 3), S14–S22.

Braak, H., & Braak, E. (1991). Neuropathological staging of Alzheimer-related changes. *Acta Neuropathologica (Berlin), 82,* 239–259.

Braak, H., & Braak, E. (1997). Diagnostic criteria for neuropathologic assessment of Alzheimer's disease. *Neurobiology of Aging, 18* (Suppl. 4), S85–S88.

Braak, H., Braak, E., Bohl, J., & Bratzke, H. (1998). Evolution of Alzheimer's disease related cortical lesions. *Journal of Neural Transmission, 54* (Suppl.), 97–106.

Breslaw, L. (1999). Aricept® and Alzheimer's—an early stage Alzheimer's patient writes of his personal experiences. *American Journal of Alzheimer's Disease, 14,* 317–319.

Broca, P. (1861). Remarques sur le siège de la faculté du langage articulé, suivies d'une observation d'aphémie [Remarks on the seat of the faculty of articulated language following observation of aphasia]. *Bulletin de la Société Anatomique 6,* 330–357.

Broca, P. (1865). Du siège de la faculté du langage articulé dans l'hémisphére gauche du cerveau [On the seat of the faculty of articulated language in the left hemisphere of the brain]. *Bulletin de la Société d'Anthropologie 6,* 377–393.

Brumback, R. A., & Leech, R. W. (1994). Alzheimer's disease: Pathophysiology and the hope for therapy. *Journal of the Oklahoma State Medical Association, 87,* 103–111.

Buell, S. J., & Coleman, P. D. (1981). Quantitative evidence for selective dendritic growth in normal human aging but not in senile dementia. *Brain Research, 214,* 23–41.

Cohen-Mansfield, J. (1986). Agitated behaviors in the elderly: II, Preliminary results in the cognitively deteriorated. *Journal of the American Geriatrics Society, 34,* 722–727.

Cole, M., & Dastoor, D. (1983). The Hierarchic Dementia Rating Scale. *Journal of Clinical and Experimental Gerontology, 5,* 219–234.

Cummings, J., Mega, M., Gray, K., Rosenberg-Thompson, S., Carusi, D. A., & Gornbein, J. (1994). The Neuropsychiatric Inventory: Comprehensive assessment of psychopathology in dementia. *Neurology, 44,* 2308–2314.

Cummings, J. L., & Benson, D. F. (1984). Subcortical dementia: Review of an emerging concept. *Archives of Neurology, 41,* 874–879.

Diagnostic and statistical manual of mental disorders. (DSM-IV). (1994). 4th edition. Washington, DC: American Psychiatric Association.

Evans, D. A., Funkenstein, H., Albert, M. S., Scherr, P. A., Cook, N. R., Chown, M. J., et al. (1989). Prevalence of Alzheimer's disease in a community of older persons: Higher than reported separately. *Journal of the American Medical Association, 262,* 2551–2556.

Evans, D. A., Smith, L. A., Scherr, P. A., Albert, M. S., Funkenstein, H. H., & Hebert, L. E. (1991). Risk of death from Alzheimer's disease in a community population of older persons. *American Journal of Epidemiology, 134,* 403–412.

Foley, D., Masaki, K., White, L., Ross, G. W., Eberhard, J., Dubinsky, R. M., et al. (2001). Practice parameter: Risk of driving and Alzheimer's disease. *Neurology, 56,* 695.

Folstein, M. F., Folstein, S. E., & McHugh, P. R. (1975). "Mini-mental state": A practical method for grading the cognitive state of patients for the clinician. *Journal of Psychiatric Research, 12,* 189–198.

Fratiglioni, L., Grut, M., Forsell, Y., Viitanen, M., Grafstrom, M., Holmen, K., et al. (1991). Prevalence of Alzheimer's disease and other dementias in an elderly urban population: Relationship with age, sex, and education. *Neurology, 41,* 1886–1892.

Gauthier, S. (Ed.). (1996). *Clinical diagnosis and management of Alzheimer's disease.* Boston, MA: Butterworth-Heinemann.

Good, D. C., & Couch, J. R., Jr. (Eds.). (1994). *Handbook of neurorehabilitation.* New York: Marcel Dekker.

Gottfries, C. G., Brane, G., Gullberg, B., & Steen, G. (1982). A new rating scale for dementia syndromes. *Archives of Gerontology and Geriatrics, 1,* 311–330.

Grundman, M., & Thal, L. J. (2000). Treatment of Alzheimer's disease: Rationale and strategies. *Neurologic Clinics, 18,* 807–827.

Hebert, L. E., Scherr, P. A., Beckett, L. A., Albert, M. S., Pilgrim, D. M., Chown, M. J., et al. (1995). Age-specific incidence of Alzheimer's disease in a community population. *Journal of the American Medical Association, 273,* 1354–1359.

Heilman, K. M., & Valenstein, E. (Eds.). (1993). *Clinical neuropsychology* (3rd ed.). New York: Oxford University Press.

Kaye, J., Swihart, T., Howieson, D., Dame, A., Moore, M. M., Karnos, T., et al. (1997). Volume loss of the hippocampus and temporal lobe in healthy elderly persons destined to develop dementia. *Neurology, 48,* 1297–1304.

Knopman, D., Knapp, M. J., Gracon, S. I., & Davis, C. S. (1994). The Clinician Interview-based Impression (CIBI): A clinician's global change rating scale in Alzheimer's disease. *Neurology, 44,* 2315–2321.

Kukull, W. A., & Ganguli, M. (2000). Epidemiology of dementia: Concepts and overview. *Neurology Clinics, 18,* 923–950.

Lezak, M. D. (1995). *Neuropsychological assessment* (3rd ed.). New York: Oxford University Press.

Lucas, J. A., Ivnik, R. J., Smith, G. E., Bohac, D. L., Tangalos, E. G., Kokmen, E., et al. (1998). Normative data for the Mattis Dementia Rating Scale. *Journal of Clinical and Experimental Neuropsychology, 20,* 536–547.

Malloy, P. F., Cummings, J. L., Coffey, C. E., Duffy, J., Fink, M., Lauterbach, E. C., et al. (1997). Cognitive screening instruments in neuropsychiatry: A report of the Committee on Research of the American Neuropsychiatric Association. *Journal of Neuropsychiatry and Clinical Neuroscience, 9,* 189–197.

Mesulam, M. M. (2000). Behavioral neuroanatomy: Large-scale networks, association cortex, frontal syndromes, the limbic system, and hemispheric specializations. In M. M. Mesulam (Ed.), *Principles of behavioral and cognitive neurology* (2nd ed.) (pp. 1–120). New York: Oxford University Press.

Milberg, W. (1996). Issues in the assessment of cognitive function in dementia. *Brain and Cognition, 31,* 114–132.

Miner, G. D., Winters-Miner, L. A., Blass, J. P., Richter, R. W., & Valentine, J. L. (1989). *Caring for Alzheimer's patients: A guide for family and healthcare providers.* New York: Plenum Press.

Morris, J. C. (1993). The Clinical Dementia Rating (CDR): Current version and scoring rules. *Neurology, 43,* 2412–2414.

Morris, J. C., Storandt, M., Miller, J. P., McKeel, D. W., Price, J. L., Rubin, E. H., & Berg, L. (2001). Mild cognitive impairment represents early-stage Alzheimer disease. *Archives of Neurology, 58,* 397–405.

Nagy, Z., Hindley, N. J., Braak, H., Braak, E., Yilmazer-Hanke, D. M., Schultz, C., et al. (1999a). Relationship between clinical and radiological diagnostic criteria for Alzheimer's disease and the extent of neuropathology as reflected by "stages": A prospective study. *Dementia and Geriatric Cognitive Disorders, 10,* 109–114.

Nagy, Z., Hindley, N. J., Braak, H., Braak, E., Yilmazer-Hanke, D. M., Schultz, C., et al. (1999b). The progression of Alzheimer's disease from limbic regions to the neocortex: Clinical, radiological, and pathological relationships. *Dementia and Geriatric Cognitive Disorders, 10,* 115–120.

Overall, J. E., & Schaltenbrand, R. (1992). The SKT neuropsychological test battery. *Journal of Geriatric Psychiatry and Neurology, 5,* 220–227.

Oxford English Dictionary. (1971). Compact Edition, Volume 2. Glasgow: Oxford University Press.

Reisberg, B. (1988). Functional assessment staging (FAST). *Psychopharmacology Bulletin, 24,* 653–659.

Reisberg, B., Borenstein, J., Salob, S. P., Ferris, S. H., Franssen, E., & Georgotas, A. (1987). Behavioral symptoms in Alzheimer's disease: Phenomenology and treatment. *Journal of Clinical Psychiatry, 48,* 9–15.

Reisberg, B., Ferris, S. H., de Leon, M. J., & Crook, T. (1982). The Global Deterioration Scale for assessment of primary degenerative dementia. *American Journal of Psychiatry, 139,* 1136–1139.

Riva, D., Bova, S. M., & Bruzzone, M. G. (2000). Neuropsychological testing may predict early progression of asymptomatic adrenoleukodystrophy. *Neurology, 54,* 1651–1655.

Rosen, W. G., Mohs, R. C., & Davis, K. L. (1984). A new rating scale for Alzheimer's disease. *American Journal of Psychiatry, 4,* 1356–1364.

Ross, E. D. (1996). Hemispheric specialization for emotions, affective aspects of language and communication, and the cognitive control of display behaviors in humans. *Progress in Brain Research, 107,* 583–594.

Ross, E. D., Homan, R. W., & Buck, R. (1994). Differential hemispheric lateralization of primary and social emotions: Implications for developing a comprehensive neurology for emotion, repression, and the subconscious. *Neuropsychiatry, Neuropsychology, and Behavioral Neurology, 7,* 1–19.

Sabat, S. R. (2001). *The experience of Alzheimer's disease: Life through a tangled veil.* Malden, MA: Blackwell.

Savage, C. R. (1997). Neuropsychology of subcortical dementias. *Psychiatric Clinics of North America, 20,* 911–931.

Schmitt, F. A., Ashford, W., Ernesto, C., Saxton, J., Schneider, L. S., Clark, C. M., et al. (1997). The severe impairment battery: Concurrent validity and the assessment of longitudinal change in Alzheimer's disease. The Alzheimer's Disease Cooperative Study. *Alzheimer Disease and Associated Disorders, 11* (Suppl. 2), S51–S56.

Schneider, L. S., Olin, J. T., Doody, R. S., Clark, C. M., Morris, J. C., Reisberg, B., et al. (1996). Validity and reliability of the Alzheimer's Disease Study-Clinical Global Impression of Change (ADCS-CGIC). *Alzheimer Disease and Associated Disorders, 11* (Suppl. 2), S22–S32.

Shader, R. I., Harmatz, J. S., & Salzman, C. (1974). A new scale for clinical assessment in geriatric populations: Sandoz Clinical Assessment-Geriatric (SCAG). *Journal of the American Geriatrics Society, 22,* 107–113.

Spiegel, R., Brunner, C., Ermini-Funfschilling, D., Monsch, A., Notter, M., Puxty, J., et al. (1991). A new behavioral assessment scale for geriatric out- and in-patients: The NOSGER (Nurses' Observation Scale for Geriatric Patients). *Journal of the American Geriatrics Society, 39,* 339–347.

Stringer, A. Y. (1996). *A guide to adult neuropsychological diagnosis.* Philadelphia, PA: F. A. Davis.

Tariot, P. N., Mack, J. L., Patterson, M. B., Edland, S. D., Weiner, M. F., Fillenbaum, G., et al. (1995). The Behavior Rating Scale for Dementia of the Consortium to Establish a Registry for Alzheimer's Disease. The Behavioral Pathology Committee of the Consortium to Establish a Registry for Alzheimer's Disease. *American Journal of Psychiatry, 152,* 1349–1357.

Terry, R. D., Katzman, R., Bick, K. L., & Sisodia, S. S. (Eds.). (1999). *Alzheimer disease* (2nd ed.). Philadelphia, PA: Lippincott Williams & Wilkins.

Tröster, A. I. (Ed.). (1998). *Memory in neurodegenerative disease: Biological, cognitive, and clinical perspectives.* Cambridge: Cambridge University Press.

Weinberg, W. A., Harper, C. R., Emslie, G. J., & Brumback, R. A. (1995). Depression and other affective illnesses as a cause of school failure and maladaptation in learning disabled children, adolescents, and young adults. In *Secondary education and beyond: Providing opportunities for students with learning disabilities* (pp. 234–264). Pittsburgh, PA: Learning Disabilities Association of America.

CHAPTER THREE

The Clinical Challenge of Uncertain Diagnosis and Prognosis in Patients with Dementia

David A. Bennahum, M.D.

Alzheimer disease (AD) is most often thought of by the general public as being characterized by memory loss. But most humans experience a loss of memory with illness or old age, and in my years as a clinician I have learned that it can be difficult to distinguish a dementia from common age-related forgetfulness, although recent research would suggest that the latter might predict future disease. I have also found that as the number of people with dementias increases, clinicians must become more and more skilled in distinguishing among the different types. Dementia, described by Brumback in the preceding chapter, can be the result of more than fifty-five conditions, among them Huntington disease, vitamin B_{12} deficiency and pernicious anemia, hypothyroidism, Parkinson disease, Pick disease, syphilis, AIDS, arteriosclerosis, strokes, Down syndrome, and, of course, Alzheimer disease. Most of these conditions affect memory, behavior, and overall health. The dementia associated with them, if untreated, or inappropriately treated, can result in premature death.

In this chapter, I provide the reader with some typical cases that a clinician might see and then briefly summarize the most common conditions that result in dementia by distinguishing the presenting symptoms, how each diagnosis is made, whether predictive genetic testing is now available, treatment, and what is known about the physiologic basis of each disease. It is noteworthy that the diagnosis and prognosis for a patient may depend more on the clinical experience and acumen of the physician than on any particular test or procedure. Discovery of the genes that correlate with Alzheimer and Huntington diseases have improved not only the physician's diagnostic ability but also may make it possible to predict the probability of disease in a patient's children and other relatives. Recently, positron emission tomography (PET) scanning has been suggested as a potentially accurate tool for the diagnosis of AD, but further corroboration still is required.

❧ Aging and Dementia

Confusion and loss of memory are increasingly common as people age (Byrne, 1994). The prevalence of dementia increases with age: "It occurs primarily late in life; the prevalence is about 1% at the age of 60 and it doubles every five years, to reach 30% to 50% by the age of 85" (Geldmacher & Whitehouse, 1996, p. 330). By the age of sixty-five, 2 to 3 percent of the population in the industrialized world have probable AD—a percentage as noted above that doubles every five years thereafter. At age seventy-five, between 12 and 14 percent have AD, and at age eighty the probability of AD is closer to 25 percent. After age eighty-five, somewhere between one-third and one-half of all individuals may be affected (Post, 2000).

Alzheimer disease "affects over 4 million people in the United States, resulting in over 100,000 deaths per year and costing the nation more than $60 billion annually" (Martin, 1999, p. 1970). It is predicted that the number of persons with dementia will rise throughout the world. As population growth declines in both the developed and the underdeveloped world, the problem of caring for so many fragile elders will become enormous.

❧ Assessing Patients Who Are Confused

In any geriatric practice, one sees many patients who have memory loss and are confused and disoriented. It is equally important to recognize and respond to the fears and needs of families and caregivers. The following are typical examples.

Case 1. A seventy-five-year-old retired physician is brought to the clinic by his wife. He looks well and states that he feels fine and that he has not noticed any loss of memory. His wife states that he has trouble accomplishing simple tasks such as shopping at the supermarket and that, the week before, he became lost while driving. On the Folstein Mini-Mental State Examination (see table 2.1), the patient scores 22 out of a possible 30. The normal range is 25 to 30 (Folstein, 1975). When asked to draw a clock, he places all the numbers on one side. The rest of the history and the physical examination are normal. The patient is not anemic, he has normal B_{12} and thyroid tests, and an MRI (magnetic resonance imaging) of the brain that reveals generalized tissue loss without enlargement of the ventricles. His syphilis test is negative. The physician is therefore able to rule out normal pressure hydrocephalus, a hypothyroid state, and B_{12} deficiency. He then advises the patient and the wife that the patient probably has Alzheimer disease.

Case 2. A lady of sixty-two has been forgetful, confused, and disoriented, and recently became incontinent of urine. On entering the examining room, the physician notes that the patient has an unsteady gait. Ten years ago she had a concussion after a motor vehicle accident. An MRI reveals greatly enlarged ventricles due to obstruction to free flow of the cerebrospinal fluid. A diagnosis of Normal Pressure Hydrocephalus was made and a shunt was placed from the brain to the venous system to drain off the fluid. Her condition then stabilized.

Case 3. A seventy-year-old retired college professor is in a panic. He can no longer remember the names of some of his students and forgets various items when shopping at the supermarket. He is convinced that he has AD, but no member of his family has ever had a dementia except for a cousin. All of his tests except the thyroid stimulating hormone are normal, and he scores a 28 on the Mini-Mental State Examination. He is treated with thyroid hormone, and six months later his memory has improved.

Case 4. A thirty-two-year-old biochemist tells his physician that he fears he will develop dementia since both his mother and father, as well as two uncles, have AD. He has heard that there is a genetic test to diagnose the disease. He asks the physician to order the test. The physician fears that if the patient learns that he carries one or more alleles for the disease, this may provoke a depression or even suicide. The physician does not know if she should acquiesce to the patient's request.

Case 5. The daughter of a man with severe dementia is designated as the decision maker for health care in the patient's advance directive. She asks the physician to end her father's life on the grounds that he would not have wanted to live in a confused state that she thinks is without dignity. The patient is unaware of her request. The physician points out that the patient appears to enjoy his meals and the outings at the nursing home where he now lives. The physician says she is uncomfortable with the daughter's request on ethical grounds. The physician and daughter agree to discuss the request again in a month.

In each of these cases, one could assume that the patient has Alzheimer disease. In truth, 85 percent of patients with symptoms of dementia will turn out to have AD, but 15 percent will have another explanation for their symptoms. It is very important to rule out treatable causes of dementia such as B_{12} deficiency and hypothyroidism. Other patients have dementia that is due to other degenerative diseases of the brain such as Parkinson disease, Huntington disease, Creutzfeldt-Jacob disease, and Pick disease. A common cause of dementia is multiple small infarctions of the brain. When multiinfarct dementia coexists with AD, the course of the dementia is more severe. In the past, syphilis was a common cause of dementia, and it is still found on occasion; and, though rarely, an elderly person may present with dementia due to AIDS.

❧ Clinical Symptoms and Pathological Findings

Although the clinical symptoms are very similar, each disease that can cause a dementia has a different pathology at autopsy. Additionally, an elderly patient might have more than one disease—for example, Parkinson disease and AD, either of which could be causing the dementia. The following are the most common conditions that result in dementia:

Vascular dementias can be due to large-vessel disease, as when a clot separates from the carotid artery and causes a large stroke or when multiple small emboli produce small infarctions of brain tissue over time. When this occurs in the setting of Alzheimer disease, the dementia tends to accelerate and the symptoms to increase in severity. The patients often have a history of cardiovascular disease and may have hypertension, heart failure, and a history of small or large strokes. The progression of multiinfarct dementia tends to be step-like, with long periods of stable symptoms and then an abrupt worsening. Patients present with loss of short-term memory and confusion very much like that found in Alzheimer dementia.

Lewy body dementia tends to be less severe than AD and includes a triad of fluctuating symptoms, including memory loss, visual hallucinations, and spontaneously arising Parkinson disease. The pathology presents characteristic intraneural inclusions that are pathological aggregations of neurofilaments, known as Lewy bodies (LBs). "Indeed, LBs represent yet another example of intracellular and extracellular proteinaceous aggregates that are a common neuropathological feature of several different sporadic and hereditary neurodegenerative diseases" (Vogelsberg-Ragaglia, 1999, p. 364).

Binswanger disease is a dementia found in relatively young patients—patients in their fifties. They are often hypertensive patients who on an MRI have cerebral white matter changes and arteriosclerosis. The patients often appear apathetic, although language skills are preserved. Often the patient will have problems sequencing ideas and will have a loss in executive functions. Gait changes are an early clue, as is the slowly progressive nature of the disease.

Frontal lobe dementias are a varied group of diseases of adult life that include focal cortical dementias and Pick disease. These can be mistaken for AD and are characterized by an "early deterioration in social conduct, personality, initiative, insight and attention with jocularity, rudeness, loss of emotional warmth, disinhibition and distractibility" (Pryse-Phillips, 1999, p. 80).

Normal pressure hydrocephalus is usually the result of brain trauma or infection resulting in fibrous tissue that obstructs outflow of the central nervous system fluid from the ventricles of the brain. The patient usually presents with a triad of ataxia, dementia, and incontinence. The buildup of fluid that enlarges the ventricles, thereby placing pressure on the brain, can be diagnosed with a CAT scan or MRI and treated by placing a shunt from the ventricles to the vascular system. Treatment slows or stops progression, but rarely cures the disease. After age seventy-five, shunts usually are not recommended since the benefit decreases with age.

Subcortical dementias include progressive supranuclear palsy (PSP), Huntington disease (HD), and several other conditions. In PSP there is widespread loss of nerve cells and the presence of tangles that have straight filaments that are therefore different from the tangles of AD. Patients with PSP have dementia, rigidity, and problems with eye movement. HD can be predicted with genetic testing and is characterized by the insidious onset in late midlife of uncontrolled movements and a gradually worsening dementia.

Parkinson disease can be expected to cause a dementia in up to 30 percent of patients. Patients who are over seventy and have severe rigidity and gait disorder, but only a mild tremor, are more at risk. The patients exhibit decreased cognitive function and difficulty drawing and solving problems. Parkinson disease with dementia can be associated with three conditions: (1) idiopathic dementia; (2) dementia with cortical Lewy bodies; and (3) some cases of Alzheimer dementia (Foster, Minoshima, & Kuhl, 1999). More than 1 million people are affected in North America. "In fact, neurodegenerative diseases are projected to surpass cancer as the second most common cause of death among the elderly by the year 2040" (Lang, 1998, p. 1044).

There are also the prion disorders. The infectious prion protein has become famous as the cause of mad cow disease after animal protein was fed to cattle, but it is also associated with scrapie in sheep, kuru, due to the practice of ritual cannibalism by the Fore People in the highlands of New Guinea, and Creutzfeldt-Jacob disease. The patients develop spongiform changes in the brain with a normal spinal fluid, and progressive neurologic changes characterized by a dementia that has a relatively rapid onset and is accompanied by myoclonus and leads eventually to death.

Toxic and metabolic causes, while relatively rare, are important because they include the treatable dementias caused by vitamin B_{12}, folate, or thyroid insufficiency. In patients with B_{12} deficiency, a subtle dementia with loss of short-term memory and cognitive skills may develop, preceding the anemia and that may be mistaken for AD. The same is true for thyroid deficiency. Alcohol and various drugs and chemicals can also result in loss of memory, judgment, psychosis, and dementia.

Infectious diseases such as syphilis, Whipple disease, and AIDS may be associated with a dementia.

It is now thought that dementia of the Alzheimer type (DAT) is one disease, rather than several. The severity of the disease and the age at which it begins may reflect a genetic predisposition. Women may be affected slightly more frequently than men, the frequency increasing as people age. Alzheimer dementia is characterized by a gradual and progressive course. Patients with DAT demonstrate loss of short-term and long-term memory. They lose their orientation for time and, soon, for place. They have difficulty learning new information. Eventually they lose the ability to name things, and at the end stages of the disease no longer speak. An early sign may be the inability to copy two superimposed pentagons or to draw a clock face. In the Mini-Mental State Examination, one can detect the loss of many of these abilities with simple questions such as: What is the date today? Do you know the season we are in? Where is the place we are right now? Can you subtract seven from one hundred and then continue to subtract seven from each answer? Often a patient will not remember the sequence of objects—ball, flag, tree—or how to spell the word *w-o-r-l-d* backwards. It is important to recognize that education, native language, and culture may aid or inhibit the person being tested. As the disease progresses, the patient may become uninhibited and speak loudly, get angry, have paranoid ideas or visual hallucinations such as seeing insects on the floor, or become sexually aggressive. Motor skills are preserved until very late in the disease. In the end, the patient no longer speaks, no longer recognizes friends and family, and may become incontinent and without appetite.

For the family, the loved one dies before their eyes. The family is bereaved while the patient still lives, and that is terribly difficult to bear. It is important that the family and friends as well as the patient receive support and care—issues that are raised in several chapters of this book. Many institutions have bereavement counselors who hold sessions and provide counseling for family members of DAT patients.

When a pathologist examines the brains of patients who were presumed to have died of AD, the most striking findings are aggregates of amyloid protein and neurofibrillary tangles. Whether the amyloid precedes or follows the neurofibrillary tangles is not clear. The presence of amyloid, a protein usually found in inflammatory states, has led to the suggestion that anti-inflammatory drugs such as ibuprofen might be effective in AD.

While AD is the disease most commonly found at autopsy in patients who had dementia, there are a number of other conditions, as noted above, that must be considered in the evaluation of a person with memory loss. A few of these conditions respond to treatment; for example, vitamin B_{12} deficiency, hypothyroidism, normal pressure hydrocephalus, Parkinson disease, and depression. There are also numerous degenerative neurological diseases such as Pick disease and Huntington disease that often cause loss of memory, confusion, and dementia for which no treatment exists. In some of these diseases, such as Huntington disease, genetic testing can be used to identify carriers who may then decide not to have children (Harper, 2000). Tragically, there is a high suicide rate in patients with chronic degenerative diseases such as HD or amytrophic lateral sclerosis (Ganzini, 1998).

The principal risk factors for AD are age and family history. The disease is more common in individuals with little education. Traumatic head injury is also more frequent in those who develop AD. The observation that individuals with Down syndrome who lived beyond the age of forty invariably developed AD led to an examination of the chromosomes of these individuals (Mayeux, 1999). And indeed Down syndrome patients with AD have amyloid deposits and neurofibrillary tangles in the brain that look like those of AD patients (Poirier, 1999). Brain imaging has been very helpful in research, but much less so in clinical application. New techniques such as PET and SPECT scanning, however, hold great promise (Gilman, 1998).

Recent research has identified a number of genetic markers for AD that include two genes for amyloid and one for apolipoprotein E (Bedlack, 2000). Chromosome 1 carries the presenilin gene II, chromosome 14, the presenilin gene I, and chromosome 21, the APP gene or amyloid precurser protein gene. All three genes are necessary for the production of amyloid. These genes are thought to be responsible for the rare form of autosomal dominant, early onset AD that includes only about 1 to 5 percent of all Alzheimer dementia patients. Chromosome 19 carries the apolipoprotein E gene. This is responsible for 50 percent of AD. Three alleles of this gene, numbered 2, 3 and 4, can be inherited from one's parents in various combinations. If one inherits number 4, the probability of AD rises dramatically. Chromosome 12 has recently been studied and is thought to be associated with AD in 30 percent of the cases.

The apolipoprotein alleles have been used to predict the probability of disease occurrence in relatives of patients with AD (Boss, 2000). These alleles can be tested for, and the results can raise difficult questions. In the current situation, when there is no curative treatment for the disease, should one inform a relative that he or she is at risk for AD? Will insurance companies refuse to insure carriers of these genes? Will testing lead to the termination of some pregnancies? Predictive genetic testing in AD, as in other diseases such as breast cancer, is bound to create a host of ethical and legal dilemmas (Grady, 1999). Now that genetic testing will identify those at risk for AD, society must decide how such information will be handled and how to avoid harming individuals who are carriers of pathologic genes (Panegyres, 2000).

✌ Treatment and Care of Alzheimer Patients

Alzheimer disease involves family, friends, and society more than do most other serious conditions. Diagnosis is often delayed because the early symptoms appear gradually. A change in personality or behavior, forgetfulness, and inattention to self-care or the home are early warning signs that spouses, children, and friends may not immediately understand. It may take months and visits to a number of physicians before the diagnosis can be made, and even then, in the absence of a diagnostic test, the diagnosis of AD is always presumptive. First the physician must exclude treatable causes of dementia, as outlined above. The care and education of the family can be most important. In this context, providing a case manager, home visits, and a well-planned care plan is very helpful. The loved ones, family, and friends of a patient with AD will become bereaved while the patient is still alive, and this slow process of loss needs to be recognized and support provided.

The health professions team, working with the family, must direct attention to the patient's general health. If possible, while the patient retains decisional capacity, an advance directive should be discussed, written, and signed; and a durable power of attorney for health care should be executed, identifying a decision maker for health care decisions in the future when the patient is no longer able to do so (a point that Scheirton elaborates in chapter 16). Some challenges surrounding the use of such directives are discussed in part IV of this book. Preventive therapies should include antioxidants such as vitamin E. A nonprescription medication from the *Ginkgo biloba* tree is popularly advocated, but rigorous studies of its efficacy have yet to be completed. A recent study suggested that two years of NSAIDs (nonsteroidal anti-inflammatory drugs) dramatically reduced the development of AD in its later stages. Estrogen was until recently considered a preventive strategy, but new research has thrown doubt on the estrogen hypothesis. Another treatment that is unsubstantiated and some suggest may actually accelerate progression is the use of cholinesterase inhibitors that enhance cholinergic transmission. These include tacrine, donepezil, rivastigmine, metrifonate, and galantamine (Knopman, 2000). As the reader knows from the newspapers, radio, and television, a fierce battle has emerged about the ethics of using

stem cells derived from human embryos to develop possible treatments for neurodegenerative diseases, including AD (Begley, 2001).

✿ The Challenge of Alzheimer Disease: A Clinician's and Medical Educator's Perspective on the Ethical Issues

A prolonged disease of old age that at great cost robs the individual of pleas-
ure, identity, and dignity and for which there is neither prevention nor treatment
is an enormous challenge to any society. For the United States, the problem of
AD is compounded by the lack of universal health insurance and the for-profit
nature of the long-term care industry. AD can impoverish a family that desper-
ately tries to pay for long-term care while watching the person they knew disappear before their eyes. Despair can lead patients to depression and requests for
aid-in-dying. Until recently, most of the concern about patients suffering from
AD has been centered on issues of care and respect, themes further developed in
this book. As Stephen Post has argued movingly, AD presents a moral challenge
in that we need to care deeply for such patients. Not only must we avoid prejudice against the elderly and the forgetful, also we must protect them against burdensome and invasive treatments. Respect for persons includes attempts to
address very simple, but basic, needs, such as those for cleanliness, stimulation,
touching, and laughter. Post points out that our society emphasizes rationality
and memory to a fault and that this disenfranchises this most vulnerable of all
groups (2000).

At present there is no cure for Alzheimer dementia, and few preventive strategies have been clearly proven to provide long-term benefit. Taking the various
concerns discussed in this chapter, how, then, should we approach this tragic disease? First, we must acknowledge that it is not the patient alone who requires
treatment, but rather the patient and the patient's family. Second, it is imperative
that a care model, rather than a cure model, of treatment be proposed and explained to patients and families, even as research for prevention and curative
treatments continue. Perhaps it is even more important to educate physicians,
nurses, and other health professionals to advocate a palliative care model for the
treatment of these patients and, as part II of this book highlights, to shape palliative measures to ameliorate the specific symptoms of AD. A palliative care
model discourages inappropriate hospitalization, tube feeding, cardiopul-

monary resuscitation, and the use of restraints. Third, whenever possible, an advance directive and durable power of attorney for health care should be executed by patients while they still retain decisional capacity. To summarize, comfort, dignity, affection, and stimulation are what Alzheimer dementia patients need. Every effort should be made for their provision (Volicer, 2001).

The new ethical challenge is also societal and involves confidentiality, the privacy of medical records, the financing of research on diseases of the elderly, the right of individuals to health care (a right that is not presently recognized in the United States), and creative thinking about the artistic and spiritual potential of the elderly. The health insurance system in the United States needs to be modified to embrace basic coverage for everyone and to encourage and finance home care. The respectful care and treatment of these, among the most fragile members of society, is the measure of a just and humane community.

I would like to leave the reader with three principles that should guide health professionals and society alike in their approach to people with AD:

1. Respect individuals as equals and honor their inherent autonomy and previously expressed wishes
2. Provide care that enhances each patient's dignity while instilling comfort and stimulation and recognizes the individual's life-long personality and style
3. Do not prolong life by artificial means if it does not enhance the quality of life and the dignity of the individual

In short, if respect for the dignity of each person is at the core of our personal and professional ethics, we will have moved a long way in the right direction with Alzheimer dementia patients being treated in a just and caring manner.

REFERENCES

Bedlack, R., Strittmatter, W. J., & Morgenlander, J. C. (2000). Apolipoprotein E and neuromuscular disease. *Archives of Neurology, 57,* 1561–1565.
Begley, S. (2001). Cellular divide. *Newsweek, July 9,* 22–25.
Boss, M. A. (2000). Diagnostic approaches to Alzheimer's disease. *Biochimica et Biophysica Acta 1502,* 188–200.
Byrne, E. J. (1994). *Confusional states in older people.* London: Edward Arnold.

Folstein, M. F., Folstein, S. E., & McHugh, P. R. (1975). "Mini-mental state": A practical method for grading the cognitive state of patients for the clinician. *Journal of Psychiatric Research, 12,* 189–198.

Foster, N. L., Minoshima, S., & Kuhl, D. E. (1999). Brain imaging in Alzheimer's disease. In R. D. Terry, R. Katzman, K. Bick, & S. S. Sisodia (Eds.), *Alzheimer's disease* (pp. 83–84). Philadelphia, PA: Lippincott Williams & Wilkins.

Ganzini, L., Johnston, W. S., McFarland B. H., Tolle S. W., & Lee, M. A. (1998). Attitudes of patients with amyotrophic lateral sclerosis and their caregivers toward assisted suicide. *New England Journal of Medicine, 339,* 967–973.

Geldmacher, D. S., & Whitehouse, P. J. (1996). Evaluation of dementia. *New England Journal of Medicine, 335* (5), 330–336.

Gilman, S. (1998). Imaging the brain. *New England Journal of Medicine, 338* (12), 812–820.

Grady, C. (1999). *Ethics and genetic testing in advances in internal medicine.* St. Louis, MO: Mosby.

Harper, P. S., Lim, C., & Crawford, D. (2000). Ten years of presymptomatic testing for Huntington's disease: The experience of the UK Huntington's disease prediction consortium. *Journal of Medical Genetics, 37,* 567–571.

Knopman, D. S. (2000). Implications of early diagnosis for the development of therapeutics for Alzheimer's disease. In L. F. M. Scinto & K. R. Daffner (Eds.), *Early diagnosis of Alzheimer's disease* (pp. 297–316). Totowa, NJ: Humana Press.

Lang, A. E., & Lozano, A. M. (1998). Parkinson's disease. *New England Journal of Medicine, 339* (15), 1044.

Martin, J. B. (1999). Molecular basis of neurodegenerative disorders. *New England Journal of Medicine, 340* (25), 1970.

Mayeux, R., & Christen, Y. (1999). *Epidemiology of Alzheimer's disease: From gene to prevention,* Berlin: Springer-Verlag, 19–31.

Panegyres, P. K., Goldblatt, J., Walpole, I., Connor, C., Liebeck, T., & Harrop, K. (2000). Genetic testing for Alzheimer's disease. *Medical Journal of Australia, 172,* 339–343.

Poirier, J., Danik, M., & Blass, J. P. (1999). Pathophysiology of the Alzheimer syndrome. In S. Gauthier (Ed.), *Alzheimer's disease* (p. 23). London: Martin Dunitz.

Post, S. G. (2000). *The moral challenge of Alzheimer disease.* Baltimore, MD: Johns Hopkins University Press.

Pryse-Phillips, W., & Galasko, D. (1999). Non-Alzheimer dementias. In S. Gauthier (Ed.), *Alzheimer's disease* (pp. 73–79). London: Martin Dunitz.

Vogelsberg-Ragaglia, V., Trojanowski, J. Q., & Lee, V. M-Y. (1999). Cytoskeletal pathology in Alzheimer's disease. In R. D. Terry, R. Katzman, K. Bick, & S. S. Sisodia (Eds.), *Alzheimer's disease* (p. 364). Philadelphia, PA: Lippincott Williams & Wilkins.

Volicer, L., McKee, A., & Hewitt, S. (2001). Dementia. In A. C. Carver & K. M. Foley (Eds.), *Palliative care* (pp. 867–885). Neurologic Clinics of North America, volume 19, no 4.

Part II / European Voices on U.S. and European Models of Palliative Care

CHAPTER FOUR

Expanding the Scope of Palliative Care

Henk A.M.J. ten Have, M.D., Ph.D.

The number of persons with Alzheimer disease will increase substantially over the forthcoming decades, as O'Brien illustrated in the first part of this book. A report of the Health Council of the Netherlands, for example, estimated that in the year 2000, one in every ninety-three people in the country had dementia. In 2050, the prevalence will be one in forty-four (Gezondheidsraad, 2002).

Potential methods of prevention are not yet adequately explored. The report also concludes that genetic diagnosis is not worthwhile: a negative predictive test result will not imply that the person will remain free from AD, and a positive outcome does not mean that a person will develop the disease. Furthermore, it is stated that antidementia drugs so far are unsuccessful; one of the conclusions of the report is that in the foreseeable future it is unlikely that medication that is capable of controlling all of the symptoms of dementia will be discovered. Given the lack of preventive and curative approaches, as well as the increasing prevalence of the disease, an atmosphere of powerlessness and even desperation may arise. The personal, social, and economic burdens of AD may become overwhelming, as documented by O'Brien (chapter 1.) This makes patients, families, caregivers, and health care professionals vulnerable to the "therapeutic illusion"—the unfounded belief that remedies are almost at hand and certainly available in the very near future.

On the other hand, what are the options? With a growing number of persons requiring care, the only option indeed is to provide adequate care. In 2000, approximately 35 percent of dementia patients were in nursing homes or residential care facilities. In order to maintain a comparable level of professional care with the increasing prevalence of dementia, six new nursing homes per year should be established in the Netherlands (creating an annual 1,300 institutional places). This estimation, of course, presupposes that, at present, treatment, care, and support are adequate. In the report it is acknowledged that this is not the case. Therefore, if in the current situation providing care is the only feasible option, it is clear that an enormous effort will be required, not only as far as family and professional caregivers are concerned but even more on a social and cultural level, where better, as well as many more, care service arrangements should be created.

However, what is rarely discussed is what type of care is most adequate for persons with AD. It is suggested that palliative care is the preferred type of care. Palliative care should be expanded so that it will include care for AD patients (George & Sykes, 1997; R. Janssens et al., 2002). It is no longer defensible to restrict palliative care to people with cancer; we should develop palliative care beyond cancer, and people with AD clearly are at the moment a disadvantaged group. The question, however, is how palliative care as it has evolved recently, with its particular conceptual, philosophical, and ethical framework, relates to care for people with AD.

❧ The Development of Palliative Care

During recent decades, the development of palliative care has been impressive. During the 1970s, the ideas of the hospice movement were disseminated. In Canada, Balfour Mount established in 1975 the first in-patient palliative care unit in Montreal's Royal Victoria Hospital, introducing the new term *palliative care*. In the 1980s, the modern ideas of hospice and palliative care were gaining ground in various European countries (ten Have & Janssens, 2001; Jacquemin, 2001). For example, in 1987 the first palliative care unit in France was founded in the international hospital of the University of Paris. Years before, palliative home care services had begun in Sweden (in 1977) and Italy (1980). Germany, Spain, and Belgium initiated palliative care services in the first half of the 1980s. In the

Netherlands, palliative care arrived rather late, with the establishment of the first hospice in 1991 and academic palliative care centers in 1999. The need for palliative care is similar in both developed and developing countries. Every country is confronted with demographic changes leading to an aging population.

At the same time, the character of medical problems is changing, with an increasing burden of chronic illnesses in which the possibilities of cure are limited. The prolonged lifespan is associated with longer average stays in medical institutions and an increasing need of care and assistance. Also, the general nature of dying has changed from acute, sudden death to a long process of dying, often with mental and physical deterioration and suffering. New and different medical services need to be developed in order to have an appropriate response to these changes. However, the organizational forms of palliative care in various countries are different. A range of services, from hospices, home care services, and consultation teams to palliative care units in nursing homes, oncology clinics, and hospitals can be distinguished. The establishment of palliative care services is adapted to the characteristics of the health care system, depending on the focus, whether it be on specialist hospital-based medicine or on home care services and general practice.

It is also relevant that palliation has always been a goal of medical care. Although the current emphasis on palliative care is more articulated and identified as a separate activity, the development of palliative care services often starts from existing structures. This implies that palliative care is developing from various settings—for example, oncology, geriatrics, anesthesiology, or nursing home medicine. This heterogeneity is leading to different concepts of palliative care in different countries.

The variety of palliative care also flows from an ambiguity in the palliative care movement itself. Initially, hospices were established because of dissatisfaction with the medical care provided in the usual hospital setting, with insufficient attention to the needs of dying persons. Separate institutions were considered necessary in order to focus on this particular category of patients. Palliative care in this view was seen as a complementary arrangement that could make the health care system more encompassing and attentive to the needs of modern patients. However, at the same time, the hospice and palliative care philosophy also emphasized that care and compassion cannot only be provided in a separate setting but need to be basic components of all health care. Instead of establishing another system of services, it is necessary to introduce the ideas of palliative care in other health care services and transform medicine into a human activity of caring.

❧ Concepts of Palliative Care

The hospice movement in the United Kingdom has been a paradigm for many palliative care services in other European countries. From the beginning, advocates of palliative care have argued that palliative care is first and foremost a concept of care that is different from standard (medical) practice. The concept, it is argued, is different because it is related to specific moral values (concerning life and death, pain and suffering, individual person and social context); but at the same time, the concept is homogeneous since the same moral values are shared regardless of the specific palliative care setting. Yet, as the comparison of different countries has shown, the concept of palliative care is shaped in different institutional forms (ten Have & Janssens, 2001). It is unclear whether this range of organizational systems is the expression of an identical concept or whether different concepts of palliative care are at work.

Currently, palliative care is in a crucial phase of development in many countries. Although palliative care has been recognized as a medical specialty in the United Kingdom, most other countries are struggling with the issue of how to relate palliative care to the health care system. Palliative care is increasingly organized within the setting of the formal health care system, but it is still open whether this implies specialization (developing a specific discipline with university departments and chairs, in-patient units, with all the paraphernalia of a medical specialty) or integration (incorporating palliative care in established clinical departments, and cooperating with existing medical disciplines). In view of this dilemma, the concept of palliative care has become ambivalent. The philosophy of palliative care emphasizes care and communication rather than intervention and treatment. Mainstream medicine still is largely dominated by the values of technology and active intervention.

In such antagonistic contexts, development as a distinct new discipline apparently is more feasible than permeating all medical disciplines with a new ethos. At the same time, the increasing interrelations with mainstream medicine have also changed the initial concept of palliative care. First, the identification of palliative care with the terminal phase of illness is rejected now by most participants in the debates. This majority holds, instead, that palliative care starts from the time of diagnosis. Second, the identification of palliative care with cancer care is put more and more under critique. It is widely acknowledged that patients suffering from Alzheimer disease, heart failure, AIDS, multiple sclerosis, and other chronic diseases have been neglected by palliative care practitioners for too long. Third, the moral notions initially motivating palliative care practitioners have been strongly associated with the Western Christian tradition ("love," "sympathy," "sanctity of life"); these notions are now "translated" into universal, bioethical notions ("quality of life," "human dignity," "total care"). Fourth, the ethical norms that should prevail in palliative care practice are more and more subject to debate. In the Netherlands, the majority of physicians providing palliative care accept euthanasia as a means of last resort and in other countries there is no consensus that euthanasia should be excluded from palliative care. Debates on the validity of the doctrine of double effect, on withholding and withdrawing life-prolonging treatment, on terminal sedation, and on research in palliative care have intensified during the past three decades, and a consensus cannot be expected. The integration process of palliative care into mainstream health care systems has made the concept of palliative care ambiguous and ambivalent.

The scope of palliative care has expanded mainly as a result of three processes:

1. It is no longer connected to a specific institution such as a hospice or a palliative care unit; in fact, we notice a range of diverging practices, all under the "palliative care" umbrella.
2. It no longer focuses on a specific category of patients—that is, cancer patients.
3. It is no longer applied within a particular time frame in the disease trajectory (i.e., the terminal phase).

As a result of these processes, the scope of palliative care may become unclear. Its demarcation from other medical practices may become problematic. The expanding scope of palliative care at the same time raises the question "What is the distinctive core of palliative care?" It is argued that the concept(s) of palliative care primarily are determined and motivated by a common core of moral values (Janssens, 2001).

❧ The Underlying Value Structure

Clarification of the underlying value structure of palliative care is facilitated if it is remembered that the concept(s) of palliative care are morally motivated. Characterizations of palliative care in the professional literature always emphasize the following four determinants:

1. *Specific goals.* Palliative care first of all is special because it has particular goals, different from the more usual goals of cure and prevention. Although there is a lot of debate regarding the meaning and implementation of these goals, four goals are frequently connected with palliative care: (a) improvement of quality of life; (b) symptom control and relief of pain; (c) accomplishment of a good death; and (d) prevention of euthanasia.

2. *Specific attitudes.* Palliative care practice is requiring a set of typical attitudes—for example, the acceptance of human finiteness. Palliative care will do nothing to prolong the dying of the patients, but also nothing to hasten the death of the patient. The fact that the patient is nearing death is accepted. This also implies an attitude of restraint. Palliative care is death-accepting but life-enhancing. Contrary to the active interventionism of medicine in other circumstances, palliative treatment is restricted to symptom control and relief of suffering. Palliative care should also be "total comfort care," requiring compassion and openness as well as a focus on all the needs of the patient, not only the physical, but also social, psychological, and spiritual needs.

3. *Integral care.* The totality of the patient is in focus. Palliative care implies holistic or whole-person care. It is patient-centered, not disease-focused. This requires not only an interest in biopsychosocial and spiritual dimensions but also multidisciplinary teamwork. The crucial notion of responsibility is of as much importance here as that of practical wisdom (what Aristotle called *phrónesis*) (Randall & Downie 1996).

4. *Involvement of patients as well as relatives.* Palliative care is characterized more by the notion of interpersonal relationships than one of individual autonomy. It also implies partnership with the patient and is therefore based on shared decision making.

All four of these determinants point to the relationship of palliative care and ethics. This area of health care is distinctive because it has a specific set of underlying values. Clarifying these underlying values is important for the future development of palliative care.

❧ Ethics and Palliative Care

Interesting connections exist between palliative care and ethics, many of which have not been fully analyzed and explored. In the context of palliative care practice, specific moral dilemmas and problems arise that need clarification, explanation, and resolution from the perspectives of ethical theory and methodology. And, looked at from the other direction, ethics itself may benefit from the peculiarities of palliative care as a movement and philosophy of care—one that introduces new moral notions particularly relevant in the context of health care. These fascinating interactions and possible mutual benefits are now beginning to be discovered and explored by scholars and professionals in both palliative care and ethics (Clark & Seymour, 1999; Jennings, 1997; Randall & Downie, 1996; Webb, 2000; ten Have & Clark, 2002).

This rather late interest is surprising. Palliative care and ethics have at least three features in common. First, both have a long-standing tradition in health care; they have been part and parcel of medicine since its origins. Until the recent development of effective therapies and preventive strategies, palliation was the most significant goal of medical care. Ethics has been an essential component of medical practice since Hippocrates established medicine as a profession separated from religion and philosophy.

Second, although palliative care and ethics have always been intrinsic to medicine, since the 1960s both have enjoyed a resurgence of interest. Modern medicine developed rapidly in the decades following World War II. For the first time in the profession's history, effective treatment was available to eradicate many life-threatening diseases. Innovative technologies expanded the diagnostic and therapeutic abilities of physicians. Life-saving technologies and advanced surgery not only could counteract the impact of emergencies but also prevent acute death. This explosion of medical innovations, technologies, and therapies instigated the emergence of bioethics in the late 1960s. There were controversial cases and public scandals in relation to medical research, dialysis treatment, and resuscitation policies, first in North America and somewhat later in Europe. At the same time, death and dying have been the special focus of critical attention because the expansion of medicine has increasingly transformed not only the location of the process of dying (from the home to the hospital) but also its management (from care to intervention). Palliative care, and especially the hospice movement, developed as an effort to improve health care for dying patients and to redirect the emphasis of therapy- and technology-driven medicine. Therefore, the new interest in ethics as well as palliative care was not simply a reiteration of long-existing but forgotten dimensions but also an attempt to redefine the core of medicine itself, to influence its development, and to at least remedy a one-sided interest in technological interventions primarily aimed at curing illness and prolonging life.

This observation points to the third common feature: bioethics and palliative care seem to have a similar basic objective—that is, to maintain or, if necessary, reinstitute a humane medicine, primarily focused on the human person in need. Instead of being driven by technology and the possibilities and promises of science, medicine should first of all be committed to the patient and the patient's particular interests. Medicine should also acknowledge that technology and science can easily distort the proper view of what is really appropriate in certain circumstances—for example, when frail and vulnerable patients are admitted to the intensive unit, when patients with advanced cancer are included in another clinical trial, or when medical interventions for elderly persons with dementia are continued without critical assessment.

Notwithstanding this shared background in history, recent interest, and general objective, until recently a disjunction of ethics and palliative care has been noticeable. Bioethics developed as a separate discipline, interested in death-and-dying issues—particularly controversies in regard to euthanasia and foregoing medical treatment, but not specifically focused on the area of palliative care. At the same time, palliative care emerged as a new approach and philosophy of care, creating new structures and arrangements of care, and developing into a new discipline, with textbooks, chairs, departments, educational programs and special services. In journals devoted to palliative care, moral dilemmas and issues have been discussed regularly, but participation by professional bioethicists has been limited (Hermsen & ten Have, 2001). The literature shows that palliative care practitioners frequently have to deal with moral issues. Not only do they encounter many moral queries that arise in other health care areas, but they also experience moral problems specific to the palliative care setting. Bioethics can contribute to analysis and clarification of these problems and to the develop-

ment of practical approaches and methods to support palliative care practitioners in coping with these queries.

In this regard, palliative care presents itself, albeit late, as a new area of bioethical research and consultation. As medical knowledge grows and medical practice evolves, new areas and topics require ethical analysis, and we tend to see
technology and science as generators of these new moral queries (e.g., in stem
cell research, genetic screening technologies, xenotransplantation). Palliative
care, however, is an example that shows that transformation and innovation
of health care practice can introduce new moral issues. Rather than being driven
by the necessities of science and technology, practice changes come about because of new perceptions of patient needs, demographic changes, the increasing
burden of chronic disease, and the need to improve the quality of care. This is
particularly the case in Alzheimer disease. If new curative and preventive technologies cannot be expected in the near future, innovations and improvements
in the care of patients with AD are badly needed.

However, what is more important than the opening up of new areas for
bioethical research is the inspiration that palliative care may give to reconsider
some of the basic notions and approaches of bioethics itself. The moral values
incorporated in palliative care practice are not easily compatible with the dominant conception of bioethics. Bioethics can learn from the experiences of palliative care practitioners.

❧ Ethics *in* and *of* Palliative Care

Pellegrino (1976) introduced a distinction that can clarify the various connections between ethics and palliative care. Explaining how philosophy can engage with medicine, Pellegrino distinguished two modes of engagement: philosophy *in* medicine and philosophy *of* medicine. The first mode refers to "the
application of the traditional tools of philosophy—critical reflection, dialectical
reasoning, uncovering of value and purpose, or asking first-order questions—to
some medically defined problems" (1976, p. 20). Similarly, we can refer to ethics
in palliative care as the application of the tools of ethics to the problems of palliative care. The bioethicist can illuminate and examine critically what palliative
care practitioners do in everyday practice. This specialist can make contributions
in teaching, research, and consultation that can enhance the further development of palliative care.

This mode of engagement is important since in the context of care for incurably, and often terminally, ill persons, particular moral problems emerge more frequently than in other health care settings. Four problems that have been analyzed most are sedation, euthanasia, research, and futility (ten Have & Clark, 2002). Terminal sedation frequently is used, for example, in palliative care in Spain. It is frequently associated with the hastening of the patient's death, but thorough moral analysis shows that it is primarily a means of relief of refractory pain. However, making a suffering patient unconscious in the face of death is not easily acceptable in some other countries. For example, in the Netherlands a debate on terminal sedation is almost absent. On the other hand, that same country has in practice, under specific conditions, legalized euthanasia and physician-assisted suicide, while the practice of palliative care there has only recently started to unfold. This raises the issue: Are palliative care and euthanasia compatible? Research in palliative care is also an issue of increasing debate. Palliative care will only improve if clinical research continues to be executed. At the same time, research with severely ill and dying patients is ethically problematic. The current guidelines and standards for clinical research need to be adapted to the necessities of better palliative care, but moral reflection has hardly begun.

A final, and not frequently addressed, issue is the question of the limits of palliative care. It is often taken for granted that care itself is unlimited. Palliative care in particular starts at a time when medical interventions have become futile: cure is no longer a feasible goal, and other goals should prevail. However, improving quality of life or relieving suffering cannot be restricted in principle. The notion of futility therefore has a limited use in the context of palliative care. On the other hand, it is imperative to make specific arrangements and policies for withholding and withdrawing treatment (ten Have & Janssens, 2002).

Philosophy *of* medicine examines the conceptual foundations, the ideologies, the ethos of medicine. Medicine generates philosophical issues in regard to its meaning, its nature, concepts, purposes, and value to society. In this critical examination, the practical context of medicine is no longer taken for granted but is considered as the object of philosophical inquiry. Analogously, ethics of palliative care can be regarded as the critical examination of the meaning of palliative care, its nature, concepts, purposes, and value to society.

This analysis assumes that palliative care as a practical human activity has a transmedical meaning that has important implications for bioethics itself. Reflection on experiences in palliative care may produce insights that influence and change current notions and approaches in bioethics. The question, for example, is whether the dominant conception of bioethics is adequate when faced with the dilemmas in palliative care practice. The actual experiences of patients and health care practitioners, as well as the context in which physicians, nurses, patients, and others experience their moral lives (e.g., the roles they play, the relationships in which they participate, the expectations they have, and the values they cherish) should be taken into moral consideration. The physician-patient relationship is neither ahistorical, acultural, nor an abstract rational notion; persons are always persons-in-relation, are always members of communities, are immersed in a tradition, and participants in a particular culture, and perhaps even more so when they are dying and suffering. Experiences in palliative care also create interest in alternative conceptions of ethics in order to better explain the moral experiences of patients and professionals. For example, narrative ethics emphasizes the stories of individual patients (Newton, 1995); care ethics focuses on the context of support and care (Tronto, 1993); responsibility ethics and virtue ethics articulate qualities of character in both individuals and communities (Gracia, 2002; Pellegrino & Thomasma, 1993). These conceptions attempt to provide a more comprehensive understanding of the nature, scope, method, and application of ethics in the contemporary health care context.

In sum, palliative care aptly illustrates the contemporary criticism of the principlism approach in bioethics. It demonstrates that a proper understanding of the moral problems and dilemmas of health care practice requires, first, a conception of interpretative ethics (Svenaeus, 1999). Within this conception, notions and perspectives different from those in the current conception of ethics will be emphasized (ten Have, 1994). For example, consider the notion of experience. Taking the experience of the patient as a starting point is particularly important in the context of palliative care since the comfort and quality of care of the patient is a directive for care. Other important notions are attitudes and emotions. Randall & Downie argue that in palliative care we have to recognize not only the cognitive dimension but the affective as well: "The morally good person is not just principled, but also compassionate" (1996, p. 13). An argument can be made that, for ethics, the fundamental question is not so much "What to do?" but "How to live?" This seems particularly significant for palliative care since it is not focused on action and doing but on creating the conditions for living unto death. The moral relevancy of our actions should not be reduced to their effects; it is also determined by an evaluation of what we do in executing our actions. For example, the problem of experimenting with terminal patients should not be settled by reference to future results but should raise the question: Why are we interested in scientific research? The problem of euthanasia should not be reduced to the question of whether it will eliminate suffering or respect the autonomy of the patient; it should also focus attention on how we deal with suffering and what the meaning is of medicine that saves the lives of patients and at the same time terminates human life. Is it ever possible for medicine not to act? This change of focus implies a reorientation from activity to passivity, from acts to attitudes and emotions.

Finally, the notion of community is particularly relevant (Street, 1998). The interpretative reading of a patient's situation is not only a doctor's affair. The medical prior understandings that orient the interpretation are the sediments of traditional cultural assumptions concerning the nature of the world, the body, life and death, and the results of a specific historical evolution of medical knowledge. This is especially true for palliative care, where we have the identification of goals such as "a good death" and "quality of life." Interpretation presupposes a universe of understanding. This is a consequence of the so-called hermeneutic circle: in order to interpret a text's meaning, the interpreter must be familiar with the vocabulary and grammar of the text and have some idea of what the text might mean (Daniel, 1986). For man as a social being, understanding is always a community phenomenon: understanding in communication with others. The continuous effort to reach consensus through a dialogue with patients, colleagues, and other health professionals induces us to discover the particularities of our own prior understanding and, through that, to attain a more general level of understanding.

Using these notions, an interpretative conception of bioethics can be further developed. Experiences in palliative care can help not only to underline the need for such a new conception but also to clarify and expand the characteristic parameters of this conception.

❧ The Palliative Approach: Authentic Relationships

In the dominant conception of bioethics, individual autonomy has a peculiar role. Respect for autonomy is one among usually four moral principles, but at the same time it often is considered to override the other three. This emphasis on individual autonomy is understandable since it seems to be the only effective counterbalance to medical power. Moral issues arise from an almost exclusively technological orientation to the world and a predominant scientific conceptualization of human life. Human beings resist the tendencies of medicine to focus primarily on their bodies and biological existence. They protest against the overwhelming power of health professionals and health care institutions that reduce patients to cases, numbers, and objects. They object to the lack of involvement of individual beings within decision-making processes and to the lack of respect for the authenticity and subjectivity of individual patients. Bioethics has emerged as a movement to reintroduce the subject of individual patients into the health care setting, emphasizing patients' rights, respect for individual autonomy, and the need to set limits on medical power (ten Have & Gordijn, 2001).

However, the emphasis on individual autonomy has two consequences that in the context of palliative care are continuously criticized. First, it is associated with a mechanistic view of the human body (whereas palliative care is whole-person care). Second, it focuses on the individual person (whereas palliative care also includes family members, relatives, or others close to the patient).

The role of the human body in bioethical discourse is paradoxical. Bioethics as a critical movement originated from the recognition that medicine separates the individual person into subject and object. The best way to focus attention on the patient as a whole person and as an agent being in control of his or her life is to stress the autonomy of the individual subject and to demand moral respect for this autonomy. However, the emphasis on individual autonomy tends to neglect the significance of the human body. In most ethical discourse, there is no recognition of the special experiences of embodiment: it seems as if the autonomous subject is not embodied. The body is merely the instrument through which the subject interacts with the world. The subject is in full control of the subject's body. It is imperative that the integrity of the body should be respected since it is the prime vehicle of the autonomous person. The moral principle of respect for autonomy in health care ethics apparently is associated with a popular image of the body as property (ten Have & Welie, 1998). When the individual is regarded as autonomous subject, then the body is that individual's private property. And the person is the sovereign authority with property rights over that body.

At the same time, the concept of body ownership is morally problematic. The distinction between person and body is contrary to our existential identification with our bodies and the self-experience of ourselves as embodied selves. In making such a distinction between autonomous subject and an object—more specifically, between an owner and a body, or private property—bioethics seems to proceed from the same dualism that was criticized in its earlier days. Moreover, it is apparently using a dualistic distinction between person and body, subject and object—a distinction that has led to the emergence of bioethics itself. Whereas medicine tends to neglect the subject, bioethics tends to neglect the body (ten Have, 1998; Zwart, 1998).

When palliative care and the hospice movement emerged, this dualism was rejected. The dualism promotes a view that medical interventions should focus on the human body since the body is the vehicle for prolonging life; as long as the body is functioning, medical interference and activities will be justified. Separating object and subject, differentiating between an objective, real world independent of an isolated, individual subject, leads to an almost exclusive preference for the methods of the natural sciences in the context of health care. These methods are focused on intervention, control, and manipulation, introducing the technical point of view of the engineer into the domain of disease, suffering, and death. A dualistic view leads to a one-sided approach of suffering and symptoms in general because these are merely regarded as bodily phenomena. Cicely Saunders (1967) opposed this approach by introducing the concept of "total pain." Pain is having physical, emotional, social, and spiritual components; unless each of these is tackled, relief of pain is unlikely. Also, since a dualistic view is unwarranted, the primacy of the medical approach, primarily targeted on the human body, will disappear; instead, a multiprofessional approach to the dying patient and his family will be necessary.

The focus on individual autonomy is, of course, central in palliative care, too. Autonomy, however, tends to isolate the person as sovereign decision maker. It neglects dimensions of human vulnerability, dependency, and fragility that are characteristic of human existence and that are particularly experienced when confronted with serious illness, suffering, and debilitating conditions. In an ethics of care, these dimensions are recognized. It is suggested that the notion of authenticity better conforms to moral experiences in palliative care than the notion of autonomy (Janssens, Zylicz, & ten Have, 1999). Authenticity underlines that the individual's decisions need to be interpreted within the perspective of that individual's personality and biography. It also acknowledges that the individual existence is fragile and dependent (Welie, 1998).

But authenticity needs to be fostered and sustained. Patients should be aware that they can be themselves despite all suffering because vulnerability and dependency is shared with caregivers, both professional and nonprofessional, as conditions common to all human beings. This awareness also links authenticity with community. Individuals are social beings; they can be autonomous decision makers only because the community provides the proper conditions and adequate circumstances. Palliative care aims at creating such conditions and circumstances in order to let the patient experience that he or she is a fellow human being, a member of a community, particularly at the moment of death. The patient is not an "unencumbered self" as postulated in the liberal tradition emphasizing individual autonomy (Sandel, 1996). On the contrary, the cloak of palliative care demonstrates that the patient is essentially related to others and situated in a community.

Palliative care therefore can make contributions to bioethics. Not only does palliative care demonstrate the inadequacy of the current conception of bioethics (the one-sidedness of the principle of respect for autonomy) and the need for alternative approaches, it also indicates that in health care an image of human beings is necessary that is more comprehensive than the images dominating in everyday life. In the palliative care approach, particular emphasis is put upon notions such as authenticity and community, as well as those of responsibility and engagement. Human beings are dynamic beings who adapt to the world; they reconstruct and redefine their identity in order to keep it solid and stable and to give meaning to life's various stages and experiences. This is the image of human life as pilgrimage (Bauman, 1994; 1995). For the human being as pilgrim, the true place is always some time away, some distance away. What makes human life worthwhile is the proximity between the true world and this world; men and women are destined to be elsewhere; the pilgrim's life is worthwhile to the extent that the individual still journeys, but because the pilgrim actually wishes to attain a goal or destination, the closer he or she is to that goal, the more worthwhile is that individual's life. Because life has been transformed into a pilgrimage, it has meaning. The destination makes a whole out of the fragmentation—that lends continuity to the episodic. Human life, therefore, is a continuous story, and although it is an individual project it is carried out in an orderly, determined, predictable world. And health care, especially, aims at providing care and shelter for this journey through life. The hospice movement developed a discourse that focuses on life as journeying, as pilgrimage, and on the meaning of suffering (Clark & Seymour, 1999). Although this image of the human being as pilgrim can be criticized, it seems necessary as an antidote to the notion of fragmentary existence that is projected by postmodern philosophy. It delineates specific characteristics that are basic to human life: goal-directness; the deliberate choosing of successive steps in life—life in a world that, as it slowly changes, requires men and women to adapt and to bring unity and continuity to the life project. It may be more difficult for postmodern human beings to realize these characteristics, but that does not diminish their relevancy. Perhaps it is the essential function of health care, especially when someone faces chronic, incurable, and terminal illness, to provide a niche within today's hectic, disengaged social environment that will allow "wandering," vulnerable people to find peace and tranquility, and finally to be "home" (Dekkers, 2001; Rumbold, 1998).

❧ Conclusion

The scope of palliative care nowadays is expanding. This is not only an expansion that includes new organizational forms, new patient categories such as persons with AD, and new disease trajectories: the scope of palliative care is expanding because it also can give an incentive to ethical reflection and stimulate the development of new conceptions and approaches in ethics itself. Palliative care and ethics are entering into a new and fascinating phase of interaction and cooperation. The increasing challenge of how to organize and provide (future) care for a growing population of Alzheimer patients also demands new reflection upon concepts and models of palliative care.

On the one hand, many moral issues and dilemmas arise in the practice of palliative care. Ethics can help to analyze and elucidate these particular problems. Ethics can also provide models and methods to address and discuss practical cases systematically in order to facilitate clinical decision making. This level of interaction is ethics *in* palliative care. On the other hand, bioethics may be enriched by the experiences in palliative care practice. This second level of interaction is ethics *of* palliative care. Here the approaches, concepts, and values in palliative care may be relevant to a critical reflection of bioethics itself and may provide new ideas and richer views.

In three areas, palliative care may give significant inspiration to enrich bioethics. First, the practice of palliative care demonstrates the inadequacy of the current dominant conception of bioethics as applied ethics. It shows the need for an interpretative ethics that is better accommodated to health care practice.

Second, palliative care illustrates the one-sidedness of the major moral principle of today (i.e., the moral principle of respect for autonomy). From the perspective of care, although individual autonomy is important, it is necessary not to disconnect the autonomous subject from the objective human body, with its ailments, deficiencies, and suffering. It is also necessary to regard the individual patient as a member of a supportive community. Third, palliative care points attention to certain images of human beings that tend to be neglected in postmodern society, particularly the image of the human person as pilgrim. In short, palliative care is more than another context of health care in which moral issues emerge. It is an incentive for philosophers, theologians, and ethicists to evaluate the notions and models of present-day bioethics.

REFERENCES

Bauman, Z. (1994). *Alone again: Ethics after certainty.* London: Demos.

Bauman, Z. (1995). *Life in fragments: Essays in postmodern morality.* Oxford: Blackwell.

Clark, D., & Seymour, J. (1999). *Reflections on palliative care.* Buckingham, UK: Open University Press.

Daniel, S. L. (1986). The patient as text: A model of clinical hermeneutics. *Theoretical Medicine, 7,* 195–210.

Dekkers, W. (2001). Coming home: On the goals of palliative care. In H.A.M.J. ten Have & M.J.P.A. Janssens (Eds.), *Palliative care in Europe: Concepts and policies* (pp. 117–125). Amsterdam: IOS Press.

George, R., & Sykes, J. (1997): Beyond cancer? In D. Clark, J. Hockley, & S. Ahmedzai (Eds.), *New themes in palliative care* (pp. 239–254). Buckingham, UK: Open University Press.

Gezondheidsraad. (2002). *Dementie* [Dementia]. The Hague: Gezondheidsraad (pub. no. 2002/04).

Gracia, D. (2002). From conviction to responsibility in palliative care ethics. In H.A.M.J. ten Have & D. Clark (Eds.), *The ethics of palliative care: European perspectives* (pp. 87–105). Buckingham, UK: Open University Press.

ten Have, H.A.M.J. (1994). The hyperreality of clinical ethics: A unitary theory and hermeneutics. *Theoretical Medicine, 15* (2): 113–131.

ten Have, H.A.M.J. (1998). Health care and the human body. *Medicine, Health Care and Philosophy, 1* (2), 103–105.

ten Have, H.A.M.J. (2001). Theoretical models and approaches to ethics. In H.A.M.J. ten Have & B. Gordijn (Eds.), *Bioethics in a European perspective* (pp. 51–82). Dordrecht: Kluwer Academic Publishers.

ten Have, H.A.M.J., & Clark, D. (Eds.). (2002). *The ethics of palliative care: European perspectives.* Buckingham, UK: Open University Press.

ten Have, H.A.M.J., & Gordijn, B. (Eds.). (2001). *Bioethics in a European perspective.* Dordrecht: Kluwer Academic Publishers.

ten Have, H.A.M.J., & Janssens, M.J.P.A. (Eds.), (2001). *Palliative care in Europe: Concepts and policies.* Amsterdam: IOS Press

ten Have, H.A.M.J., & Janssens, R. (2002). Futility, limits, and palliative care. In H.A.M.J. ten Have & D. Clark (Eds.), *The ethics of palliative care: European perspectives* (pp. 212–232).Buckingham, UK: Open University Press.

ten Have, H.A.M.J., & Welie, J. V. M. (Eds.). (1998). *Ownership of the human body: Philosophical considerations on the use of the human body and its parts in healthcare.* Dordrecht: Kluwer Academic Publishers.

Hermsen, M., & ten Have, H.A.M.J. (2001). Moral problems in palliative care journals. *Palliative Medicine, 15* (5), 425–431.

Jacquemin, D. (Ed.). (2001). *Manuel de soins palliative* [Handbook of palliative care] (2nd ed.). Paris: Dunod.

Janssens, M.J.P.A. (2001). *Palliative care: Concepts and ethics.* Nijmegen: Nijmegen University Press.

Janssens, M.J.P.A., Zylicz, Z., & ten Have, H.A.M.J. (1999). Articulating the concept of palliative care: Philosophical and theological perspectives. *Journal of Palliative Care, 15* (2), 38–44.

Janssens, R., & ten Have, H.A.M.J., Broeckaert, B., Clark, D., Gracia, D., Illhardt, F., et al. (2002). Moral values in palliative care: A European comparison. In H.A.M.J. ten Have & D. Clark (Eds.), *The ethics of palliative care: European perspectives* (pp. 72–86). Buckingham, UK: Open University Press.

Jennings, B. (Ed.). (1997). *Ethics in hospice care: Challenges to hospice values in a changing health care environment.* New York: Haworth Press.

Newton, A. Z. (1995). *Narrative ethics.* Cambridge: Harvard University Press.

Pellegrino, E. D. (1976). Philosophy of medicine: Problematic and potential. *Journal of Medicine and Philosophy, 1* (1), 5–31.

Pellegrino, E. D., & Thomasma, D. C. (1993). *The virtues in medical practice.* New York: Oxford University Press.

Randall, F., & Downie, R. S. (1996). *Palliative care ethics: A good companion.* Oxford: Oxford University Press.

Rumbold, B. D. (1998). Implications of mainstreaming hospice into palliative care services. In J. M. Parker & S. Aranda (Eds.), *Palliative care: Explorations and challenges* (pp. 3–20). Sydney: MacLennan & Petty.

Sandel, M. J. (1996). *Democracy's discontent: America in search of a public philosophy.* Cambridge, MA: Belknap Press.

Saunders, C. (1967). *The management of terminal illness.* London: Hospital Medicine Publications.

Street, A. (1998). Competing discourses with/in palliative care. In J. M. Parker & S. Aranda (Eds.), *Palliative care: Explorations and challenges* (pp. 68–81). Sydney: MacLennan & Petty.

Svenaeus, F. (1999). *The hermeneutics of medicine and the phenomenology of health: Steps towards a philosophy of medical practice.* Linköping, Sweden: Linköping University.

Tronto, J. C. (1993). *Moral boundaries: A political argument for an ethic of care.* New York: Routledge.

Webb, P. (Ed.). (2000). *Ethical issues in palliative care.* Manchester, UK: Hochland & Hochland.

Welie, J. V. M. (1998). *In the face of suffering: The philosophical-anthropological foundations of clinical ethics.* Omaha, NE: Creighton University Press.

Zwart, H. (1998). Medicine, symbolization, and the "real" body—Lacan's understanding of medical science. *Medicine, Health Care and Philosophy, 1* (2), 107–117.

CHAPTER FIVE

Hospital-based Palliative Care and Dementia, or What Do We Treat Patients For and How Do We Do It?

Marcel G. M. Olde Rikkert, M.D., Ph.D.

Anne-Sophie Rigaud, M.D., Ph.D.

This chapter focuses on hospital-based palliative care in dementia. The symptoms of dementia are not of course limited to Alzheimer disease (AD), but almost all of what we offer applies well to the specific situation of AD.

Palliative care in dementia may have to be redefined, starting from the general definition of palliative care given by the World Health Organization (WHO): integral, active, and multidimensional care for patients with incurable diseases, aimed at optimizing quality of life both for the patient and the family. As elaborated elsewhere in this book, the concept of palliative care comes primarily from medical oncology and has some major characteristics (Sipsma, 2001):

- dying is regarded as an intrinsic part of life
- acceleration or postponement of death is not an aim of palliative care
- palliative care aims at lessening pain and other burdensome symptoms
- palliative care is designed to help patients become as active and autonomous as possible
- palliative care supports the family in coping with the disease of their loved one

There is a controversy regarding the stages of chronic diseases to which palliative care should be restricted. A limited view on palliative care restricts this type of service to the terminal stage (i.e., the last twelve months of life). Palliative care according to the WHO definition, when applied to dementia, may start early in the natural course of the disease and is not restricted to the final stage— because at present the majority of dementia syndromes are incurable from the start. More than 95 percent of all patients suffering from dementia, and 100 percent of patients with AD, have an irreversible and incurable disease. Ultimately they will die from their dementia or from their co-morbidity. However, there is a controversy about the duration of AD from diagnosis till death. For a long time, a median duration of from 5.0 to 9.3 years has been accepted, but a recent report showed a median duration of only 3.0 years (with probable AD, 3.1 years) (Wolfson et al., 2001). These recent data on the natural history have had considerable impact on our thinking about dementia, changing it from an incurable, slowly progressive disease to an incurable disease with a rapidly progressive evolution. However, because of the large differences in survival reported so far, more data is needed. In the final stages of dementia, in which patients cannot walk, swallow, sit, stand, or toilet, patients usually are cared for in nursing homes, and in cases of concurrent disease most often are no longer referred to a hospital.

Given both the differences in interpretation of palliative care as a specific model and expertise in health care and the highly variable, individual course of dementia, we support an individualized decision on when the leading principle in the management of a patient with dementia should be palliative care. This decision should be a team decision, agreed on by all the health care professionals actively involved in the patient's treatment. Reasons to decide to turn to a strict palliative treatment may be that other treatment does not serve a reasonable goal anymore or that the burdens of treatment outweigh the benefits.

In the final stages of dementia, palliative care may be limited to symptomatic care, which in the Netherlands is regarded as even more restrictive than palliative care. Symptomatic care aims at lightening the burden of symptoms, but the agents used to this end are not used if they would prolong life; in other words, in symptomatic care prolongation of life is considered a worse course than optimal treatment of symptoms. For example, under palliative care, shortness of breath caused by a bronchitis may be treated with antibiotics and, in treating the infection, life extension is taken for granted. In symptomatic care, the bronchitis should not be treated with antibiotics because this might cure the bronchitis and extend survival time, which would no longer be in accordance with the patient's wishes. In such a case, only anti-cough agents, such as oxygen and opiates, should be given. In Dutch hospitals, palliative care for patients with AD generally is limited to the group of patients who are in a terminal stage of life because of co-morbidity.

☙ Dementia in General Hospitals

The kind of patients with dementia who are referred to general hospitals fall into five main categories.

1. Patients at a mild stage of dementia in whom the *diagnosis of cognitive decline* is uncertain or unknown. In many countries in and outside Europe, specialized memory clinics have been founded. In the main, these are places in outpatient or day hospital facilities. Patients may be under observation (or treatment) until the diagnosis is clear. In these cases, there is no hospital-based palliative care model.

2. Family practitioners may refer patients for *treatment trials or well-accepted therapy* (e.g., cholinesterase inhibitors). When cholinergic drugs are given, and probably also in most drug trials, this does not mean cure or modification of the underlying pathology but only symptomatic treatment for cognitive decline. This symptomatic treatment is part of palliative care. Some authors clearly describe a cholinergic drugs regimen as (part of) palliative care (Moss et al., 1999); however, most do not. In monitoring these patients, other aspects of palliative care—for example, psychosocial guidance—should also be implemented. However, especially in trials, the nondrug aspects of the treatment may be omitted to prevent unwanted effects on the end points of the trials.

3. Patients with *acute care problems due to social network breakdown.* For all kinds of reasons (disease of patient, of spouse, or of caregiver; dementia progression; limited availability of professional caregivers; burnout of primary caregiver, etc.) professional or nonprofessional care may stop or become insufficient. Shortage of care often cannot be solved by general practitioners (for instance, because of waiting lists for nursing homes). The only solution sometimes is to send such patients to a hospital emergency ward, with or without an acute care diagnosis. From the hospital point of view, there is enormous reluctance to take care of these patients, who are often sent home without even proper examination or history taking. In this group of patients (sometimes pejoratively known

as GOMERS—the acronym for Get Out of My Emergency Room) a large number of existing diseases will not be diagnosed correctly.

4. Patients with *complications of dementia.* In the various stages of dementia, different complications may occur. Behavioral complications are very important in disease management, and these mostly occur in the stages of moderate and severe dementia; however, because of substantial differences among individuals in the natural history of AD, they are not confined to these stages. Peaks are found in the incidence of different behavioral problems. First, one may encounter psychomotor activity disorders and diurnal rhythm disorders; later in the natural history, depression and paranoia may occur, followed by an increasing incidence of wandering and aggression (Eastwood & Reisberg, 1999). These conduct disorders are called behavioral and psychological symptoms in dementia (BPSD). They have a large impact on the quality of life and need for care of patients' families and caregivers. The most important complications of dementia are delirium, dehydration, falls (and subsequent fractures), incontinence, immobility, and weight loss (i.e., malnutrition and/or sarcopenia) (Hogan & McCraken, 1999). These psychological and physical complications of dementia ask for a specific medical or palliative care policy in hospital.

5. Patients with *dementia and co-morbidity.* In co-morbidity one can differentiate between associated co-morbidity (e.g., peripheral artery disease in vascular dementia) and nonassociated co-morbidity (e.g., breast cancer in AD). For a long time, it has been thought that co-morbidity might be less frequent in dementia or in AD than in other groups of elderly subjects without dementia. Dementia might have protective effects on the prevalence of other diseases. However, in a retrospective study, Holstein, Chatellier, and Moulias did not find a decline in incidence nor prevalence of co-morbidity (1994). On average, they found 3.3 associated diseases in the Alzheimer dementia group and 4.7 in the vascular dementia group, which is similar to the 3.9 diseases in the group without dementia. These findings are confirmed in a pathological case study carried out by Thorpe et al. (1994). In their study, cancer, diabetes, myocardial infarction, and stroke were remarkably common in patients with AD. It may be that certain diseases have higher prevalence (e.g., atrial fibrillation, diabetes mellitus, hypertension), while others have lower prevalence in AD (e.g., seizures, arthritis, headaches). Both progression of chronic diseases and acute exacerbations or acute incident diseases (e.g., pneumonia; hip fracture) probably have a large

impact on homeostasis, functional performance, and cognition, in the case of dementia. Therefore, prognosis of co-morbidity is worse in dementia. For example, with similar orthopedic treatment, six-month mortality for hip fracture was 55 percent in end-stage dementia patients compared with 12 percent in cognitively intact patients (Morrison & Siu, 2000). Similarly, when patients were treated similarly with antibiotics, after six months there was a big difference in pneumonia-associated mortality between patients with dementia and patients without dementia (Morrison & Siu, 2000). The substantial impact and worsening prognosis caused by this kind of co-morbidity, in patients already seriously handicapped by loss of independence in activities of daily living, often calls up the question of whether palliative care or curative care for the co-morbid condition is the most appropriate. Living wills with statements concerning treatment of co-morbidity in the case of dementia require a decision with regard to the choice between curative and palliative treatment.

It will be clear from the description of the several categories of patients that palliative care policy may differ substantially among the various kinds. Though there are large, qualitative differences between the interventions needed, only limited data are available on their efficacy and effectiveness in clinical practice. The recent study by Nourashémi et al. (2001) is, as far as we know, the only one to present empirical data on the incidence of a wide range of reasons for patients with cognitive impairment to be referred to emergency departments and acute Alzheimer care units. Complications such as behavioral problems (26.3%) and falls (18.6%) were the most important, followed by co-morbid gastrointestinal problems (14.4%), fever (11%), neurological disorders, whether or not the patient is conscious (11.8%) and social grounds (2.5%).

In Nourashémi et al.'s study of geriatric admission policy, 118 patients were admitted over a four-month period (2001). The reasons for referral of course differ between subacute and nonacute admissions. Since the number of people age sixty-five and over is increasing, it is likely that more and more of those admitted to acute care hospitals will be suffering from cognitive decline. Tolson, Smith, and Knight (1999) found that 66 percent of the admissions to wards for acute care of elderly people involved patients who suffered from cognitive impairment, 40 percent experiencing severe problems.

In our description below of the principles of palliative care in dementia, we focus on patients from categories 4 and 5 because those are the most clear and urgent cases in which questions concerning palliative care have to be answered.

❧ Empirical Data

In this era of evidence-based medicine, one should start a review of hospital-based palliative care with the description of current practice and add a summary of trial-based evidence on efficacy, effectiveness, and efficiency of different models and treatment. However, there is a great lack of data in the field. As far as we know, no randomized controlled trial (RCT) is available. Not one. The evidence base therefore has to be limited to clinical experience and to the small number of articles that analyze current practice of palliative hospital-based care for patients with dementia, generally as compared with cancer patients. None of the more than sixty papers published in the "Study to Understand Prognoses and Preferences for Outcomes and Risks of Treatment in the Elderly" (SUPPORT) and the "Hospitalized Elderly Longitudinal Project" (HELP) for the very elderly focuses on the description of the last months of patients with dementia or on palliative care for these patients (Freeborne, 2000). Furthermore, the *Oxford Textbook of Palliative Medicine,* which mentions dementia as a set of symptoms that accompany organic brain disease, does no more than pay a little bit of attention to delirium (Doyle, Hanks, & MacDonald, 1993). Fortunately, a few empirical, though non-RCT, studies have addressed aspects of hospital-based palliative care in dementia (if palliative care is defined in a broad sense as care for incurable diseases). Those studies we focus on later.

Morrison and Siu (2000) compared the treatments given for pneumonia and hip fracture in patients with severe dementia (i.e., those with short-version Mini-Mental State Exam score <18 of 24; unable to recall names of close relatives or spouse; complete dependence in all activities of daily living) with the same treatments given to elderly persons without dementia. In sum, included in the study were 216 patients with pneumonia (n=126) and hip fracture (n=97), older than seventy, who were admitted to a large hospital in New York. Patients with hip fracture received intravenous antibiotics, those with pneumonia received hip surgery. The prognosis was worse in dementia. The diagnostic and therapeutic procedures used were valued as equally burdensome (painful or uncomfortable, such as arterial blood gas measurement, central line placement, indwelling catheter placement, use of restraints, nasogastric tubes, daily phlebotomy, etc) in patients with dementia compared with patients without dementia. In hip fracture patients, opiates were used less: daily doses of morphine equivalents were

1.7 mg per day for patients with dementia versus 4.1 mg per day for the patients who did not have dementia. Moreover, only 9 percent of the patients with dementia received a standard order for an analgesic. Finally, in 90 percent of the charts of 118 patients with severe dementia, no documentation was found of any staff discussion about goals of care. As recognized in Riesenberg's (2000) editorial on this paper, the study clarifies that palliative care was neither a leading nor a minor principle in the treatment policy in these patients with severe dementia. With regard to the effectiveness of pneumonia treatment, it would be very important to know more about the differences in outcome between patients with and without dementia. However, the end points registered in this study cannot tell us.

Another landmark study in this field, Fabiszewski, Volicer, and Volicer (1990), showed no difference in survival between patients with severe dementia with pneumonia who were treated with antibiotics and those who were not treated (in both groups there was only ± 50% survival after thirty months). Antibiotic treatment for pneumonia in patients with moderately severe dementia who were still able to walk, had no eating problems and no contractures, were not mute, and had only intermittent muscle rigidity, improved in survival from 60 percent to 100 percent survival in thirty months. Unfortunately, neither quality of life nor dyspnea severity were end points in this study; therefore, it is still unknown whether antibiotic treatment made a difference in symptom severity in patients with dementia suffering from pneumonia. Recent data from a nursing home study in the Netherlands show that those patients with dementia not receiving antibiotics for pneumonia already had a lower quality of life before the pneumonia episode, and the difference with those patients treated with antibiotics stayed the same following pneumonia (Van der Steen, 2002). In both groups, pneumonia caused considerable loss of quality of life.

Ahronheim et al. (1996) retrospectively compared treatments offered to patients with metastatic tumor malignancy (n=84) with treatments offered to patients with advanced stage of dementia (n=80). Overall, 47 percent of the patients received invasive nonpalliative treatments (e.g., hemodialysis, enteral tube feeding, mechanical ventilatory support, etc.). There was no difference between the two groups in the total number of procedures when controlled for age, length of stay, and type of insurance. However, patients with dementia were more likely to receive feeding tubes (21% versus 8%), but less likely to get invasive or noninvasive diagnostics tests. Moreover, patients with dementia were more likely to receive antibiotics, but less likely to get analgesics, hypnotics, and antidepressants. Overall, 88 percent of the patients received antibiotics. In both groups, 24 percent had cardiopulmonary resuscitation, which is also a remarkably high number for end stages of life. Only a minority of the patients (31% of cancer patients; 8% of patients with dementia) had advance directives—which, moreover, did not make any difference in the treatment policy. The surprisingly high prevalence of nonpalliative treatment options in this large tertiary center teaching hospital may be clarified partly by the very strict standards for withdrawing treatment and nutritional support in terminally ill patients set by regional state jurisdiction (New York). Probably another reason for the high prevalence of feeding tubes in advanced dementia is the failure to recognize patients who have dementia, with or without co-morbidity, as terminally ill.

Another comparison of the end stage of life of patients with dementia with the end stage of cancer patients' lives was carried out by McCarthy, Addington-Hall, and Altman (1997). Retrospectively, they compared the symptoms, level of care, and feelings of caregivers of 170 patients with dementia with 1,513 cancer patients in their last twelve months. The global spectrum of symptoms expressed by the two groups was similar. Comparable numbers of patients experienced mental confusion (80%), urinary incontinence (70%), pain (65%), depressed mood (60%), constipation (60%), and loss of appetite (60%). Dementia patients suffered from these symptoms longer. They also lost more of their activities of daily living and needed more supportive care. Hospital care was used more often by cancer patients (90% versus 67%), but patients with dementia stayed much longer in hospital (three months during their last year). In their conclusion, McCarthy, Addington-Hall, and Altman state that patients dying from dementia have symptoms and health care needs comparable with those of cancer patients. They plead for more attention to the needs of patients with dementia and for a concrete model of hospital-based palliative care for such patients.

Hospital admission and diagnostic and therapeutic procedures for patients with dementia may be valued differently compared with those for patients who do not have dementia. Morrison et al. (1998) developed a valid and reliable scale on which patients with dementia can rank hospital procedures according to pain and discomfort. Procedures such as arterial blood gas measurements, central line placement, nasogastric tube placement, intramuscular injection, and so forth were valued as quite burdensome. In another study on patients with dementia and fever, it was shown that diagnostics and treatments were globally valued as being less burdensome on a "Dementia Special Care Unit" of a general hospital, compared with a traditional, longitudinal care institution (Hurley et al., 1993).

In the field of nursing research, the impact of palliative care on individual professional caregivers and palliative care teams is also empirically studied. In a large-scale Scandinavian study, proneness to burnout was correlated with a less-empathic behavior (Astrom et al., 1990). This accords with other authors who suggest that the burnout experience leads to lower empathy in nursing staff. Another study showed that exhaustion in staff may be related to overwhelming experiences when staff have been close to patients with dementia and also to feelings of guilt at, nevertheless, not being sufficiently close to patients (Kuremyr et al., 1994). These alarming findings might be directly related to current problems of not being able to attract sufficient nursing staff to work in geriatric departments. These vacancies are themselves a threat to palliative care for hospitalized patients with dementia. Intervention studies that focus on improvement of the quality of current work with patients with dementia are of great importance (Berg, Hansson, & Hallberg, 1998). Tedium and burnout among nurses decreased significantly when systematic clinical supervision and individualized planned care were introduced. These approaches increased nurses' creativity. It may be that such staff-centered interventions are of direct beneficial effect on quality of patient care.

In sum, the picture that emerges in these empirical studies is that patients with dementia in general hospitals are a severely diseased group. They are frail because of the stage of dementia, the complications, and the co-morbidity. The prevalence of behavioral problems in dementia has been shown to be high, and the prevalence of co-morbidity is found to be similar to other groups of elderly subjects.

The general physical and mental condition of hospitalized patients with dementia is reflected in the poor prognosis with regard to survival and functional performance; this differs little from that for cancer patients. Working with these vulnerable patients is shown to be burdensome, and it increases the nurses' risk for burnout. Moreover, treatment policies are valued as burdensome by the patients themselves. Therefore, every investigation carried out should have clear and important implications for each individual patient, should mean a chance for improvement of quality of life, and should be part of an individualized palliative care plan. Careful and creative planning of palliative management policies appears to be beneficial, both for patients and staff (Astrom et al., 1990).

❧ The Practice of Hospital-based Palliative Care

Fortunately, with regard to advanced dementia and behavioral complications, a body of knowledge is evolving that guides symptomatic treatment in hospitals (Shuster, 2000; De Deyn et al., 1999; De Deyn, 2000). This expertise plays an important role in palliative care for patients at this stage, close to the end of life. This chapter does not aim to present the state of the art on all possible symptomatic treatments for dementia, drug and nondrug, but we refer readers to the excellent papers of Inouye et al. (2000) and Shuster (2000) for detailed descriptions of hospital-based palliative care for dementia.

Two important reasons that palliative care for patients with dementia can be given much better in geriatric departments than in other parts of hospitals have to do with architecture and the provision of other specific facilities. Other departments are not designed and developed to fit closely to the needs of elderly patients. Additional reasons for preferring treatment in a geriatric department are the greater availability of high technical expertise in the symptomatic treatment of AD and the need for multidisciplinary care. Shortage of beds and staff at geriatric departments, however, make it impossible to treat all the patients with dementia from other hospital departments. Such shortages similarly prevent admission of some patients referred by general practitioners or nursing home physicians for this kind of palliative care. The shortage of resources, including the greater lack of expertise of treatment and care for patients with dementia, begs for hospital-wide education and implementation of geriatric principles of care. This can be realized only with an appropriate implementation plan and a strongly developed, multidisciplinary geriatric consultation service. Inouye et al. (2000) recently described a blueprint of such a strong consultation service—a blueprint that has successfully been turned into practice at Yale.

We here focus on a hospital-based decision-making process in palliative care—a process for both the AD patient and the patient's family—and on some practical guidelines to translate palliative policy into geriatric practice. The evidence is primarily drawn from our own clinical experience and from Dutch and American statements of adequate palliative care and medical decision

TABLE 5.1.   Deciding Whether to Implement Palliative Care
for Patients with Dementia

Compare life expectancy for the patient's stage of dementia with the impact of co-morbidity on this life expectancy

Assess the effects of frailty and other physical impairments on the patient's potential to tolerate optimal therapy

Weigh evidence of the natural course of the co-morbid disease(s) and evidence on the effects of curative treatments

Assess the risks, burdens, and advantages of available palliative care options and weigh them against the curative treatment options

Assess the risk for new iatrogenic health problems because of co-morbidity, polypharmacy, functional decline, and severity of dementia

Carefully assess the patient's decision-making capacity, because suffering from dementia does not in itself mean incapacity to consent

Individualize treatment by striving for palliative care that is multidisciplinary and goal guided, and that reflects the informed consent of family

Structure the decision-making process as a consensus-building process grounded in dialogue among a patient's proxy and other professional team members

Strive toward a clear idea of the patient's preferences in daily living and preferences for end-of-life decisions, and see how these fit into the patient's life history

---

making in patients with dementia (Hertogh & Ribbe, 1996; Katz, 1993; Van der Steen, 2002).

With the patient in mind, we can describe some practical guidelines in treating and caring for these patients. First, it has to be stressed that, with regard to symptoms of the previous days or weeks, a medical history from a patient is unreliable. A patient with dementia is generally very able to enumerate his complaints during the moment we are talking to him; depending on the severity of dementia, however, symptoms of an earlier date may be forgotten. Too often, the taking of medical history is skipped in the case of dementia. For example, complaints of abdominal pain may well point to infection of the gall bladder.

In general, we should talk several times with a patient with dementia who is severely ill. Patients still are the ones who give us the most important clues for goal setting of palliative treatment. Before starting these talks, to stress that we care and to maximize communication we should at least optimize vision and hearing—for example, by assisting the patient in the correct use of eyeglasses and hearing aids—and also use physical contact whenever appropriate. With such aids, a patient with dementia may very clearly state her current feelings and complaints.

In the quest for consensus on the diagnostic and therapeutic procedures to be carried out, one has to take into account the person's evaluation of the burden of diagnostic procedures. Individualized evidence on risks and burdens concerning the relevant medical procedures should ideally guide the decision about the initial management. Factors that should generally be considered in deciding whether or not to start palliative care in elderly patients are summarized in table 5.1. One can picture a triangle that determines the success of palliative care in dementia: the sides of this triangle are the patient, the patient's family, and the professionals (physician, nurse, and team). To have it work, all three parties have to agree to the palliative management policy since palliation is meant to be healing for both the patient and the family. These three parties should seriously consider each other's needs and wishes. When the wishes and needs of the family seem extreme, every effort must be exerted to make the situation agreeable for all.

It must also be remembered that, while palliative care for the patient stops at death, the family may need support beyond that time. The need for postmortem support is well recognized in pediatrics, but probably not always adequately addressed in geriatrics.

There is enormous heterogeneity among patients with AD and other dementias, but there are also similarities in frailty, cognitive decline, social dependency, and communicative disorders. These cognitive disabilities, put into the context of a progressive, incurable disease with a limited lifespan, are so important in the palliative care management that there is a need for an explicit and concrete description of palliative care principles and practical guidelines.

We have presented some of the practical issues: first, on when and how to change the treatment policy that aims for cure into a palliative treatment policy; second, on how to formulate the content of a palliative treatment program and individualize treatments. Such individualized policies should be both evidence-based and ethics-based. Berg, Hanssib, and Halberg (1994) showed that implementation of individualized treatment plans will also improve the job satisfaction of the nursing staff, who have to accomplish the hard job of fulfilling the cognitive, social, emotional, and somatic care needs of their hospitalized, elderly patients. We also have demonstrated that there is hardly any evidence on palliative care in patients with dementia, especially the ones treated in hospitals. So far, this area is neglected, but at the same time it probably is an area where the classical instruments of clinical epidemiology, such as randomized controlled trials, cannot be used to solve relevant questions. A combination of quantitative

TABLE 5.2.   Practical Application of Principles of Palliative Care
in Hospitalized Patients with Dementia

Be aware that dementia makes it more difficult to monitor effects of palliative care for many reasons including:
- increased frailty/worsening prognosis
- insufficient reporting and recall of symptoms by patient
- increased burden of diagnostic procedures
- decreased cooperation during treatment procedures
- decreased stress tolerance
- difficult interpretation of pain behavior, which might express a mixture of pain and coping problems and/or behavioral disturbances
- difficult goal setting for the palliative care period, because of absence of awareness of dementia and the other co-morbid diseases

Take the patient's medical history several times during the week, with special focus on complaints and wishes/preferences

Ask for observation of complaints by a nurse or family member and monitor drug compliance and drug side effects

Evaluate burden-benefit ratio of all diagnostic and therapeutic procedures, in which the burden has to be assessed for frail patients with dementia

Reduce all drugs used, especially preventive drugs (e.g., for prevention of cardiovascular events)

Consider all options for treating symptoms, no matter how technical and no matter how expensive

Develop palliative care plans by consensus among patients, families, and staff

Assume that discussions about planning end-of-life care do not have to be completed in one session but should be an agenda item in consecutive meetings

If they are not already available, advance directives should be discussed

Palliative care for the family does not necessarily stop immediately after the death of the patient and the family's bereavement; take into account the family's factual, medical, and spiritual needs

Nonabandonment principle: Palliative care of a patient with dementia and of his/her family is not handed over to a colleague. This treatment model is the most effective—but most rarely offered—palliative care model in dementia

and qualitative studies is probably most appropriate, most informative, and therefore most successful, in conducting research in these patients. These studies should address patients' satisfaction with the process of diagnostics and their assessment of the burdens and risks of treatment options.

Synthesis of scientific data from palliative care studies and the patients' individual care preferences, possibly clearly expressed earlier in the life history, should be used in a palliative care plan. Hospital-based palliative care models probably should adapt hospice care models and create special care units for patients with dementia. Luchins and Hanrahan (1993) have shown that physicians, family members, and gerontologists would strongly prefer palliative care, when it is asked for, in end stages of dementia. In their study, hospice care models seemed most attractive to 90 percent of all three groups (this model is described in chapter 15 by Furlong). However, only a small minority of professionals (22%) and family members (15%) were aware where such hospice-based care models could be found in their region (Luchins & Hanrahan, 1993).

As long as data are lacking, we may try to generalize data coming from other patient groups. But because of lack of evidence, we should focus on defining the dilemmas and try, by all means, to reach consensus on how to answer the relevant treatment questions. General principles of "doing good," "do no harm," "*in dubio abstine*" may be the best to rely on. In the drama of complicated dementia, without evidence that guides us, no professional has the knowledge nor the position to fight preferences or choices of patients or their families. In such cases, even questionable capacity to consent might be enough to make decisions. Engaging in a harmonious quest for the best treatment, in close cooperation with the patient and the patient's family, is probably more important than the outcome of this quest. In fact, for the professionals, this joint venture itself may provide at least a partial solution to a clinical problem or palliative care dilemma. A formal, multidisciplinary meeting should be organized to prepare for such discussions, and of course patient and family involvement should be secured.

The implementation of practical guidelines on hospital-based palliative care for patients with dementia will probably improve quality, ethics, and aesthetics of care for this vulnerable group of patients. Fortunately, this improvement of quality of care is possible without implementing the whole set of end-of-life decisions (such as euthanasia, assisted suicide, and urging elderly patients into starvation). Though a lot of elderly patients are willing to talk about their death and sometimes wish to be dead, this does not mean that the best palliative treatment is to help them die rapidly. Often when patients are longing for the end of their lives, this longing may become bearable by an agreement being made to come back to that issue at regular times during the week. Compassionate stimulation of other aspects of daily life may diminish the wish for urgent death, which may even evaporate if life is accepted again. However, the most important remedy, and also probably the hardest to meet, is the principle of nonabandonment (table 5.2). The security of having one physician (or nurse practitioner) who will care for the patient until death, without delegating this responsibility, is a strong argument against leaving life and leaving this patient-physician relationship prematurely. Nonabandonment should be an important goal in health services for patients with dementia, and also in services for their families.

Striving toward and acting according to a palliative care model for patients with dementia in hospitals would be a major step forward in current health care for elderly persons. The demographic transition we are confronted with urges us to write and accept guidelines that will allow us to orchestrate the last stages in the lives of patients with dementia. Were we to succeed, patients and responsible professionals may hear the touching requiem of harmoniously orchestrated end-of-life care.

REFERENCES

Ahronheim, J., Morrison, S., Baskin, S., Morris, J., & Meier, D. (1996). Treatment of the dying in the acute hospital care: Advanced dementia and metastatic cancer. *Archives of Internal Medicine, 156,* 2094–2100.

Astrom, S., Nilsson, M., Norberg, A., & Winblad, B. (1990). Empathy, experience of burnout, and attitudes towards patients with dementia among nursing staff in geriatric care. *Journal of Advanced Nursing, 15,* 1236–1244.

Berg, A., Hansson, U., & Hallberg, I. (1994). Nurses' creativity, tedium, and burnout during one year of clinical supervision and implementation of individually planned nursing care: Comparisons between a ward for severely demented patients with dementia and a similar control ward. *Journal of Advanced Nursing, 20,* 742–749.

De Deyn, P. (2000). Treatment of Alzheimer's disease. *New England Journal of Medicine, 342,* 821.

De Deyn, P., Rabheru, K., Rasmussen, A., Bocksberger, J. P., Dantzenberg, P. L., Eriksson, S., et al. (1999). A randomized trial of risperidone, placebo, and haloperidol for behavioral symptoms of dementia. *Neurology, 53,* 946–955.

Doyle, D., Hanks, G., & MacDonald, N. (1993). *Oxford textbook of palliative medicine.* Oxford: Oxford University Press.

Eastwood, R., & Reisberg, B. (1999). Abnormal behavior in Alzheimer's disease. In S. Gauthier (Ed.), *Clinical diagnosis and management of Alzheimer's disease* (pp. 197–210). Malden, MA: Blackwell Science.

Fabiszewski, K., Volicer, B., & Volicer, L. (1990). Effect of antibiotic treatment on outcome of fevers in institutionalized Alzheimer patients. *Journal of the American Medical Association, 263,* 3168–3172.

Freeborne, N. (2000). The collected reports from SUPPORT and HELP: An annotated bibliography of manuscripts in print as of December 31, 1999 and SUPPORT prognostic formulas. *Journal of the American Geriatric Society, 48,* 222–233.

Hertogh, M., & Ribbe, M. (1996). Ethical aspects of medical decision-making in patients with dementia: A report from the Netherlands. *Alzheimer Disease and Associated Disorders, 10,* 11–19.

Hogan, D., & McCracken, P. (1999). Associated medical conditions and complications. In S. Gauthier (Ed.), *Clinical diagnosis and management of Alzheimer's disease* (pp. 279–286). Malden, MA: Blackwell Science.

Holstein, J., Chatellier, G., & Moulias R. (1994). Prevalence of associated diseases in different types of dementia among elderly institutionalized patients: Analysis of 3,447 records. *Journal of the American Geriatric Society, 42,* 972–977.

Hurley A., Volicer B., Mahoney M., & Volicer L. (1993). Palliative fever management in Alzheimer patients: Quality plus fiscal responsibility. *Advanced Nursing Science, 16,* 21–32.

Inouye, S., Bogardus, S., Baker, D., Leo-Summers, L., & Cooney, L. (2000). The hospital elder life program: A model of care to prevent cognitive decline in older hospitalized patients. *Journal of the American Geriatric Society, 8,* 1697–1706.

Katz, P. R. (1993). Antibiotics for nursing home residents: When are they appropriate? *Post Graduate Medicine, 93,* 173–180.

Kuremyr, D., Kihlgren, M., Norberg, A., Astrom S., & Karlsson, I. (1994). Emotional experiences, empathy, and burnout among staff caring for demented patients at a collective living unit and a nursing home. *Journal of Advanced Nursing, 19* (4), 670–679.

Luchins, D., & Hanrahan, P. (1993). What is appropriate health care for end-stage dementia? *Journal of the American Geriatric Society, 41,* 25–30.

McCarthy, M., Addington-Hall, J., & Altman, D. (1997). The experience of dying with dementia: A retrospective study. *International Journal of Geriatric Psychiatry, 12,* 404–409.

Morrison, R., Ahronheim, J., Morrison, G., Darling, E., Baskin, S., Morris, J., et al. (1998). Pain and discomfort associated with common hospital procedures and experiences. *Journal of Pain and Symptom Management, 15,* 91–101.

Morrison, R., & Siu, A. (2000). Survival in end-stage dementia following acute illness. *Journal of the American Medical Association, 284,* 47–52.

Moss, D., Berlanga, P., Hagan, M., Sandoval, H., & Ishida, C. (1999). Methanesulfonyl Fluoride (MSF): A double-blind placebo-controlled study of safety and efficacy in the treatment of senile dementia of the Alzheimer type. *Alzheimer Disease and Associated Disorders, 13,* 20–25.

Nourhashémi, F., Andrieu, S., Sastres, N., Ducassé, J., Lauque, D., Sinclair, A., et al. (2001). Descriptive analysis of emergency hospital admissions of patients with Alzheimer disease. *Alzheimer Disease and Associated Disorders, 15,* 21–25.

Riesenberg, D. (2000). Hospital care of patients with dementia. *Journal of the American Medical Association, 284,* 87–90.

Shuster, J. (2000). Palliative care for advanced dementia. *Clinical Geriatric Medicine, 16,* 373–386.

Sipsma, D. (2001). Dementia in the terminal stage. In F. Alkema, M. Kootte, & D. Sipsma (Eds.), *Dementia: Disease and care* (pp. 192–206). Assen, Netherlands: Van Gorcum.

Thorpe J., Widman, L., Wallin, A., Beiwanger, J., & Blumenthal, H. (1994). Co-morbidity of other chronic age dependent diseases in dementia. *Aging Clinical Experimental Research, 6,* 159–166.

Tolson, D., Smith, M., & Knight, P. (1999). An investigation of the components of best nursing practice in the care of acutely ill hospitalized older patients with coincidental dementia: A multi-method design. *Journal of Advanced Nursing, 30,* 1127–1136.

Van der Steen, J. (2002). *Curative or palliative treatment of pneumonia in psycho geriatric nursing home patients: Development and evaluation of a guideline, decision-making, and disease course.* Thesis, VU Medical Centre at Amsterdam.

Wolfson, C., Wolfson, D. B., Asgharian, M., M'Lan, C. E., Østbye, T., Rockwood, K., et al. (2001). A reevaluation of duration of survival after the onset of dementia. *New England Journal of Medicine, 344,* 1111–1116.

CHAPTER SIX

Elderly Persons with Advanced Dementia

An Opportunity for a Palliative Culture in Medicine

Pierre Boitte, Ph.D.

For the last twenty to thirty years in the history of Western medicine, the risks of neglect because of therapeutic powerlessness have been endured by two categories of patients: patients who were going to die and those with dementia.

The development of the palliative care movement has tried for about twenty years to respond to the first risk, "demanding that the physical, psychological and spiritual needs of patients are met at the end of their life" (Basset et al., 1992, p. 95). The development of geriatrics has promoted the less-well-publicized trend to demand a high quality of care and services for patients with advanced dementia—a position emphasized by Rigaux (1998). Geriatrics tries to make certain that those patients "are understood, recognized in their desires, that their needs are met, their handicaps are adapted to the shape of their lives and above all that they are not put aside from life" (Basset et al., 1992, p. 95).

But what happens to these patients with dementia, of which Alzheimer disease (AD) is one good example, when they come to the end of their lives? In this context where neither palliative care medicine nor geriatrics is really completely integrated, even if these two movements each now have a strong foundation, these patients are at risk to suffer, in a cumulative way, from the double exclusion of the dying and of being old and having dementia.

It could be possible in our societies to unite these two movements in order to ensure a palliative care approach for persons with dementia. If such a union were to come true, it would be to the honor of a medicine that too often is said to be dehumanizing because of too much reliance on technique. It would prove itself equal to the existential challenges created nowadays by our aging societies, especially the increasing prevalence of AD.

In order to become effective, such potential requires taking a departure from a too-ideal model of palliative care as is at times administered by some professional bodies.

❧ An "Ideal Model" of Palliative Care

The palliative care movement, introduced in France in the late 1970s, has been developed and strengthened mainly thanks to the experience of the St Christopher Hospice, created in London in 1967. From its English origin, the palliative care movement, supported by Cicely Saunders, has had three parts (Lamau, 2001, p. 11):

1. To protest against medicine's indifference to what those who are going to die go through
2. To attest that the end of life, given certain conditions, is an experience worth being fully lived
3. To invite a larger conception of care, linking technical approaches with the relational dimensions

On this basis, certain concepts and notions become imperative:

- Take into account the *total pain* of the person at the end of life, physical pains and psychological sufferings being closely linked
- Implement an *ethics of relationship* by the caregiving team so that fears, anxieties, and questions can really be listened to
- Adopt a holistic conception of the human being that does not separate body, psyche, and mind

The supporting humanistic philosophy for the palliative movement, whatever its variants were historically (i.e., first, North American variants, and then worldwide ones) include the following:

- Death is part of human destiny, and to be against death when it comes, by using all the resources of medical technology, proves to be inhuman and unreasonable.
- The last moments of life have worth just as they are. They are to be respected by encouraging the autonomy of the dying person, "his deepest expectations, honored in all its dimensions."
- The patient is considered as a relational being in his or her organic and psychic entirety, which invites "a certain quality of *inter-human solidarity*" (Lamau, 2001, p. 17). This solidarity requires that the dignity of every human being, even at the end of life when death is imminent, must be respected.

Such a conception of care at the end of life begs for a different approach by caregivers. Actions of the different members of the professional teams (e.g., doctors, nurses, nurse's aides, psychologists, physical therapists, social workers) stepping into their work with people at the end of life cannot be distinguished or divided in practice. The *interdisciplinarity*, or at least "the complementarity of the roles and qualifications," is a new way of approaching the person, accompanying him and his family, and it allows the caregivers to meet the ill person in the singularity of his history (Jacquemin, 2001, p. 102), while satisfying all his needs—physical, psychological, social, and spiritual.

One of the main aims of palliative practice is to relieve pain and suffering in a person facing death. Instead of the expression "total pain," which tends to articulate the person's moral, physical, spiritual, and social types of pain, we prefer the expression *global pain* (Richard, 2001), which adds a notion of solitude to the notion of physical pain (C. Jasmin, quoted by Richard, p. 119). The ambition of the palliative care approach consists in striving to preserve the best possible living till death by accompanying the global pain: "Palliative care, in the notion of accompanying, defends the idea of a care which recognizes the human dimension of the patient in extreme situations. The experience of palliative care in different locations has shown the capacity of this approach to ensure a high quality of living, sometimes unexpected, till death" (Pourchet, Guillot, & La Piana, 2001, p. 274). Some steps are required to accompany a human being who is suffering at life's end. There must be

- listening to the patient's cries, fears, and silences
- respect for the other, in her body, in its beliefs, mystery, and unshakable solitude

- honoring of the imperative that the highest level of competence be maintained toward this person (Richard, 2001, pp. 120–124)

This accompanying is by all means a relationship of helping, understood as an "interpersonal therapeutic process" that is established between the ill person and the caring team (Nectoux et al., 2001, p. 126). Instead of interesting the patient in a solution that would be judged good for them from an outside point of view, such a relation of help consists in "helping the person to have her own resources emerge so that one can be motivated to have their own way in responding to the life which is coming to an end" (p. 130).

Working in teams is one of the prominent details of the palliative care approach: "The principle of team work has become obvious in medicine and is now imperative" (Girardier, 2001, p. 364). Care directed to the multiple aspects of the patient's suffering serves to legitimate that the suffering warrants the health professionals' deep concern because so many of them are paying attention to it. Each of them has a precise role to play, none having at first a more important role than another's. In palliative care, the challenge is to introduce *interdisciplinarity* into the usual functioning of a multidisciplinary team. Medical knowledge does not play the main part automatically and systematically; rather, the exchange of points of view, of different looks at the same situation, is warranted in order to have "a collective care" (Mallet, Chekroud, & Frank, 2001, p. 379). Family and relatives must take part, too. "Interdisciplinarity shows the dynamics between the people who exchange their different knowledge. It is no longer a question of joining side by side a series of knowledges but-thanks to the dialogue-a question of mixing them so that they change each other. The expected result is an enrichment of the competence of persons and an understanding of a situation" (Girardier, 2001, p. 369).

The charge given to the palliative care team, beyond the exchange of points of view, consists in exchanging words, not as a confrontation of "experiences of knowledge" (Lassaunieres & Plages, quoted by Girardier, 2001, p. 369) but as a reply "to the order of life," as a discovery of "the impossibility to have a set formula for compassion (to suffer and to love)" (Bounon, quoted by Girardier, p. 369).

The spiritual approach in accompanying persons who are ill plays a very important role in palliative speech and practice. The notion of "spiritual needs" of ill persons spread in France even before the palliative movement appeared. This notion has been developed with regard to serious diseases and has gained a higher stature with the development of palliative care.

There are several realities in this notion of "spiritual needs": the need to be recognized as a person; the need to understand one's life, to search for a meaning of life; the need to free oneself from a guiltiness (why this pain? why to me?); the desire to make peace with oneself and/or with others; the desire to become open to transcendence and to perceive a "beyond" when the end of one's life comes (Thieffry, 2001, p. 546). These needs and desires, without necessarily being the object of a specific religious approach, deserve attention as means of showing "spiritual support" (p. 554). They can be addressed through the care given to the body, in the one-to-one listening relationship, in making the steps of reconciliation easier, in helping to maintain the person's social and family roles. Supporting and accompanying the patient's needs and desires set into action the words and subjectivity of team members involved in such support.

To respond to the spiritual needs of a patient at the end of his life is one of the main points in the palliative approach. Indeed, what is proposed in such an approach is not an all-out response to a certain need, but "a space for getting on the fundamental desire which is inside each human being: the fulfillment quest" (Frings, 2001, p. 570). This quest is probably the most personal aspect of a human being. Offering at the same time "the necessary conditions so that life will carry on till the end and there is an absolutely necessary relation for it—that is to say presence to the other, real attention to the needs, compassion—a certain 'atmosphere' is created, allowing to carry on life, allowing the human potential to develop" (p. 571). Here is the prospect of a palliative care approach in which a humanistic philosophy is eminently revealed. This is

- a global approach that strives to face global suffering, the spiritual dimension of which seems essential
- spiritual support that does its best to provide "a breath of life" until the end (Frings, 2001, p. 573)
- recognition of a patient for whom the team must respect the freedom to carry on—must leave her the responsibility as far as her life is concerned.

The expectation is that such an approach will make the passage from life to death more human, an expectation, too, that "a road to humanization of medicine will also be taken" (Thieffry, 2001, p. 557).

❧ Advanced Dementia at the End of Life: Questions for Palliative Care

What happens to such a prospect when patients with dementia—more precisely, patients with AD—must be accompanied at the end of their life? Is it possible for those people to profit from palliative care and so to "have a good dying," as is done for other categories of patients at the end of life? Just to assume the contrary does not seem legitimate, but it is worth underlining the complexity of the existing situation concerning dementia and the difficulties of looking after such persons even before they come to the last stage of the disease. Then the question of palliative care for patients with advanced dementia will be tackled as clearly as possible.

❧ Difficulties of Looking after Patients with Dementia

The global situation in the care of patients with dementia is proved nowadays to be more complex than it was ten or fifteen years ago. There are multiple reasons for that complexity: "a constant progression of the number of affected persons, quite a long evolution of the affliction, its more and more precocious evocation with the development of 'memory consultations' and the improvement of diagnostic strategies" (Michel et al., 2000, p. 307). Individual situations often seem quite complicated. Among the main elements of difficulty are the heterogeneity of problems and their progressive nature, the importance of the social interaction, especially with the primary caregiver, the changes in communication, the appearance of a true amnesiac syndrome, and sometimes the appearance of a patient's failure to perceive his own cognitive problems or even awareness of his own identity (p. 307).

The burden of care can often be heavy because of the intensity of the downward progression, the absence of any hope of improvement: "This kind of patient drives us to failure: they have a fixed gaze, emptied of any meaning, their face has a mask set in a rictus, impossible to guess any reply" (Basset et al., 1992, p. 97). In course of time, "death wishes can appear" in the caregivers' mind, and "the feelings of guiltiness and of aggressivity are sometimes badly repressed" (Coppex, 1997, p. 16). These feelings are described in several chapters of this book.

The caregivers of such patients often express their difficulty in communicating with the patient. How is it possible to build an interpersonal relationship when there is no recognition, due to the loss of memory that prevents the person from recognizing others—when the words, pronounced only moments ago, are forgotten? For those caregivers, knowing that the patient does not necessarily identify them, that he seems to forget what has just been said, can in the course of time be disturbing and lead them to question the possibility of establishing a relationship, even a thin one. Indeed, being sure that they are recognized and invested in a relationship is probably not required for the work of the caregivers: at the very time when we talk to someone, even a person with dementia, a relationship exists, and there is no evidence that it disappears without trace in the patient's mind. Moreover, the nonverbal communication used at this time (touch, massage) gains yet greater importance. Nevertheless, the caring work in such a context requires real effort, which increases with the length of the experience.

What about the autonomy of persons with dementia, an autonomy that is so valued today in the therapeutic relationship? The patient's own conscience being disturbed, her own history being more or less forgotten, and given her inability to converse, in some cases a patient's autonomy can be extremely relative.

❧ Difficulties of a Palliative Approach to Alzheimer Disease

A main problem with palliative care for patients with Alzheimer disease is its long development (on average, ten years) and its always being fatal, whatever improvement recent, mainly symptomatic, treatments can provide. Knowing that these types of pathologies seem to be incurable, the approach of caring cannot but be palliative, although on many points it does not correspond to the ideal plan of providing palliative care.

A first point that poses a problem is that of suffering and its management and control. The notion of global suffering seems relevant to the situation of patients with dementia, although we do not know anything precise about what this suffering can be. For example, what about the utter solitude that must face a person whose mind is demented and who at the same time is dying? More generally, does this type of elderly patient suffer when she thinks of death? Does she suffer from having dementia? Pragmatically speaking, how can we evaluate the pain felt by a person with dementia—a person who cannot express the pain herself in the usual ways, especially if "physical pain is neither a classic symptom nor a specific one in Alzheimer's Disease"? (Lefebvre-Chapiro, Legrain, & Sebag-Lanoë, 1998, p. 18). If it is not possible to question a patient directly, scales for measuring pain self-assessment cannot be used. In such situations, it is extremely difficult to assess whether the persistence of the symptomatology, supposedly linked to pain, corresponds to insufficient treatment or to an error in diagnosis.

Another point concerns the bereavement work of the patient, aimed at preparing him for the coming death that in the traditional palliative approach is affirmed to exist at the end of life. Do these patients know they are going to die? Are they unconscious of the situation they are in, or are they partly conscious, the unconsciousness being illuminated by bits of consciousness? Do they go through times of denial or through "the crisis of the end of life" (De Beir, 2001, p. 324), corresponding to the bereavement of their own life, accompanied by many losses and fears? Is this very notion of bereavement work linked to the coming end of life relevant for patients with dementia? Some people hypothesize that such patients' dementia "can be explained by stopping the bereavement work in their work of getting old" (Coppex, 1997, p. 17; Maisondieu, 1993).

How, in such a context, can the caregivers put into place an ethics of relationship, so important in palliative care, especially by listening to the fears, anxieties, and questions of the person at the end of life? What can it mean to show care by encouraging the autonomy of the patient with AD, especially by showing respect for the needs and desires the patient would express? For example, the patient's nonconsciousness may prevent him from being clear about his situation and from expressing his desires regarding the end of his life. Is the conception of a relationship of help as a therapeutic interpersonal process still relevant in such a situation? The person with dementia still owns her human possibilities and capabilities, as all of us do. The challenge for the caregivers is to be able to bring out the dying person's capacities in ways that will help her forge her path.

Another point, in connection with the two above, concerns spiritual support. In such cases, in comparison with the possibilities offered to patients who are still conscious, this support clearly is reduced. If care of the body is to be privileged, what about interpersonal listening and maintaining social and family roles? What about the fulfillment quest: the desire that quickens any way of getting on humanly? Is this quest always present in the mind of a patient with AD? Who could say so? In other respects, "the lucid thoughts of a person, their feelings about his or her coming death can be lost in confused and disordered words" (Benbow & Quinn, 1991, p. 12). How can these thoughts be recognized and how can these questions be answered?

Finally, a number of serious considerations come up regarding therapeutic relationships during the palliative process, induced by all the previous difficulties (generally or more directly linked to palliative care). First, those with regard to the patient:

- There is the challenge of informing him about his condition when the disease first is discovered, hopefully at an early stage (when nonconsciousness of the person is rare).
- From that time on, there are challenges of communicating with the patient about his desires regarding his future.
- There is the need not to give inadequate life-extending treatment, thus preventing unnecessary suffering for patient, family, and caregivers and not incurring the expenses of useless care.
- Issues of nutrition must be considered carefully: is it necessary to implement artificial nutrition if such methods do not change the progression of the disease and are difficult to use?
- There will also be a need to evaluate the movement, inevitably progressive, from light, moderate stages of the disease to more advanced ones (when concurrent pathologies, especially infectious ones, do not have to be treated, except symptomatically).

With regard to the family, other issues come up.

- The family may have difficulty in accepting the situation if it is immediately presented by the doctor as one that is clearly palliative—a difficulty that is increased by lack of understanding of what a probable dementia entails.
- The family may have difficulty in recognizing the physical and psychological downward course of a loved one, and accepting it.
- There is risk of early bereavement work by the family if there is a succession of states, the patient sometimes being conscious sometimes not conscious. There is the risk that the patient will be put aside, abandoned, or be the recipient of reactive overinvestment.
- The family has to deal with the lack of assurance that can be promised them by health professionals with regard to accompanying a loved one from the time the diagnosis is announced to after the patient's death.

For professional caregivers there are other considerations.

- It is necessary to provide psychological bereavement work for caregivers after the patient's death: the deceased person may have been known to the geriatric or psychiatric unit for months, and sometimes for years.
- There is difficulty for the whole team in providing a coherent approach to care. The nurses can have very different interpretations from those of physicians or social workers of what the patient understands of her disease, of her consciousness about it, and of her possible wishes. These varied concerns are discussed in other chapters of this book.

Palliative Practice in Cases of Advanced Dementia

The preceding considerations and questions are not, of course, designed to question the necessity of palliative care for patients with advanced dementia. They stress the kinds of presence that should be brought to the person at the end of life, including the presence of loved ones, especially the family. These patients insist on a constant search for a quality of living until the last breath and so they set up a way of being and doing relevant to facing their tragic situation. Therefore, it is possible, in the name of the interhuman solidarity that is defended by a palliative approach, to show respect for the patients' dignity as they end their lives. More and more teams are giving attention to the task. But with this kind of patient, respect is more difficult to achieve. In carrying out their accompanying and supporting roles, caregivers have to be creative. In other regards, the difficulties that caregivers face can stimulate critical renewal of normative ideals of the palliative movement and palliative practices.

The Experience of Palliative Care for AD Patients

Some teams have tried to be creative in treating advanced dementia and have outlined responses to the above concerns and questions. These teams hope to leave "an open door" (Masson, 1998, p. 154)—a door to imagining that there is meaning in apparently meaningless situations. In spite of the difficulty of understanding the psychic or behavioral syndrome, in its shape as well as in regard to a situation, the team says: "This symptom is the expression of the person, it is for him meaningful; it must be listened to and taken as a means of communication" (Coppex, 1997, p. 19). On this basis, caring for the body is probably a privileged moment to have a relationship with the person—in touching her, in looking at her. This care can help, in some cases, to give back "a way of speaking to the cared as being the equal of the caregiver, who shows an interest for that life in order that the person herself can carry on feeling interesting to others" (p. 19). Even at advanced stages of the disease, the issue is to take the chance that the person still potentially has an affective life and that, in spite of cognitive troubles, can apprehend the reality of the situation for a long time and can express opinions, needs of care, and spiritual desires.

In the same vein, it is worth trying to give meaning to the present again in a life that seems to be without meaning. The presence of family and relatives is very desirable: this validates the fact that each patient has his own singular and original history. Taking into account his former times, such a patient can be more easily helped to remain nearest to what he has been and what he is now.

The caregivers' experience shows that "death, bereavement and end of life are not negligible elements in caring for the demented patient" (Benbow & Quinn, 1991, p. 12). For example, it is not rare to see a person with dementia reacting violently to the loss of wife or husband, close friend, or roommate. Bereavement therapy can sometimes be started—for example, if it is clear enough that there is a link between the behavioral problems or a deep grief and the bereavement itself (p. 12). This type of accompanying and the actual results issuing from it in favor of the patient show that it is worth "joining the demented person in his suffering, listening to her speaking even shortly about his fear, her death, helping him as much as possible in the psychic organization of this passage from life to death" (Masson, 1998, p. 151).

The importance of the global nature of such care and the accompanying are underlined even more than they are with the "usual" palliative care. There should be

- a warm and individualized welcome
- knowledge of the patient's past
- constant watchfulness for changes of behavior (suffering, pain, worsening of psychic state)
- analysis by the team of those behaviors, and respect for them
- attention to physical needs and bodily care
- development of team dynamics

- listening to families
- when the time comes, time left for words about death
- continuity in care relationships until the terminal phase
- attention to funerary rites (Masson, 1998, p. 152)

In these ways, despite the apparent meaninglessness of the situation and the person's approaching death, a relationship is built, day-by-day—a choosing of the option of global care that assumes there is meaning.

All these approaches need to acquire a specific savoir-faire and competence—for example, in attention being given to cutaneous care; to difficulties with taking nourishment and with bowel and bladder functions; periods of confusion; deficits in verbal communication and judgment and reasoning problems. These situations require recognition of the patient's psychological state as a message of what can work. To succeed requires very fine observations on the behavior of the patient (George, Blique, & Penin, 1998, p. 39). The ability of *doing* goes with the ability of *being* in the communication: it is important to develop a therapeutic attitude based on the quality of listening and presence.

The importance of the team is proving crucial in this setting. There is indeed a greater necessity of teamwork than in *stricto sensu* palliative care. Collectively, the pressures form a triangle of care: patient/family entourage/professional caregiver. Only excellent coordination allows "the coherent taking in charge of the patient, the family and the team of care" (Michel et al., 2000, p. 307). It also allows the team during the whole evolution of the disease to "wonder about the appropriateness between the given care, the psychological state of the patient, the patient's expressed desires and the opinion of the family and the caregivers" (Lefebvre-Chapiro, Legrain, & Sebag-Lanoë, 1998, p. 20).

An Ethical Reflection

The great ideal of palliative care comes up against difficulties in the experience of caring for persons with advanced dementia, and Alzheimer disease is a good example of these difficulties. The undeniable, wonderful creativity of most caregivers in accompanying these persons to their death must not hide the need for further development and adaptation of palliative care in geriatric or psychogeriatric units. The ideal model refers back to the palliative care movement's beginnings and to the conviction of the founders. For there to be success in the treatment of persons with AD, we must acknowledge a need for adaptation.

To allow palliative care to continue to develop beyond its established boundaries and, little by little, to spread in hospital units, we must propose appropriate changes so as to avoid "useless situations of suffering" for caregivers, who often face the impossibility of reaching this ideal in their practice; and at the same time we must aim at "allowing the ideal of palliative care to carry on its critical aim" (Jacquemin & Mallet, 2000, pp. 128–129). One key adaptation is to acknowledge the usefulness of palliative care in situations that go beyond the traditional idea that it should be used only at the end of life (Boitte, 2001).

To propose changes means, more particularly, to identify tensions in current palliative care practices that question the practical legitimacy of palliative care when the purpose is to apply these ideals to the situation of patients with dementia. Let us simply think of the global nature of the intent to care, the concern for well-doing, in the act of accompanying. From this position, "power attitudes" for the patient or his family can emerge. This identification can be done indirectly by analyzing clinical ethics issues with palliative care teams. At the same time, it can be done by using "control and limit"—a double category: What, in its practice, does palliative care want to control? In cases of looking after weak patients, what limits should be established to the power that caregivers have? How do we ensure that this power is not exceeded?

This book is important because it starts an ethical evaluation of palliative care for elderly patients with dementia. This evaluation must be done remembering that the ethical approach—its aim, its involvement—must permeate the whole of palliative practices. In doing so, questions (those asked above and some others) must be raised. The obvious will be brought to consciousness—namely, that "it is impossible for human rationality to integrate, in a definitely well-ordered way, this always single, always tragic, event of the subject's death" (Cadoré, 2000, p. 14).

REFERENCES

Basset, P., Hamon, B., Passarelli, P., Boutrelle, J., & Hohn, C. (1992). Soins palliatifs, démence et dements [Palliative care, dementia, and the demented]. In D. J. Roy and C. H. Rapin, *Les Annales de Soins Palliatifs: Les Défis* (pp. 95–99). Montreal: Institut de recherches cliniques de Montréal.

Benbow, S. M., & Quinn, A. (1991). Démence, deuil, et fin de vie [Dementia, bereavement, and the end of life]. *Info-Kara, 21*, 11–16.

Boitte, P. (2001). Les derniers moments de la vie: Un temps à maîtriser? [The last moments of life: A time to master?]. In D. Jacquemin (Ed.), *Manuel des Soins Palliatifs* (2nd ed.) (pp. 343–349). Paris: Dunod.

Cadoré, B. (2000, June 23–24). Des champs éthiques ouverts par les soins palliatifs [Ethics fields opened by palliative care]. *Actes du 7ème Congrès national de la Société française d'accompagnement et de soins palliatifs, 9–14.*

Coppex, P. (1997). Les soins palliatifs: Un attachement et un cheminement dans la séparation des personnes souffrant de démence avancée [Palliative care: An attachment and slow progression in the separation of people suffering from advanced dementia]. *Info-Kara, 47,* 16–21.

De Beir, C. (2001). La phase ultime [The final phase]. In D. Jacquemin (Ed.), *Manuel des Soins Palliatifs* (2nd ed.) (pp. 322–342). Paris: Dunod.

Frings, M. (2001). La dimension spirituelle des soins palliatifs chez Cicely Saunders [The spiritual dimension of palliative care in the work of Cicely Saunders]. In D. Jacquemin (Ed.), *Manuel des Soins Palliatifs* (2nd ed.) (pp. 569–578). Paris: Dunod.

George, M. Y., Blique, S., & Penin, F. (1998). Démence et fin de vie . . . en quête de sens: Quel projet de soin en unité de longue durée? [Dementia and the end of life . . . in search of meaning: What kind of long-term care project?]. *Info-Kara, 51,* 37–44.

Girardier, J. (2001). Le travail en équipe de soins palliatifs [Working in a palliative care team]. In D. Jacquemin (Ed.), *Manuel des Soins Palliatifs* (2nd ed.) (pp. 365–372). Paris: Dunod.

Jackson, A. (2001). Histoire et rayonnement mondial [History and worldwide spread]. In D. Jacquemin (Ed.), *Manuel des Soins Palliatifs* (2nd ed.) (pp. 21–31). Paris: Dunod.

Jacquemin, D. (2001). Place des soins palliatifs dans l'évolution d'une philosophie du soin [The place of palliative care in the evolution of a philosophy of care]. In D. Jacquemin (Ed.), *Manuel des Soins Palliatifs* (2nd ed.) (pp. 99–109). Paris: Dunod.

Jacquemin, D., & Mallet, D. (2000, June 23–24). Discours et imaginaire des soins palliatifs: Nécessité et modalité d'une distance critique [Discourse and imagination in palliative care: Necessity and modality of critical distance]. In *Actes du 7ème Congrès national de la Société française d'accompagnement et de soins palliatifs, 127–136.*

Lamau, M. L. (2001). Origines et inspirations [Origins and inspirations]. In D. Jacquemin (Ed.), *Manuel des Soins Palliatifs* (2nd ed.) (pp. 8–20). Paris: Dunod.

Lefebvre-Chapiro, S., Legrain, S., Sebag-Lanoë, R. (1998). Les soins palliatifs se développent chez les patients atteints de maladie d'Alzheimer évoluée [Palliative care develops for patients struck by advanced Alzheimer's disease]. *La Revue du Praticien-Médecine générale, 12* (406), 18–20.

Maisondieu, J. (1993). La démence: Manque de savoir-vivre ou manque de savoir mourir? [Dementia: A lack of wisdom to live or a lack of wisdom to die?]. In C. Montandon-Binet & A. Montandon (Eds.), *Savoir mourir* (pp. 233–244). Paris: Editions L'Harmattan, 3–4 April.

Mallet, D., & Chekroud, F. C. (2001). Le médecin [The physician]. In D. Jacquemin (Ed.), *Manuel des Soins Palliatifs* (2nd ed.) (pp. 379–383). Paris: Dunod.

Masson, M. (1998). Démence sénile et mort [Senile dementia and death]. *Actes du 6ème Congrès national de la Société française d'accompagnement et de soins palliatifs,* 1:151–154.

Michel, J. M., Leval, M., Wirrmann, D., Hild, J. (2000, June 23–24). Maladie d'Alzheimer et soins palliatifs [Alzheimer's disease and palliative care]. *Actes du 7ème Congrès national de la Société française d'accompagnement et de soins palliatifs,* 307–311.

Nectoux, M., Bernard, M. F., Guillaume, O., & Delorme, A. (2001). La relation d'aide [The care relationship]. In D. Jacquemin (Ed.), *Manuel des Soins Palliatifs* (2nd ed.) (pp. 126–137). Paris: Dunod.

Pourchet, S., Guillod, M., & La Piana, J.-M. (2001). SIDA et soins palliatifs [AIDS and palliative care]. In D. Jacquemin (Ed.), *Manuel des Soins Palliatifs* (2nd ed.) (pp. 263–274). Paris: Dunod.

Richard, M. S. (2001). La souffrance globale [Global suffering]. In D. Jacquemin (Ed.), *Manuel des Soins Palliatifs* (2nd ed.) (pp. 115–125). Paris: Dunod.

Rigaux, N. (1998). *Le pari du sens: Une nouvelle éthique de la relation avec les patients âgés déments* [A wager for meaning: A new ethics for the relationship with elderly patients with dementia]. Le Plessis-Robinson, France: Institut Synthélabo pour le progrès de la connaissance.

Thieffry, J. H. (2001). Les besoins spirituels au cours des maladies graves [Spiritual needs in the course of serious illness]. In D. Jacquemin (Ed.), *Manuel des Soins Palliatifs* (2nd ed.) (pp. 546–557). Paris: Dunod.

Part III / Philosophical and
Theological Explorations

CHAPTER SEVEN

Autonomy and the Lived Body in Cases of Severe Dementia

Wim J. M. Dekkers, M.D., Ph.D.

In many countries, physical restraints and other coercive measures are daily practice in the care for persons with dementia. Mechanical measures that must guarantee the safety of the patient and of fellow patients are frequently taken, and these necessarily restrict the freedom of the patient. Psychogeriatric institutions also experience another common problem: having to decide whether or not to start, or continue, tube feeding of patients with dementia. In both situations, patients often resist these interventions, using verbal protest, agitated behavior, or bodily defensive movement.

- Mr. M., aged seventy-two, with unspecified dementia, was admitted to a nursing home when his wife was no longer able to care for him. Mr. M. is frequently upset after his wife's visits, and when she leaves he often strikes out at the staff. As a result, he is placed in a geriatric chair, and one day his wife found the chair tied to a railing near the nurses' station. A staff member explained that this is necessary to keep Mr. M. from "wheeling around" (Strumpf & Evans, 1991).
- Mrs. G., a ninety-year-old with AD, has been a resident of a nursing home for thirteen years. Recently she has refused to eat, and for three years her wrists have been restrained to prevent her from pulling out a nasogastric

tube. A decision to place a gastrostomy tube is now pending (Strumpf & Evans, 1991).

Situations like these raise two kinds of problems. First, there is the practical moral problem of what to do. Must verbal utterances, agitational behavior, and defensive movements be disregarded or overridden in the best interest of the patient or others? How can coercive measures be justified when they are obviously against the will of the patient? Here it is worth emphasizing that persons with advanced dementia are vulnerable to medicalized dying with a nasogastric tube or percutaneous endoscopic gastrostomy. Post writes: "If it is the wisdom of nature that people with profound dementia forget how to swallow, if it was wise when Plato wrote that to the dying food 'appears sour and is so,' I wonder about our technological audacity and readiness to 'play God' by inserting tubes" (Post, 1995, p. 7). Is it true that we "play God" if we start tube feeding against the obvious will of the patient?

Second, there is the philosophical problem of how agitational behavior and defensive movements must be understood. Are bodily defensive movements to be explained from a purely biomedical perspective as automatic reflex movements that can be ignored? Or must they be interpreted as a meaningful bodily expression that may tell us something about the person's wishes? Another most important theoretical question is whether persons with severe dementia actually have wishes and desires. And to widen the scope even further, what, in such situations, does it mean to adhere to the ideal of taking persons with (severe) dementia seriously and to treat them with respect and dignity?

This chapter focuses primarily on the second type of question, though it also presents some practical consequences that may be derived from these theoretical considerations. The chapter's first aim is to describe and interpret bodily defensive movements of persons with severe dementia. The search here for an interpretation of the concepts of autonomy and the human body results in one that in many ways differs from current interpretations. Especially when the concept of autonomy is dealt with, I go off the beaten track. The second aim of this chapter is philosophically to underpin the often intuitively felt hesitation and resistance to prolong the life of persons with severe dementia by tube feeding them. First, before focusing on autonomy and the lived body, I describe what it is to be severely demented.

❧ What Is It Like to Have Severe Dementia?

Generally, dementia—for example, Alzheimer disease—is a long-lasting and gradual process. While the body of the person with dementia often remains strong for a number of years, mental capacities as well as the accumulated competencies and memories of a lifetime gradually slip away. People with advanced dementia generally do still have fears and longings, even if these are limited to the immediate present, but in cases of severe dementia, the self (or call it the mind, the soul, the will) that constitutes the central locus of humanity is severely affected or may even be lost. The self is, so to speak, increasingly fragmented and scattered. In the end stage, persons with dementia lie in bed in a fetus-like position seemingly living as a vegetative organism, totally dependent on the care of others.

The difference between a first-person and a third-person perspective of this long-lasting process of mental decay and bodily deterioration is striking. In the brief second section of his book *Elegy for Iris* (1999), John Bayley describes seven episodes of his life with his wife, the philosopher and novelist Iris Murdoch. Iris Murdoch had been suffering from Alzheimer disease since the mid-1990s, and she died in 1999. Bayley's digressions will be familiar to Alzheimer's families who witness the mental and physical deteriorating process of a beloved family member, an experience that often is a nightmare. "Family members find themselves dealing with a disorder that robs their loved one of individuality and autonomy, yet leaves the physical self intact" (Binstock, Post, & Whitehouse, 1992, pp. 1–2).

The Dutch writer Bernlef, on the other hand, has tried in his novel *Out of Mind* (1988) to empathize a demented person's experiences by giving a first-person account of a process of becoming demented. The main character, Maarten, is gradually losing his grip on both himself and the world. It is typical of this narrative that it is increasingly difficult for the reader to comprehend Maarten's experiences and to understand them as expressions of a rational being. Maarten's experiences and expressions become completely confused and seem to dissolve in an entirely amorphic and incomprehensible mass. In the end, the first-person narrative simply stops. One can argue that Maarten, after the ending of his first-person account, continues to write his life story just by living and acting and that he will continue to be a part of the life story of others. But his verbal account of what it is to be demented stops. From that time on, one can only guess what is going on in his mind.

In 1974, Thomas Nagel published his article "What Is It Like to Be a Bat?" In this well-known piece, he explores the possibilities of saying something meaningful about the conscious experiences and mental states of a "fundamentally *alien* form of life" (p. 438). At the end of the article, Nagel suggests that such considerations could deal with, instead of animals, human beings. One might try, for example, to develop concepts that could be used to explain to a person blind from birth what it is like to see. Although the ontological status of people with severe dementia differs considerably from that of animals and blind persons, my belief is that it makes sense to ask the question, "What is it like to be severely demented?" People with severe dementia cannot entirely be denied a (rudimentary) form of selfhood or personhood. They definitely are not persons in the strict sense of moral agents who are self-conscious and rational and demonstrate a minimal moral sense, but at least they can be called persons in a (weaker) social sense. In many ways, they can be regarded as if they were persons (Engelhardt, 1996). However, my belief that people with severe dementia are somehow persons with a self provides no indication for knowing what it is like to be severely demented. Generally, one can try to describe the ontological status of people with severe dementia by using concepts like self, person, soul, human being, rationality, and so forth, but one still does not know how it feels to be severely demented. We have to live with the fact that we will never have a satisfying answer to the intriguing question, "What is it like to be severely demented?"

What Is Left in Severe Dementia?

What does it mean when one considers someone to be "totally demented"? Currently, the emphasis is on what is gone. It is often said that there is a loss of everything that makes a being a human being. However, one can also ask what is left? The question, then, is not what kind of capacities are absent, but what capacities are intact. Do persons with severe dementia still have a will or desires? Is there still a kind of (primitive) interrelationship? Are they, in any sense of the word, competent? Holm suggests that except in the most severe cases of dementia, incompetence is patchy and that there may be "large islands of competence" (Holm, 2001, p. 154). It is beyond doubt that persons with (severe) dementia are incompetent to make a rational, explicit, and deliberate decision, but does this lack of explicit decision-making capacity automatically imply that there is no competence left? Should a person with severe dementia be denied any kind of autonomy?

Patients with severe dementia often seem to refuse treatment (indicated by continued attempts to pull out dialysis or feeding tubes, by defensive movements, and the like). A comparison with other "incompetent" human beings forces itself upon us. Psychotic patients may refuse medical treatment, and act accordingly. Young children who are afraid of being vaccinated may make defensive movements when they realize that an injection needle will penetrate their skin; also when they hear other "victims" crying. As mentioned in the introduction to this chapter, bodily defensive movements can be considered in two ways. First, they can be explained from a purely biomedical point of view, as automatic reflex movements. From this perspective, which leans heavily upon a Cartesian, mechanistic view of the human body, it is thought that these defensive movements must be considered as being totally separated from expressions of the person or the self. Second, they can be interpreted as meaningful bodily expressions that tell us something about the person, the self, or the person's wishes.

In this regard, another comparison forces itself upon us; namely, that between the person with severe dementia, for whom death is not far away, and the severely handicapped newborn, who fights for life. When caregivers in neonatal intensive care units have to decide whether or not to continue medical treatment, it appears that the newborn infant's energy and vigor contributes to the clinician's judgments about life expectancy and the continuation or termination of treatment. In ethical decision making in a neonatal intensive care unit, the phenomenon of vitality appears to have moral significance (Brinchmann & Nortvedt, 2001). The phenomenon of vitality appears to be interwoven in the medical signs and symptoms that are used in the prognostic and clinical evaluation of infants. Vitality was also described as temperament, personality, or the ability to react to pleasant or unpleasant stimulation. From this perspective, some of the newborn's bodily signs were interpreted as: "I want to live" or "Please, continue with the treatment." These newborns tried, so to speak, to express their will and to execute their autonomy in *statu nascendi* just by demonstrating their vitality.

Another example can be derived from the practice of circumcision of male newborns. Of course, the young child cannot give or withhold his consent, but does that mean that he cannot do anything else to express his will (it being supposed that he has a will)? Goodman, a liberal Jewish author and an opponent of neonatal circumcision, writes: "Their reactions, their screams, and that they have to be held down at all, are their best and only way of indicating that they are actually *withholding* their consent" (1999, p. 24). Of course, we must differentiate between incompetent people who do not yet have a self in the sense of a life narrative (neonates) and incompetent people who once had or were a narrative self (people with dementia). But apart from this difference, the question is whether it makes sense to interpret in an analogous way the defensive movements of persons with severe dementia as expressions of their will—that is, as signs of their (declining) vitality and autonomy. Can these defensive movements possibly be interpreted as "Stop treatment" or "Let me die"? To provide at least a beginning of an answer, I now focus on the concepts of autonomy and the lived body.

❧ Autonomy and the Lived Body

In modern medical ethics, in particular in the (neo)liberal tradition, much emphasis is paid to the human being as a free, self-sufficient, rational, independent, and autonomous subject. If a human being is thought to have bodily aspects at all, these are generally not seen as having much to do with that which makes a being human. The human body is often considered to be either an "automaton" that automatically reacts to external stimuli or an instrument controlled (and owned) by the autonomous person. The human body has almost an exclusively instrumental value and does not seem to reveal much about the person himself. It is not my intention to reject the ideal of (rational, individual) autonomy altogether, but to try to enlarge the scope of its meaning.

This chapter is a search for an "alternative" view on autonomy and the human body that is in line with some of Kissell's main tenets in chapter 8. Summarizing the way in which the principle of autonomy is currently understood, Kissell speaks of "a dualistic Cartesian patient who *happens* to have a body, but who is primarily a rational agent." She also makes a plea for a vision of the human being as an embodied person. As embodied, the patient is "an intelligent, communicating, gesturing, moral being who understands, who converses, who relates, who presents herself, who judges, who suffers, who reproduces other moral subjects, by and through her body. She communes with, and learns about, the world through her eyes and ears and touch and smell. She interacts with others through movements and words."

Autonomy

There are many diverse conceptualizations of the term *autonomy* (G. Dworkin, 1988); however, often the concept of (individual) autonomy is thought to have close ties to the concepts of decision-making capacity and competence. It is often presupposed that the person who makes a decision ideally should be a fully rational and autonomous subject who can act independently. Independence means autonomy, and autonomy means self-governance, independence from controlling influences. The autonomous individual freely acts in accordance with a self-chosen plan. Beauchamp and Childress describe what they take to be essential to personal autonomy as "personal rule of the self that is free from both controlling interferences by others and from personal limitations that prevent meaningful choice, such as inadequate understanding" (1994, p. 121).

It is beyond dispute that persons with (severe) dementia do not fulfill the standard criteria of being an autonomous person. It generally also goes without argument that they do not meet the four requirements that are needed for a judgment of competence to decide about one's health care (S. P. K. Welie, 2001). Persons with severe dementia do not possess (1) the ability to acquire and retain cognitive content, and (2) the ability to manipulate cognitive content critically. Moreover, one will be inclined to argue that they also do not possess (3) a freedom of will, and (4) the ability to express themselves. However, the last two requirements raise questions. First, persons with severe dementia certainly do not possess a freedom of will, but can they be denied any kind of will? Second, they indeed cannot express themselves verbally and rationally, but does this mean that all capability of expression of their self is lost?

Beauchamp and Childress suggest that the principle of respect for autonomy should cover only autonomous persons. R. Dworkin (1993) recognizes respect for autonomy as an important principle in the care for people with dementia, but only insofar as it regards the former autonomous, not yet demented person. Dworkin endorses "precedent autonomy," which takes into account the person's past wishes as genuine (p. 226). In the case of the person with severe dementia who is emotionally well-adjusted and seems to be happy, Dworkin still endorses the authority of extended autonomy through advance directives such as living wills. The decisions that the person expressed prior to become demented should be honored, even though that person has not yet experienced dementia. The former decisions of a person with severe dementia remain in force because he lacks the necessary capacity for a fresh exercise of autonomy. No new decision by a person capable of autonomy has annulled those decisions (R. Dworkin, 1993).

In the slowly deteriorating process of dementia, an "erosion of real autonomy" takes place (Moody, 1992, p. 87). The question I wish to pose is whether and when this process of erosion stops. Should persons with severe dementia (though not autonomous in the current sense) be denied any form of autonomy from a certain point in time? Can bodily defensive movements be interpreted as a kind of "bodily autonomy"?—can they be seen as a remnant of what once was "real" or "rational" autonomy? The moral dilemmas that emerge in the practice of physical restraints and artificial tube feeding thus raise the problem of the relationship between the person and the body. From a nondualistic, phenomenological perspective, bodily defensive movements can be considered a meaningful answer to extreme circumstances from "somebody" who once was a "real" person.

The Lived Body

In an attempt "to take the body seriously," as Toombs (1997, p. 39) puts it, I now draw insights from a phenomenological understanding of the human body. As the French philosopher Merleau-Ponty (1962) argues, our lived body—*"le corps-sujet"*—is our only access to the outside world, the only way of being-to-the-world (*"être-au-monde"*). The lived body is the body as it is given in direct experience. It is immediately and often unconsciously felt, sensed, tasted, heard, and seen. The lived body is the expression of one's existence and is concretely lived by oneself. It is through one's lived body that one manifests oneself to the world. All structures and functions of the lived body (perceiving, moving, acting, sexual behavior, etc.) are modes of being of the person. Whether we are consciously aware of it or not, the lived body is present as a "true companion" in our personal existence. The lived body possesses its own knowledge of the world, which implies the existence of a "tacit knowledge," a silent knowledge that functions without conscious control. On a subconscious level, my body provides me with a lot of information about the world.

This Merleau-Pontian idea of the lived body can be further explained by means of the metaphor of "the body as a text" (Dekkers, 1998, 2001). The human body can be seen as a subject—that is, as an interpreter (writer or reader) of texts—and as an object—that is, as a text to be interpreted. The body is a *subject* of experience when it functions as an interpreter in its own right—when it speaks for itself, so to speak. The body interprets not only itself but also everything in the outside world with which it is confronted via the senses. This is what Merleau-Ponty means by the notion of prereflective, "tacit" knowledge. The content of these bodily interpretations of the world does not necessarily need to be known by the person. The human body may be considered the author of a text (of bodily signs), but also the reader of the text that is constituted by what is happening in the outside world. The body is an *object* of experience when one experiences one's own body. In these situations, one is more or less aware of one's body, which then can be described as a text to be interpreted. Then the person (i.e., the I person or another person) is the reader.

A very important question to be solved now is whether the Merleau-Pontian idea of the lived body is at all applicable to persons with severe dementia. Merleau-Ponty's focus was primarily on patients with brain damage and other neurological abnormalities. As far as I know, he did not deal with persons with severe dementia. However, his concept of the lived body makes sense here because the Merleau-Pontian way of thinking regards the ontological level of being human, regardless whether the human beings involved are young or old, healthy or diseased, fully rational or severely demented. The only presupposition we have to make (and it is one that I am inclined to endorse) is that persons with severe dementia do not totally lack a self or personhood. In persons with dementia, not only the mind but also the body gradually deteriorates. The person with severe dementia is extremely damaged in his mental and bodily existence. The body of such a person is in a sense a less human body than the body of a person who is not so diseased. On the basis of this empirical finding, one can argue, as the Dutch neurologist Prick (1971) does, that the unity of a mind and an animated body, which in a Merleau-Pontian way is thought to be essential to being a human being, also gradually disappears. However, if this unity of a mind and an animated body is considered an ontological characteristic of human beings, it cannot (entirely) disappear. In other words, though the body of a person with severe dementia increasingly functions as an "automaton," it still remains a lived body. "Also the human being with dementia is and remains a meaning-giving subject" (Prick, 1971, p. 558).

❧ Bodily Autonomy

In a recent study on palliative care, Lawton has criticized an "essentially 'disembodied' conception of the person/self" (2000, p. 7). Such a conception takes for granted "the presence of a healthy, autonomously functioning body; that is of a body which can actually be 'controlled' and 'fashioned' by the self" (p. 84).

Lawton challenges the conception of the person and the self as primarily or necessarily rational and autonomous. Also making use of the phenomenological notion of the lived body, she has tried to incorporate more of a bodily element by focusing on the bodily deterioration that can be found in most terminally ill patients. Her starting point is the idea that persons are not embodied in the sense that they "have" a body but in the sense that they "exist," or "live," in their body. Understanding embodiment as the experience of both being a body and living through a body provides an important conceptual perspective of understanding why a patient's self is affected when various bodily capacities are lost. An example is the (in)continence of urine and feces. Continence, considered as a form of "bodily closure" or as a "bounded body" (2000, p. 142), is a necessary means by which entry into "full person status" (p. 142) is gained. Incontinence among elderly people is, on the contrary, frequently thought to symbolize that the elderly person is no longer an adult person in the strict sense of the word *adult* (Engelhardt, 1996), but is on the road to becoming a *non*person. Expanding this way of thinking to the situation of persons with severe dementia, it is important to realize that not only the decay of bodily functions negatively influences the sense of self, but that the loss of self and of cognitive capacities also negatively influences the person's bodily functions.

Lawton introduces the term *bodily autonomy,* which apparently must be understood as a person's autonomy over his body. Bodily autonomy is considered by Lawton as a central (though not necessarily sufficient) criterion for personhood. Autonomy involves not only being able to enact one's wishes and intentions bodily, but also to maintain control of the physical boundaries of one's body. Thus, loss of "bodily autonomy" appears to have at least two different meanings: "loss of bodily mobility" and "the loss of control of the physical boundaries of the body" (2000, p. 87). Patients with "severely unbounded bodies" experience also a "loss of self" (p. 142). Patients experience considerable difficulties in maintaining a sense of self once they have lost the bodily capability to "do" and "act" in an independent way and, more fundamentally, after the physical boundaries of the body have irretrievably eroded away.

Although I, too, want to emphasize that the bodily aspects of autonomy need to be more explicitly recognized, I will, like Lawton, use the notion of bodily autonomy in a specific way, but giving it quite a different meaning. Instead of referring to control *over* the body and its boundaries, I use *bodily autonomy* in the sense of "the bodily aspect of autonomy," or "autonomy *of* the body." This is analogous to the meaning of the term *autonomic nervous system*. The autonomic nervous system consists of the sympathetic and parasympathetic nervous system. Though higher centers can control autonomic functions, the autonomic nervous system is not directly accessible to voluntary control (Berne & Levy, 2000). This means that some body parts possess an autonomy that can be controlled only indirectly, by higher brain centers.

The meaning of *bodily autonomy* that I am putting forward is a combination of the biomedical notion of bodily automatisms and the phenomenological idea of the lived body. Considered from this (combined) perspective, the human body lives its own life, to a high degree being independent of higher brain functions and conscious deliberations and intentions. The lived body demonstrates a "tacit knowledge." In a person with dementia, cognitive capabilities gradually disappear until the moment when the patient is no longer capable of exercising autonomy by making explicit decisions. This does not mean, however, that the patient's bodily knowledge, developed in the course of the patient's life, necessarily also disappears.

The question of what "bodiliness" means is therefore crucial in the practice and theory of the care of persons with dementia (De Lange, 2001). Even in advanced dementia, when rational, verbal, and emotional communication is largely absent, there are still communicative methods of importance left. The only way to communicate with these patients is via their body. This means that one must explicitly pay attention to the bodily way in which persons with dementia "are in the world." The methods of psychomotor therapy and music therapy and the practice of stimulation of the senses by means of music, light, smells and perfumes, flavors, and bodily contacts are based on these insights. By means of bodily communication, the preferences of persons with dementia (at a not too advanced stage) who can no longer express themselves verbally can be known and interpreted.

Tacit bodily knowledge is based on the sedimentation of life narratives. When the body's capability to learn gradually disappears, the body loses its capacity to build up a new repertoire of routine actions. However, though automatisms come to be lost in the course of the process of becoming demented (apraxia, abasia, astasia, etc.), persons with dementia can still have routine actions "stored" in their body. Bodily defensive movements of persons with severe dementia may be interpreted as a kind of "bodily autonomy"—as a remainder of what once has been "real" or "rational" autonomy. A person with severe dementia has, so to speak, nothing else at her disposal than these unconscious, "automatic" bodily movements. From this point of view, autonomy is not a substantial concept. Instead, as Illhardt states in chapter 12, autonomy must rather be considered a bodily way of exercising one's will as expression of one's being-to-the-world (être-au-monde). Next, I consider some practical consequences of these considerations, taking tube feeding as an example.

❧ Practical Ethical Consequences: Tube Feeding

One of the preeminent problems in caring for persons with severe dementia is deciding whether and how to provide water and food. Patients can be artificially fed by means of assisted oral feeding or by tube feeding (using nasogastric tubes and percutaneous endoscopic gastrostomy, or PEG). Mrs. G. (the patient mentioned earlier in this chapter) has been trying to pull out her nasogastric tube for three years. Placing a PEG tube is now being considered. However, this will probably cause the same problem. Even though the protruding PEG tube is short and taped over, patients with dementia, lacking insight as to why it is there, will often try to pull it out (Post, 2001). The problem that physical restraint poses is exacerbated by the fact that an otherwise minimally invasive intervention may be tantamount to an assault when it is performed on someone with dementia, who has no insight into the purposes behind the treatment. Even rather simple interventions, such as the use of a hypodermic needle or the drilling of a tooth, become much more burdensome and likely to cause agitation than they would for persons who do not have dementia.

How to act in cases like these? Respect for the autonomy of the patient (in the current sense of *autonomy*) makes sense only if there is an advance directive. But if there is no living will and if a substituted judgment of the patient's wishes is difficult (which it often is), then one must rely upon a judgment of the patient's best interest. One of the ways to assess the patient's interest is to weigh the possible benefits and risks of artificial feeding. Decisions that impose a considerable burden on the person with dementia must not be tolerated. There ought to be limits on the rights of individuals (through advance directives) and families (in cases of the incompetent person having no advance directive) to demand treatments that are significantly burdensome (Post, 1995).

Dysphagia in dementia is often multiconditional. Both biological and psychological factors may contribute to swallowing problems. However, in patients with advanced dementia, swallowing problems without specific biological or psychological causes are independently associated with mortality, whether the patients receive assisted oral feeding or long-term tube feeding. The advent of swallowing difficulties without a clear biological or psychological cause defines a dementia as so advanced that it must be loosely considered a terminal condition. Losing the ability to swallow is ultimately part of the "naturalness" of dying in persons with dementia. When tube feeding is proposed as an alternative to assisted oral feeding, its benefits are fictional. There are, however, a number of significant burdens associated with tube feeding (e.g., the increased use of physical restraints and a diminished quality of life) that can be avoided with assisted oral feeding. Also, there is growing evidence that PEG feeding provides no benefit in terms of life prolongation, maintaining weight, avoiding pressure sores, and prevention of aspiration pneumonia. It is increasingly clear that PEG feeding in persons with advanced dementia is ineffective in achieving medical goals (Post, 2001).

In chapter 10 of this book, Welie argues that, though a best-interest judgment is by no means perfect, it is an ethically more defensible decision-making strategy than either advance directives or substituted judgments by surrogates. The latter two strategies entail a severe violation of the patient's intrinsic dignity, because these strategies, unlike best-interest judgments, deny the condition from which the patient is now suffering and will suffer for the remainder of his life, and in doing so deny the patient's present personhood. Therefore, living wills and substituted judgments should be used as complements to (and not in opposition to) best-interest judgments. According to Welie, it is even virtually impossible to argue convincingly in favor of living wills without smuggling in best-interest judgments (J. V. M. Welie, 2001). Post, too, seems to underscore this point (2001). When actually confronting the decision about providing nutrition and hydration, physicians should respect autonomy by adhering to the guidelines for substitute decision making, which often includes (1) consideration of previously expressed wishes, (2) a substituted judgment of the patient's wishes, and—with my emphasis on this third point—(3) *acting in the patient's best interest,* based on the most accurate information regarding outcomes. Thus, the suggestion is that in the use of living wills and substituted judgments, best-interest considerations always play a role. Can one, however, also put it the other way around? Does it make sense to focus on the best interest of the patient by "smuggling in" respect for the patient's autonomy? I think it does, but in cases of persons with severe dementia, this is possible only if we conceive of autonomy as "bodily autonomy."

It follows that—in accordance with the extent that the self and personal qualities are gradually disappearing—we must take seriously the patient's bodily defensive movements. The person with severe dementia simply possesses no other means to express himself. He or she expresses his or her wish by constantly trying to pull out feeding tubes, and so forth. When it comes to swallowing problems, we have an even yet clearer sign that the patient no longer wishes to live.

However, if bodily defensive movements are interpreted as meaningful expressions of a person not able to express his wishes in other ways, there is still the question of whether or not to respect these wishes. The arguments must be considered. If the argument of the lived body possessing tacit knowledge makes sense (and I think it does), it must be weighed alongside other reasons for trying, or not trying, to prolong a life by inserting feeding tubes. Whatever the outcome of the debate, the argument of "unconscious, bodily expressions of one's wishes" can be added to other arguments against too activistic a treatment of patients with severe dementia: the integrity of the body, respect for the patient's dignity, the social structure in which communication takes place (wishes of family members), and the societal judgments on the boundaries of acceptable treatment decisions for persons with dementia. If the benefits of a particular intervention that causes bodily defensive movements are not clearly very large, this intervention should be stopped. In these cases, the patient "decides" by demonstrating resistance.

Post writes that "the key to an adequate ethics of dementia is full attention to the many ways of enhancing the noncognitive aspects of human well-being while not underestimating remaining capacities" (1995, p. 3). Taking the body seriously, I have interpreted noncognitive aspects of human well-being as bodily aspects, and I have taken bodily defensive movements of persons with severe dementia as examples of remaining capacities. I have challenged the current, one-sided interpretation of autonomy and have placed autonomy—letting it creep in as bodily autonomy—in the context of the best-interest standard. The only connection of the concept of bodily autonomy in persons with severe dementia with current interpretations of autonomy can be found in the notion of negative autonomy; that is, "a choice/activity that claims a right only to non-interference" (Collopy, 1988, p. 11). Bodily defensive movements of persons with severe dementia can be considered a "negative" expression of a person's autonomy—a kind of negative claim against invasion and interference. That is all that is left of their "real" autonomy. Concepts such as the naturalness of dying, (declining) vitality, and the wisdom of nature, on the one hand, and notions such as the lived body possessing tacit knowledge about the patient's wishes, on the other hand, make sense in an ethics of care for persons with severe dementia. They may support our often intuitively felt hesitancies and reservations about tube feeding them.

REFERENCES

Bayley, J. O. (1999). *Elegy for Iris.* New York: St. Martin's Press.

Beauchamp, T. L., & Childress, J. F. (1994). *Principles of biomedical ethics.* New York: Oxford University Press.

Berne, R. M., & Levy, M. N. (2000). *Principles of physiology* (3rd ed.). St. Louis, MO: Mosby.

Bernlef, J. (1988). *Out of mind.* Translated by Adrienne Dixon. Boston, MA: David R. Godine. Original Dutch title, *Hersenschimmen,* 1984.

Binstock, R. H., Post, S. G., & Whitehouse, P. J. (1992). The challenges of dementia. In R. H. Binstock, S. G. Post, & P. J. Whitehouse (Eds.), *Dementia and aging: Ethics, values, and policy choices* (pp. 1–20). Baltimore: Johns Hopkins University Press.

Brinchmann, B. S., & Nortvedt, P. (2001). Ethical decision making in neonatal units: The normative significance of vitality. *Medicine, Health Care and Philosophy, 4,* 193–200.

Collopy, B. J. (1988). Autonomy in long term care: Some crucial distinctions. *Gerontologist, 28* (Suppl.), 10–17.

Dekkers, W. J. M. (1998). The human body as a text: The interpretive tradition. In M. Evans (Ed.), *Critical reflections on medical ethics* (pp. 209–228). Advances in Bioethics, Vol. 4. London: JAI Press.

Dekkers, W. J. M. (2001). The human body. In H.A.M.J. ten Have & B. Gordijn (Eds.), *Bioethics in a European perspective* (pp. 115–140). Dordrecht: Kluwer Academic.

DeLange, P. (2001). Levensverhaal en lichaam [Life story and body]. *Humanistiek, 2,* 59–68.

Dworkin, G. (1988). *The theory and practice of autonomy.* Cambridge: Cambridge University Press.

Dworkin, R. (1993). *Life's dominion: An argument about abortion, euthanasia, and individual freedom.* New York: Knopf.

Engelhardt, H. T., Jr., (1996). *The foundations of bioethics* (2nd ed.). New York: Oxford University Press.

Goodman, J. (1999). Jewish circumcision: An alternative perspective. *BJU International, 83* (Suppl. 1), 22–27.

Holm, S. (2001). Autonomy, authenticity, or best interest: Everyday decision-making and persons with dementia. *Medicine, Health Care and Philosophy, 4,* 153–159.

Lawton, J. L. (2000). *The dying process. Patient's experiences of palliative care.* London: Routledge.

Merleau-Ponty, M. (1962). *Phenomenology of perception.* Translated by C. Smith. London: Routledge.

Moody, H. R. (1992). A critical view of ethical dilemmas in dementia. In R. H. Binstock, S. G. Post, & P. J. Whitehouse (Eds.), *Dementia and aging: Ethics, values, and policy* (pp. 86–100). Baltimore: Johns Hopkins University Press.

Nagel, T. (1974). What is it like to be a bat? *Philosophical Review, 83,* 435–450.

Post, S. G. (1995). *The moral challenge of Alzheimer disease.* Baltimore: Johns Hopkins University Press.

Post, S. G. (2001). Tube feeding and advanced progressive dementia. *Hastings Center Report, 31* (1), 36–42.

Prick, J. J. G. (1971). *Aspecten van een gerontologie en van een antropologisch-psychiatrische en neurobiologische geriatrie* [Aspects of gerontology and anthropological-psychiatric and neurobiological geriatrics]. Deventer, Netherlands: Van Loghum Slaterus.

Strumpf, N. E., & Evans, L. K. (1991). The ethical problems of prolonged physical restraint. *Journal of Gerontological Nursing, 17,* 27–30.

Toombs, S. K. (1997). Taking the body seriously. *Hastings Center Report, 27* (5), 39–43.

Welie, J. V. M. (2001). Living wills and substituted judgments: A critical analysis. *Medicine, Health Care and Philosophy, 4,* 169–183.

Welie, S. P. K. (2001). Criteria for patient decision making (in)competence: A review of and commentary on some empirical approaches. *Medicine, Health Care and Philosophy, 4,* 139–151.

CHAPTER EIGHT

The Moral Self as Patient

Judith Lee Kissell, Ph.D.

Our health care successes over the last few decades now confront us with the necessity of rethinking our model of medicine, our health care policy, and our medical ethics. We have lengthened life and prevented and controlled disease. But our mastery also presents us with the problems of elderly persons who, while they survive what might once have killed them at a younger age, now live with chronic diseases, often those of dementia. With our achievements, we have produced a growing populace of family caregivers, many of them old themselves. For these and other reasons, ethicists and clinicians are looking more and more to the issues of palliative care. But concern for caregivers and the problems that accompany diseases of dementia—notable among them, Alzheimer disease—are merely symptomatic of a far more serious disorder that afflicts medical ethics and policy.

The hospice movement, as one element of palliative care, is sensitive to patient, family members, and friends impacted by an illness. Because of their experience in working with the dying, often in the patients' homes, hospice has long recognized responsibility—officially and explicitly—not only for the patient but also for the family. On its face, this approach seems to challenge the hegemony of patient autonomy so present in other areas of health care. At the same time, no theoretical basis for hospice's nonconformist responsibility for patient *and* family has been forthcoming. As more elderly patients live longer and more family members become caught up in caregiving and decision making about end-of-life care, autonomy seems a less and less adequate response to the decisions that confront families, caregivers, and society.

The literature on decision making at the end of life is telling. A few typical titles give us the drift: "What Is the Moral Authority of Family Members to Act as Surrogates for Incompetent Patients?" (Brock, 1996); "Choosing for Others as Continuing a Life Story: The Problem of Personal Identity Revisited" (Blustein, 1999); "Alzheimer Disease and the 'Then' Self" (Post, 1995). At one level, the problem that these articles raise is about the patient's right to make decisions: how does self-determination play out for persons suffering from dementia? At another level, the problem is about the moral subject: Who is she? How does she relate to the rest of us and we to her?

The matters with which the above articles are concerned are about whether the personhood, or selfhood, of patients such as Alzheimer disease (AD) patients extends beyond competence. But this query into personal identity fails to probe in the right place. The more appropriate question is not a procedural one about decision making; nor is it a functional one about whether personhood or selfhood remains when the patient can no longer make rational decisions, communicate well, or relate to others. Rather, the issue is about how we live together, relate to and care for one another, in the midst of suffering.

Procedural approaches to decision making for these patients come to substitute for profound reflection on issues critical both to patient and to family caregivers. A psychological, functional analysis of the incompetent person's identity is both aberrant and facile. On the one hand, both the procedural approach and a functional view of personhood seek to answer a clinical question—one that the principle of autonomy and the political theory of "self-governance," introduced by Tom L. Beauchamp and James F. Childress (1994), are not equipped to handle. On the other hand, these approaches are far from the philosophical anthropology that we need to tell us more about the patient and the communities in which she lives.

The unconventional attitude of hospice toward the patient and his or her family suggests a new way to think about caring and decision making. For various reasons, we in the Western world have structured our medical ethics, and much of our public policy, on notions of liberal philosophy. We have asked only superficially whether this approach reflects reality, not confronting this question seriously enough. Michael Sandel helps us to perform just this task in his *Liberalism and the Limits of Justice* (1982). In this book, he teases out of John Rawls's *A Theory of Justice* (1971) an analysis of the "moral subjects" of Rawls's original position: those who choose the rules for a just society. It is surprising to find an American political scientist who criticizes liberalism from the standpoint of philosophical anthropology; and not only that: few critics of liberalism reach so profoundly into the problem and provide the level of insight that Sandel's thinking does.

Perhaps the most important lesson of Sandel's analysis is that moral theories, and even principles and procedures, *always* entail a philosophical anthropology, though we seldom follow them through to their logical conclusions. The question we must ask is this: does the philosophical anthropology implied by any theory disclose who we truly are? Do liberal theories based on autonomy reflect adequately who we understand ourselves to be as persons? More to the point, does the centrality we have given to patient autonomy genuinely represent patients in their hour of need?

Ironically, both our theories of medical ethics and our health care policies have adopted a philosophical anthropology that is anomalous in the world of health care—one far more political than it is medical. The principle of autonomy describes a dualistic Cartesian patient who happens to have a body but is primarily a rational agent. Beauchamp and Childress argue that in their use of the word *autonomy* they refer not to "persons," but to "choices" (1994, 68). Their disclaimer however, fails to exonerate them from Sandel's question. *What kind of moral subject* makes autonomous choices? How is that person constituted who has come to dominate—at least in principle—medical ethics policy and practice? How does "self-governance" apply to a patient entering into a system and a practice that are radically cooperative in nature? How does this patient relate to her society?

While a theoretical justification of the hospice movement and its concern for caregivers provides good reasons for this challenge to a liberal foundation of medical ethics, the more profound question of who we really are is the deeper, more important reason. My tasks are three: First, I draw from Sandel's analysis of Rawls the explicit philosophical anthropology that applies as well to other liberal thinking. In doing so, I make explicit those assumptions behind the liberal view of the person that so often remain hidden in our theory and application of medical ethics. Second, I show that autonomy-based medical ethics indeed entails this liberal moral subject. Third, I develop the contours of a subject and patient that might justify the hospice attitude toward patients and their loved ones and be more appropriate for palliative care.

❧ Sandel's Moral Subject

Sandel makes a very precise case of the term *communitarian* (Mulhall & Swift, 1996). He defines his position as follows: "At issue is not whether individual or communal claims should carry greater weight but whether the principles of justice that govern the basic structure of society can be neutral with respect to the competing moral and religious convictions its citizens espouse. *The fundamental question, in other words, is whether the right is prior to the good*" (emphasis added; 1982, p. x).

At the root of Sandel's analysis is the matter of whether we arrive cognitively or voluntaristically at our concept of ourselves. In other words, do we *construct* our selves, our values, and our relationships because we are primarily rational, choosing, and self-governing human beings? Or is there rather a sense in which we *discover* our nature and ends only by reflection? Have we a nature that defines for us, independently of our desires and preferences, what our good is? Does the good belong to us morally, logically, and epistemologically prior to our choosing it, because of *what* we are?

❧ The Critique of Rawls

To set the stage for my discussion, I begin with Sandel's critique of Rawls and deontological liberalism in general. Sandel claims that *A Theory of Justice* calls for an understanding of the liberal moral subjects who devise the rules of justice: "For what issues at one end in a theory of justice must issue at the other in a theory of the person, or more precisely, a theory of the moral subject. Looking from one direction through the lens of the original position we see the two principles of justice; looking from the other direction we see a reflection of ourselves" (1982, p. 48). Throughout his analysis, Sandel points out how the characteristics of the subject result in serious inconsistencies in Rawls's writing. Rawls thus hoists himself on his own petard, as do—I contend—other deontological liberals, including those who write about medical ethics. This liberal subject is the very one whom we have come to characterize in medical ethics: the patient whose autonomy we respect.

❧ The Moral Subject

The first characteristic of the liberal moral subject is that, logically, epistemologically, and morally, she is a self "prior" to her ends. That is, her identity and personal boundaries are established logically preceding either any ends that she selects or any characteristics that circumstances may contribute to her identity. Fundamentally, she is one who chooses and who constructs, who is capable of forging her values and of constructing, through contract, the society in which she lives. She is, says Sandel, in the most basic sense, an Agent, a capacity for choice—"a pure subject of agency and possession" (1982, p. 94). He elaborates: "It is important to recall that, on the deontological view, the notion of a self barren of essential aims and attachments does not imply that we are beings wholly without purpose or incapable of moral ties, but rather that the values and relations we have are products of choice, the possessions of a self given prior to its ends" (p. 176).

Just as the persons in Rawls's "original position" are famously "unencumbered," so, too, is the liberal subject. As subject, she might select her ends, her affiliations, and her view of the good life. She is constituted by her agency alone, and not by any circumstance of geography, birth, physiology, language, society, or family.

Sandel uses the notion of *possession* to describe how the liberal subject is attached to the objects of his choice and to the contingent circumstances that appear to make up his identity. *Possession* of particular characteristics, whether they be values, conceptions of the good, or traits of some sort, is a happenstance. Properties that we imagine to characterize this subject can be associated with him as possessions, but do not *constitute* him. Thus, neither values nor conceptions of the good, nor kinships, nor allegiances, nor other attributes are constituents of the moral subject, because his subjecthood, his identity, and his boundaries are established prior to these contingencies. Incongruously, one must suppose that physicality itself, even gender, becomes an add-on: they are mere circumstance, not part of the subject's nature. *Possession* allows the subject to *have* characteristics that are "mine rather than me" (Sandel, 1982, p. 55).

The subject as "self prior to its ends" is to be respected expressly *because* she is an Agent, capable of choosing, and not for the values she selects, the social status she enjoys, the attachments she has—all of which are matters of choice and/or chance. The point is not that we refrain from making social or moral judgments about one another, but that respect is due prior to and apart from social circumstance and moral or immoral acts, and it persists through the acts that are immoral. For example, Hitler, too, must be respected as a moral Agent. His character is underscored by the moral nature of his deeds for which, as subject, he is responsible; and that subjecthood, not the nature of his acts, is why he is respect-worthy.

Surely this fundamental human worth that precedes any of the assessments we might make about the subject is one of the most attractive features of liberal deontology. For not only do we respect the subject regardless of his moral choices, we respect him despite his economic, political, and/or social status. Deontological liberalism is responsible, theoretically at least, for the political movements that have urged liberation of ethnic groups, of women, slaves, and so forth. Applying this theory to the patient results in an important advance away from traditional medical paternalism and its consequent lack of respect for patient wishes. But it also carries with it inconsistencies and anomalies that we need to resolve.

The second characteristic of the moral subject is that she is "antecedently individuated." The most fundamental requirement for subjects to live together in an ordered (just) way is that their existence as separate persons be recognized and honored. What separates us is morally and epistemically prior to what joins us. The bounds of the self distinguish and define us before we enter into relationship (Sandel, 1982, p. 55). Because subjects within a society are individuated, they have interests that may, and often do, conflict. The idea that the Agent is capable, in relevant ways, of making choices, particularly in the matter of choosing for herself the good life, implies that she has no "nature" in the constitutive sense that either provides her with, or impels her toward, a cognitively recognized good, an identity or interests that she would necessarily hold in common with other Agents. Lacking any fundamental commonality with others, the subject stands alone. In fact, if one interprets strictly the liberal subject in this way, there is no more reason to accommodate any special relationship even among family members than for the civic society with whom such an Agent may participate in a "social contract."

Respect for the subject consists of sustaining and enhancing, through the structures of the society in which she lives, this capability to choose. The social framework takes the form it does precisely because these individuals, with their own interests and views of the good, exist as sovereign Agents. The social framework thereby protects each Agent's prerogative of determining who her community is and what is her idea of the good life (Sandel, 1982).

Third, liberal subjects are "mutually disinterested" in one another: "The parties take no interest in one another's interests" (Sandel, 1982, p. 54). But the philosophical clout of mutual disinterest does not simply mean that each Agent goes about being self-absorbed.

Mutual disinterest emerges not from a moral perspective, not from one's selfish motivations, but more importantly as an epistemological reality.

> It . . . works as an epistemological claim, as a claim about the forms of self-knowledge of which we are capable . . . The assumption of mutual disinterest is not an assumption about what motivates people, but an assumption about the nature of subjects who possess motivations in general. It concerns the nature of the self (that is, how it is constituted, how it stands with respect to its situation generally), not the nature of the self's desires or aims. (Sandel, 1982, p. 54)

The Agent, and she alone, is aware of, has access to—but more especially has charge of—those preferences, those visions of the good that move her and that serve her interests. She is *epistemologically* insulated and impervious so that the concerns and interests of others are as opaque to her as are hers to them (Sandel, 1982).

Sandel's analysis as philosophical anthropology is far more powerful than a communitarianism that explains how individualism leads to selfishness. Its efficacy lies in the explanation of how mutual disinterest and individualism are the inevitable result of the way the liberal self *is constituted*—of a philosophical anthropology. Thus the subject may have strong altruistic attachments to others whether they be family members, compatriots, or strangers. But her *motivations*—as objects of choice—are not what Sandel diagnoses here (1982). His focus on the subject helps us to understand that the self's separateness stems not from selfishness or egotism, but rather from the boundaries that define her before we consider any motives at all.

The way in which the moral self is constituted and that self's lack of epistemological access to the good and the interests of others becomes a metaphysical claim as well. Or if the term *metaphysical* is suspect, the claim ends up as one about the constitution of the self and the level at which the self is ontologically capable of relating to others. It is a statement about how people and their relationships to others exist as "furniture of the universe," in Mackie's memorable phrase (1974).

At the heart of deontological liberalism—as well as of any subject who populates that realm—lies the priority of the right over the good. For the moral subject this priority means that the dignity of the subject lies in her being an Agent rather than in her nature, the goals she chooses, the attachments she develops, or the preferences upon which she acts.

The philosophical anthropology toward which Sandel moves in criticizing this subject as he does fails to resolve all the problems of medical ethics and may, in fact, engender new quandaries. But this is not because his analysis is inadequate or unfaithful to our experience; it is due, rather, to the complexity of our nature and our identity.

❧ The Patient as Liberal Moral Subject

Just as Sandel investigates the subjecthood of those who arrive at Rawls's rules of justice, we, as medical ethicists, might also ask: What does the principle of autonomy, and the procedures and practical issues that arise from it, reveal about the subjecthood of the patient? To paraphrase Sandel: Whatever issues at one end in the principle of respect for patient autonomy must issue at the other end in a theory of the person, or, more precisely, a theory of the moral subject. Looking from one direction, we see the principle of autonomy; looking from the other direction, we see a reflection of ourselves.

The patient with whom medical ethics is concerned is strikingly similar to the liberal moral subject whom Sandel describes. At the practical level, autonomy has much to do with her ability to make a mentally competent decision, in a situation where there is no coercion or undue influence from others. Autonomy might be diminished by dementia or pain that comprises a patient's "personal limitation" (Beauchamp & Childress, 1994). Financial considerations, convenience, or the overweening influence of physician or family members might also affect the autonomy of a decision. One way or another, most autonomy problems assume the subject of liberal deontology—individuated, mutually disinterested, epistemologically opaque, an Agent. But autonomy has some strange implications for patients and their families.

Consider, for instance, the autonomy-based practices of patient confidentiality and privacy. The female relatives of the patient who suffers from BRCA1- or BRCA2-caused breast cancer are at risk for the same disease. Yet procedures of patient confidentiality dictate that this woman need not inform her mother, her aunts, her daughters, her sisters, her nieces, or her granddaughters of the condition—one that they possibly share (Deftos, 1998). Self-governance protects the patient and preserves the idea of a self whose physical connections are only incidental—a possession. Her genetic lineage neither constitutes who she is nor reflects her relationship to other human beings. Embeddedness that flows from being embodied would enervate her autonomy.

Or take the issue of end-of-life decision making for the patient who has AD. No problem draws us closer to the core of philosophical anthropology than does this one that so closely involves self-identity, personhood, and subjecthood. At the root of this issue are two ideas: (1) that the patient's moral identity is defined by her ability and prerogative to decide for herself; and (2) that only the patient, in her epistemological isolation, can truly know, and best decide, what treatment decisions constitute her interests. How, then, do we justify decisions for treatment, or withdrawal of treatment, for an incompetent patient, and particularly one whose competence has been compromised for a long time, as is often the case with a patient who has Alzheimer disease?

Because a liberal philosophy supposes that subjecthood means agency, the logical conclusion some reach is that when the patient is incapable of agency, she is either no longer a person—a moral subject—or, at least, no longer the *same* person. The question of how she is constituted becomes conflated with the psychological properties and capacities of the functioning human being. Clearly, when Beauchamp and Childress speak of autonomy and self-governance, they mean to give a moral account of the rational human being and how we are to respect her, and not a psychological analysis. Nevertheless, faced by intractable clinical problems of the incompetent but autonomous patient, some ethicists write as if this person apparently disintegrates as a subject—that is, she literally loses personal integrity, in its most profound sense. Then autonomy ceases to be an issue. This is a particularly strange predicament for a theory that views a patient as primarily rational, rather than embodied. For then the loss of her physical and psychological capabilities, though mere contingencies, do seem to count against her status as moral subject.

If the patient has an advance directive, our problems about decision making may appear to be solved. Many thinkers seem to hold that an advance directive stands by itself as a kind of entity. It best justifies treatment or its withdrawal (Dresser & Robertson, 1989; Dresser, 1995) and must be honored, regardless of any change in the patient's circumstances. For the decision the patient projects into the future for herself—the product of her agency—prevails as the emblem of her moral subjecthood. At least in this case her subjecthood remains intact. Or the patient explicitly relinquishes her autonomy to her surrogate—a strange assumption, if we assume autonomy and self-determination to be the very constitutive elements of moral subjecthood.

Or suppose, on the other hand, that the patient makes no advance directive. Then, the rationale goes, we turn to a surrogate—a "substituted judgment" by someone else. Presumably, her family is best capable of *conjecturing* what her preferences would be. In this case, we are supposed to assume that the surrogates will decide as their loved one would have done. Alternatively, the surrogate decides "in the patient's best interests." But the procedures of surrogacy bring with them a philosophical anthropology—and hence the mutual disinterest—of which Sandel speaks. Because only the patient knows what is in her best interest, only she can make a good decision for herself. If the surrogate's decisions reflect the wishes of the patient, it is only by accident. The epistemological isolation of the patient that is entailed by liberal medical ethics makes knowledge of the patient's good, as only she is capable of determining it, either an impossibility or a guess.

The policies and procedures of patient privacy and confidentiality assume the essential plurality of the society in which the relationship among its members is one of antagonism and where the interests of its members will necessarily conflict at some point. These policies anticipate a patient who is antecedently individuated: at her most basic self, she stands alone, related in no essential way to anyone else. Her illness is her own business. Likewise, surrogacy operates according to the assumption that the liberal subject-patient is *epistemologically* insulated from and opaque to others, in addition to the isolation that her dementia has produced. The practice of substituted judgment assumes that the patient and her family and caregivers are "mutually disinterested," having a shared (at best, coincidentally shared) view of the good, incapable of knowing, and limited to an "educated guess" about, what could comprise her welfare. Our policies are blind to a philosophical anthropology in which subjects share interests in any constitutive way or that a good or an end that transcends the patient as an individual might exist. The questions that permeate the literature reflect "an epistemological claim, . . . a claim about the forms of self-knowledge [as well as of other-knowledge] of which we are capable" (Sandel, 1982, p. 54).

❧ An Alternative Vision

As political creatures, we appear to be antecedently individuated, opaque to others, with impenetrable personal boundaries, having goals for our lives that are contingent to us. A formidable picture, indeed. But as patients, these characteristics seem a perversion. Without an essential relatedness to one another, a co-operative search for the common good of health, medicine would not even be possible. Science depends upon a nature that we share.

At the heart of both medicine and the philosophical anthropology underlying our medical ethics is a vision of the human being as embodied person. He or she belongs to, is part of, the physical world—his orientation to time and space, as reflected in his language, is rooted in his own bodily experience as he speaks about "in front of," "behind," "above," "below," "before," and "after," in relation to his physical orientation (Strauss, 1966). The human being's understanding of bringing about—and being responsible for, that is *causing*—evil or good is rooted in his physical power; that is, his experience of moving, throwing, hitting, crushing, and so forth. Every experience—including, if not especially, illness—is rooted in the physical. But more importantly, he is essentially social and related. He is an intelligent, communicating, gesturing, moral being who understands, who converses, who relates, who presents himself, who judges, who suffers, who reproduces other moral subjects, by and through his body. He communes with, and learns about, the world through his eyes and ears and through touch and smell. He interacts with others through movement and words (Zaner, 1981; Lakoff & Johnson, 1999).

This being is constituted as a human being by a genetic lineage that bonds her, not only with her immediate family members but with an ethnic group, with an evolution of disease and health, and with the entire biosphere. Her place in the configuration of her genealogy is not simply about ancestry, but rather about the irrevocable situatedness of time and place—of history and geography. While the *particular* person she is, and the *particular* time and place at which she finds herself, are contingent facts, *that* she is embodied, with all the connotations of genetic relationships, narrative, and location that physicality bring, is what constitutes her as a human being and as a person and what gives her her identity.

Fundamental to medicine is its existence as a science that can function only if it considers the human being as having a nature—as being a "natural kind" (Sulmasy, 2001), the knowledge of which makes possible the diagnosis and treatment of disorders, a condition that makes epistemological opacity impossible. While, as Sandel points out, human beings are never completely transparent to one another, knowledge about the embodied human being as a kind—its systems, its optimal functioning and disrupting ailments—is a critical part of knowing oneself and others. Knowledge about health care is part of the culture of every society.

We have, in addition, an identity and a transparency of ends and implications about our relationships with one another. Nature, both from the point of view of medicine as science and of health as common end, precludes our being ignorant about one another, as well as the notion that ends are merely chosen by individuals. This philosophical anthropology brings with it the need to reexamine our medical ethics as well.

Hospice has been outspoken about proclaiming that the unit of care is the patient, her loved ones, and family. This approach to care removes the adversarial nature of the decision-making process that pushes autonomy to the forefront and that could butt patient needs and interests against those of family and caregivers. This approach is a recognition of the embeddedness of the patient that more accurately portrays who she is than does the view of individuality that accompanies the predominance of autonomy.

In considering the hospice emphasis on relationships, with its ensuing attenuation of autonomy, we may find ourselves perplexed, because autonomy is, after all, not entirely negative. Self-determination has wisely counteracted the paternalism that characterized Western medicine for such a long time. It preserves the dignity of an otherwise helpless, and perhaps incompetent, patient. Moreover, families are not always the loving, comforting support systems that we would idealize them to be: often patient interests must be protected. Further, all patients do not have families. The issue, however, is not about the quality or existence of families; it is, rather, that patients—and everyone—are always and essentially related. The fundamental question here is whether treating patients, caregivers, and family members as antecedently individuated and mutually disinterested squares with our considered reflections about who we are.

The philosophical anthropology of the patient that the hospice attitude suggests is that of a person who is essentially contextual—embedded in a family, a language group, a nationality/ethnic group, and so forth. Hospice philosophy implies a patient whose "constituent nature" is to be embodied, and, thereby, fundamentally related—whether or not their memory is intact and whether or not they can communicate. This patient seeks the human flourishing possible for one in his physical state and state of human development. That is, he seeks health or comfort not as a "preference" but as the cognitively recognized end of any embodied person.

Seeing the patient as embedded makes irrelevant the question of whether the incompetent patient of today is the same person as the competent patient of a month ago. The context of embodiment, relationships, and shared nature anchor her identity. For the competent patient, as for the one suffering from dementia, her good is not some opaque preference hidden in her past or present self-awareness, but is part of a self-understanding common to embodied persons for whom illness, suffering, and death come with sharing a nature. What may seem to be the epistemological imperviousness of the wishes of the dying patient is part of the mystery of death that renders us all dumfounded.

Decision making for the terminally ill, as for all of us, is about being vulnerable within a community, whether that be the family or some other group. It has to do with surveying one's "various attachments and [acknowledging] their respective claims, [sorting] out the bounds . . . between the self and the other" (Sandel, 1982, p. 55). It means choosing in the way decisions are usually made—with regard to the other members of a family or a society, with regard to financial and emotional assets, with regard to the needs of all, with regard to medical and social resources. It need not, and should not, mean lack of dignity or care. That families might be dysfunctional or torn by disagreement does not render the patient unencumbered at death any more than selfishness and abuse render a child or a spouse encumbered during their lives. The fact of the unhappy family is not an argument for a philosophical anthropology that denies our embodiment, our connectedness, and our shared nature.

Clinical, institutional, and governmental policies and procedures follow from the "self-governance" of the unencumbered patient and the prominence of the principles of right as adjudicators of the good. In the world of the unencumbered patient/self, she is on her own. To make decisions about one's health may be a sign of dignity, but it is not the only one, nor the only way to respect a patient. We have locked ourselves into advance-directive procedures that honor a patient's wishes but that unrealistically demand foretelling the future and that allow caregivers to wash their hands of responsibility. Discussions about the personal identity of patients suffering from dementia are a modern version of how many angels can dance on the head of a pin.

Moreover, the world of liberal bioethics is one in which we need not be concerned about funding for long-term care or medication for receivers of Medicare, including medication for palliative care. We need not care about public policies that fail to provide home health care or tax policies that would protect the estimated 54 million family members who become caregivers during any given year, most of them women (National Family Caregivers Association, 2000). The big question is: Is this who we truly are?

REFERENCES

Beauchamp, T. L., & Childress, J. (1994). *The principles of biomedical ethics* (4th ed.). New York: Oxford University Press.

Blustein, J. (1999). Choosing for others as continuing a life story: The problem of personal identity revisited. *Journal of Law, Medicine and Ethics, 27,* 20–31.

Brock, D. W. (1996). What is the moral authority of family members to act as surrogates for incompetent patients? *Milbank Quarterly, 4,* 599–618.

Deftos, L. J. (1998). The evolving duty to disclose the presence of genetic disease to relatives. *Academic Medicine, 9,* 962–968.

Dresser, R. S. (1995). Dworkin on dementia: Elegant theory, questionable policy. *Hastings Center Report, 6,* 32–38.

Dresser, R. S., & Robertson, J. A. (1989). Quality of life and non-treatment decisions for incompetent patients: A critique of the orthodox approach. *Law, Medicine and Health Care, 17,* 234–244.

Lakoff, G., & Johnson, M. (1999). *Philosophy in the flesh: The embodied mind and its challenge to Western thought.* New York: Basic Books.

Mackie, J. (1974). *The cement of the universe.* Oxford, UK: Clarendon Press.

Mulhall, S., & Swift, A. (1996). *Liberals and communitarians.* Chicago: Blackwell.

Post, S. G. (1995). Alzheimer's Disease and the "then" self. *Kennedy Institute of Ethics Journal, 4,* 307–321.

Rawls, J. (1971). *A theory of justice.* Cambridge: Harvard University Press.

Sandel, M. (1982). *Liberalism and the limits of justice*. Cambridge: Cambridge University Press.

Straus, E. W. (1966). *Phenomenological psychology: Selected papers*. New York: Basic Books.

Sulmasy, D. (2001, July). The human as a natural kind: A foundation for the philosophy and ethics of medicine. International Congress on Law and Mental Health Conference, Montreal, Quebec.

Zaner, R. M. (1981). *The context of self: A phenomenological inquiry: Using medicine as a clue*. Athens: Ohio University Press.

CHAPTER NINE

The Practice of Palliative Care and the Theory of Medical Ethics

Alzheimer Disease as an Example

Rien Janssens, Ph.D.

It is far from accidental that the origins of modern medical ethics and the origins of modern palliative care both can be traced to the end of the 1960s (Janssens & ten Have, 1999). Both movements came forth out of moral discomfort with a health care system that primarily focused on cure and life prolongation, sometimes employing disproportionate technological interventions. However, whereas the discomfort was the same, the responses to it were substantially different (Saunders, Summers, & Teller, 1981).

The discomfort of the new discipline of medical ethics is related primarily to the paternalistic attitude of physicians (Katz, 1984). In the context of the technological possibilities of medicine, observers noted that under some circumstances the application of medical technology could be more harmful than beneficent to the patient's well-being. It was judged that the decision to apply such interventions should no longer be made by physicians but by patients themselves. The power of the physician to administer medical treatment where and whenever possible should be handed over to the patient. Thus, the principle of autonomy became foundational for modern medical ethics, so that the maxim of the new medical ethics no longer was to preserve human life whenever *possible*. Instead, it became to preserve human life whenever *meaningful* (Zwart, 1995; Van den Berg, 1969). Modern medical ethics thus became applied ethics intended to help physicians and nurses solve moral dilemmas in practice occasioned by the above shift in perspective. For this understanding of ethics, it does not matter much whether it is applied to acute, curative settings or to settings where long-term care is provided.

The hospice movement that stands at the basis of modern palliative care did not focus so much on the absence of the patient's voice, but rather stressed the absence of care in medicine (Gracia, 2002). Unlike medicine, it acknowledged the importance of pain control and symptom control and of psychosocial and spiritual aspects of care. The first hospices shifted attention away from technological interventions intended to prolong life to attend to the needs and wishes of dying persons for whom a lot can still be done even when cure is no longer an option. This approach acknowledged death as a part of life, not as an event to be avoided or postponed at all costs.

For some years now, the topic of palliative care has been of interest in many countries. The increasing attention given to palliative care has already done much good, inside as well as outside the formal health care system. But as this chapter indicates, the increasing attention to care practices such as palliative care not only requires a reorientation of medicine, it also requires a reorientation of medical ethics. The moral values of palliative care are to some extent different from the moral values of the curative medicine to which medical ethics directed its attention (Janssens, 2001). Caregivers in palliative care use a specific moral language that not only articulates knowledge and expertise but also stresses the importance of dispositions, attitudes, virtues, and feelings (Janssens et al., 2000). Many general ethical notions often carry a specific meaning in the context of palliative care, a meaning that asks for articulation and philosophical clarification. In other words, the material object of an ethics of palliative care is to an important extent specific, and different from the material object of medical ethics in general. This specificity is highlighted by the case of patients suffering from Alzheimer disease (AD), not only because they require long-term care but also because these patients challenge and put into question clear conceptions of competence, autonomy, and informed consent.

This background sets the context for the three aims of this chapter. The first aim here is to indicate that the moral specificity of palliative care requires a specific kind of ethic. The second aim is to propose some perspectives for a practically relevant ethics of palliative care. Before stating the third aim, it is appropriate here to explain this second aim further. It draws on the assumption that the practical relevance of ethics does not primarily consist of applying norms and principles or problem solving, because ethicists are not health professionals directly responsible for the decisions that are made: they are situated farther away from practice than those directly involved in care giving. The material with which ethicists work consists of the articulated experiences of the caregivers. What is crucial for the health professional in everyday palliative care practice? What moral values and norms are implicitly or explicitly endorsed? How are decisions accounted for? What are the arguments that prevail? Which notions and what arguments are not used? In short, there is moral practice itself and there are the *articulated* experiences of patients and caregivers. Ethical theory can occur only after all of them have articulated what is morally relevant to them. Ethics is thus mediated by their words. A practically relevant ethic of palliative care analyzes, clarifies, and enriches the articulated moral experiences of caregivers (Janssens & ten Have, 1999). Then, it matters whether caregivers work in an acute care setting or in a chronic care setting. Moreover, it matters whether caregivers care for patients suffering from AD or from other progressive diseases. Therefore, it is only such an ethic that can yield a specific account of the care process for patients with Alzheimer disease. It is especially these patients that reveal the ambiguous nature of notions such as quality of life, competence, autonomy, and dependence. They challenge their caregivers to preserve dignity, even in a situation of radical dependence, at a time when communication is no longer possible.

The third aim of this chapter is to provide some concrete challenges for an ethic of palliative care. What are important subjects that merit attention and are in need of analysis? And in what way can ethics contribute to the further development of palliative care? Each aim is addressed below.

❧ The Moral Practice of Palliative Care

In many countries, palliative care is developing rapidly (ten Have & Clark, 2002). Health policies favor the development of palliative care within the framework of the formal health care system. It is now widely acknowledged that palliative care has been underestimated in educational programs for too long. Furthermore, as Olde Rikkert and Rigaud discuss in chapter 5, expertise in the area of palliative care will need to be increased and research programs developed so that an evidence base for medical decisions is created. In short, expertise in the field of palliative care is now being promoted through education and increased through research programs. And if palliative care is to develop further, the establishment of a knowledge base and the dissemination of expertise are crucial. Complex problems are still to be dealt with, but many governments now acknowledge the need to further develop palliative care.

However, practitioners in the field argue that something more is necessary for good palliative care—something that to some extent transcends government regulations. For there to be good caregivers, it is important not only what kind of care is available but also how the care is given. To be a good caregiver, one needs specific talents that are impossible to teach explicitly. Consider the following quotation: "In my opinion, good care and good pain control are not the same as palliative care. The patient also needs a warm, beating heart in his neighborhood. Someone who gives compassion and is able to listen well. Someone who makes clear: you're one of us, we love you, you belong and we are there for you. . . . Some have it, and others don't. . . . Capability and disposition are two different things" (Bruntink, 1999, p. 15). And the director of a Dutch palliative care center writes: "It is extremely hard to express the essence of palliative care in language. . . . Within palliative care . . . we approach the limits of material and physical life. . . . The wonder of birth, life and death, has all to do with mystic . . . it is first and foremost experience and emotion" (Van Hooijdonk, 1999, p. 17).

According to many more palliative care practitioners, palliative care requires from the caregivers a specific set of talents (Barnard, 1995; Task Force on Palliative Care et al., 1998). Caregivers in palliative care need be virtuous. And though it may be possible to teach some virtues, it is impossible to teach others. Aristotle distinguished between the intellectual virtues and the moral virtues (Aristotle, 1961 trans.). The intellectual virtues may be taught. Through medical education, students gain knowledge in the scientific fundamentals of medicine and also develop a degree of professional competence. Moral virtues, however, are developed through experience, over a longer period of time. The moral virtues are based on emotions that, through practice, have been developed into habits or dispositions. They require that a person not only act in particular ways but also feel in particular ways. It is noteworthy that such moral virtues are used to describe palliative care. Palliative care is said to have a surplus value compared with other health care practices (Schotsmans, 1995). The essence of this surplus value may well lie in emotions and virtues such as love, empathy, hope, and compassion.

The works cited above seem to suggest that caregivers in palliative care look upon palliative care as an area of care that entails different, broader, moral values than does regular health care. If that is indeed the case, identifying the characteristics of palliative care requires a moral language that is different from standard medical ethical notions such as autonomy, informed consent, and the duty not to harm. In addition to knowledge and skills, emotions, attitudes, and metaphors are needed specifically, because the essence of palliative care does not lend itself to description within a scientific, objective framework (Janssens & Willems, 2001). As with any other practice, palliative care can fail, and we have to be careful not to idealize it. But if we listen closely to the voices of caregivers, it appears that scientific knowledge and medical expertise are insufficient to provide adequate palliative care. This view finds support in an empirical study demonstrating that, among a representative sample of European caregivers, a majority of 52.7 percent agree with the statement that palliative care entails a specific set of values, other than the values of mainstream health care system (Janssens & Willems, 2001). The question then is *why* the practice of palliative care requires a specific language that is different from the language of curative medicine. There are at least two important reasons.

First, this can be explained by the goal of palliative care, which is not cure but the best possible quality of life of the patient, as is emphasized time and again in part II of this book. Quality of life is a notion that is not easily described and analyzed (Cella, 1992). Instruments designed to measure the quality of life of patients have been developed, but when they are applied to a particular human person they never completely suffice. For example, a Karnofsky score, a widely used assessment tool, does not provide more than a certain clue to making the right decisions. Reading the literature on palliative care, the term *quality of life* is used in most books and articles. However, critical scrutiny is remarkably absent, and the meaning of the term usually is taken for granted. What exactly does *quality of life* denote? What is it that, in the end, makes a life worthwhile? Within the early hospice movement, care was specifically designed for cancer patients. Many cancer patients retain a degree of competence and of control, even in the terminal phase of their illness. But now that palliative care is said to include care for patients with AD (among other patient categories), difficult questions arise. In the face of a patient suffering from advanced AD, can one speak of quality of life at all? One of the maxims of palliative care has always been that if life prolongation is no longer feasible, still a lot remains to be done for the quality of the patient's life. But what if the level of awareness of such a patient passes below a certain level, so that the patient has become incompetent to have meaningful experiences or communication? Again, care for them reveals an ambiguity of notions that has been underestimated by those who hold to a certain conception of medical ethics.

Second, the presence of a specific moral language can be explained by examining the ways in which the goal of the best possible quality of life can be achieved. Whereas in curative medicine, many well-circumscribed therapies exist with a more or less predictable effectiveness, in palliative care this is hardly ever the case. What is beneficent for one patient may be harmful for another. And in order to decide what is good for *this* patient at *this* moment, authentic care is necessary for the person of the patient. Sometimes, beneficence will consist of a passive attitude. Sometimes doing nothing is better than doing something, and the virtue of prudence, or practical wisdom, may have the potential to articulate accurately when a specific act is appropriate (Pellegrino & Thomasma, 1993; Desmet, 1996). The value of simply being present is highlighted in the care for patients with advanced AD. Even though it may be impossible for caregivers and loved ones to experience any level of reciprocity, care is not futile. Contrary to prevailing anthropologies that link concepts of personhood to rationality, the experience of caregivers and loved ones at the bed of a patient far advanced in AD is that there is still a person with a life history behind him or her—a history that has evolved in the context of many social relationships. That means that the patient still has a moral appeal to the caregivers, no matter how severe the condition is. But within the currently prevailing ethical discourse, it is difficult to articulate this appeal.

The above should illustrate that the development of palliative care points to a need to reorient medical ethics. Caregivers themselves use different moral values and thus provide a specific material object for the ethicist. Clarification and demarcation of palliative care is thus not only a task of caregivers; it is predominantly an ethical task because the concept itself is morally motivated. Ethicists need, therefore, not only to solve problems but also to analyze emotions, attitudes, and metaphors. This does not imply that the language used within care practices is of higher moral quality than that within curative medicine. Put simply, it is *different*. The practice of curative medicine is as important and as necessary as the practice of palliative care, yet, differences exist, and it is imperative to articulate, explain, and analyze these differences.

The increasing attention to care practices highlights the need for the reorientation. There is, however, another reason why medical ethics is in need of a reorientation, and this has to do with not so much care practices as medical ethics itself. The next section describes how modern medical ethics is unequipped to meet the challenges posed by the increasing attention to palliative care.

❧ The Theory of Medical Ethics

Since its origins in the late 1960s, medical ethics has developed into a relatively independent discipline. In other words, it has left the philosophical and theological faculties to which it once belonged and has moved into its new home, the medical faculty (Engelhardt, 2000). Ethicists are asked for consultations in academic hospitals in order to provide solutions and develop guidelines for complex moral dilemmas (Rothman, 1991). The dominant conception of medical ethics (not all conceptions) has become applied ethics, in the sense that agreed-upon moral principles are applied to concrete cases. In other words, medical ethics has become a service to medicine, and therefore it has adopted a medical scientific methodology. Instead of theology or philosophy, medicine now prescribes the logos of ethics. With that being so, if medicine is to formulate the ethicist's tasks, a critical distance from medical practice is no longer possible. The ethicist has become a guest, and the physician is the host (Van Willigenburg, 1991). As a guest, the ethicist has to refrain from critical analyses of medicine itself since that would be considered impolite. Ethicists thus become captive in a foreign discourse that initially was not their own. Medical ethics has lost its proper theological or philosophical framework, and the metaphor of guest and host seems reminiscent of this very loss. After all, as a guest one has to adjust to one's host, like it or not.

The self-understanding of medical ethics as a guest of medicine can be further clarified by analyzing the anthropology of medical ethics. The anthropology underlying medical practice is a Cartesian dualistic anthropology (Crul, 1999). And as long as this anthropology continues to be the paradigm of medical practice, it is part of the underlying assumptions of current medical ethics as well. In this anthropology, the human being is approached as a duality of mind and body. The body is the object of the autonomous will of the person. It is an instrument, used to promote the self-fulfillment of the person. As long as the person does not give his consent, nobody is allowed to touch his body. While medicine is interested in the body, medical ethics is interested in the autonomous person who is the owner of the body. Ethics determines the conditions under which medicine may touch and invade the body. Given the self-understanding of medical ethics as outlined above, it is not considered the task of the ethicist to criticize this anthropology. The paradigm of medicine and medical ethics is the same. If the person consents, medicine is allowed to intervene. The question whether the intervention is morally allowed has thus become dependent on the right to self-determination of the person. The intervention as such is no longer scrutinized. After all, that would imply a critique of the values and goals of medicine, and that is beyond the proper scope of this understanding of the role of medical ethics.

This discourse fails when medicine's interventions are no longer successful (i.e., when cure of the defective body appears no longer possible). The paradigm that considers the body as instrumental for the person's self-fulfillment belongs to the realm of curative medicine. The instrumental notion of the body also presumes the social independence of the person. When personal development is frustrated due to a bodily defect, medicine is there to remove the defect as quickly and effectively as possible. When, however, the body has become chronically ill, the discourse of medical ethics no longer suffices. Medical ethics has difficulty in coming to terms with care practices such as palliative care and nursing home medicine (Pijnenburg, 1992). Especially in the care for patients with AD, there comes a point at which the patient is neither fully competent nor fully incompetent. The patient is able to communicate and have meaningful experiences, but it is difficult to assess whether the decisions really reflect the patient's preferences. Between competence and incompetence, there is a grey area in which the challenge is to arrive at decisions that best fit the character and personality of the patient. In this process, the voice of the patient remains crucial, but at the same time the patient's loved ones are also involved in the decision-making process. Instead of informed consent, the notion of negotiated consent has recently been introduced since it is better equipped to render account of the decision-making processes in this context (Moody, 1992; Widdershoven, 2000). Decisions are arrived at in dialogue with the patient and all those directly involved.

It was shown above that caregivers in palliative care subscribe to specific values and virtues. But in order to provide solutions that are acceptable by the majority, medical ethics wants to be rational (Engelhardt, 1991). Feelings that are difficult to render an account of within neutral, scientific language—that seem, rather, to ask for metaphors or even poetry—cannot be articulated by medical ethicists who use the traditional approaches (Roy, 1997). Two decades ago, it already was argued that the increasing number of chronically ill patients had demonstrated the urgency for an adjustment of medicine (Sporken, 1983). Now, we add that an increasing need for care practices also reveals a similar urgency for an adjustment of medical ethics.

Recently, as a reaction against the dominant conception of modern medical ethics described above, an ethics of care has been developed that has sought to abandon medicine's dualistic anthropology and instead adopt a holistic anthropology (Tronto, 1993). It not only focuses on autonomy and the (negative) right to nonintervention but also stresses more positively and dynamically how autonomy can be seen as a challenge (i.e., a dynamic process that stands out for self-fulfillment). In this notion, humans are not only rational decision makers: a human person is not conceived of as a duality, but rather as a unity with physical, emotional, social, and existential qualities, gifts, and needs. This is an ethic that is, in fact, as relevant for curative practices as it is for palliative care practices. Instead of being mutually exclusive, cure implies care. It does not pretend to provide solutions for dilemmas, but is interested in broader philosophical and theological questions. Notions such as autonomy and beneficence are not considered principles from which guidelines can be deduced. Rather, these notions are subjected to reflection, and the issue of what we actually mean by them is raised. Are we as autonomous as we think we are? as autonomous as we want to be? Are we not fooling ourselves by making our rationality and decision-making capacity so central? Are we not also radically dependent? The answer is the affirmative. Not only are we dependent on family and friends; we also depend on society, with its traditions and habits that preceded us and through which we have been shaped. Acknowledging our common interdependency creates room for care for those who have become radically dependent. Again, the radical dependency of those suffering from advanced AD does not make care giving futile. On the contrary, a society that does not provide care to those who are most dependent of all is in danger of decay.

Within the ethics of care approaches, the negative conception of autonomy, stressing the right to nonintervention as long as others are not harmed, is abandoned and replaced by a more positive and dynamic conception that stresses human capacities, qualities, and needs (Manschot & Verkerk, 1994). Alternative notions can also be proposed if they are better equipped to denote the human condition or to identify the problematic issues at stake. If common language is inadequate to formulate what is at hand, new language (neologisms) can be introduced. Note that in 1974 the term *palliative care* was a neologism.

In analyzing ethical debates and central notions such as autonomy or beneficence, this ethic of care turns away from the biomedical paradigm and assumes a critical distance toward medical practice. Seemingly self-evident assumptions are questioned, and these assumptions may subsequently appear far less self-evident than initially was suspected. A result is that ethics may make it harder for caregivers to make decisions that they never questioned before (Van Tongeren, 1988). Problems that occur may appear to be unsolvable. Situations may appear to be tragic. The practical relevance of this ethic of care is not so much associated with proposing guidelines and solving dilemmas. In their place is an emphasis on clarification and philosophical analysis of what is said by patients and caregivers so that their experiences are sensitized and a broader understanding of the everyday practice of care giving is stimulated.

✿ Some Perspectives for the Ethics of Palliative Care

In journals that deal with palliative care, there is a significant interest in ethical issues (Hermsen & ten Have, 2001). The majority of ethical articles come from the medical profession, with only a small minority written by professional ethicists. This may explain the relative absence of historical, philosophical, and theological theory in the debates on palliative care. In addition, a substantial proportion of the ethicists participating in ethical debate focus on the morality of medical decisions at the end of life and much less on conceptual analysis and clarification (Janssens & ten Have, 1999).

The debate on medical decision making at the end of life remains of interest in many countries. In the Netherlands, until recently, the debate on euthanasia focused on statistics, procedures, and an assessment of the requirements under which euthanasia would be tolerable. In the context of increasing interest in palliative care, the euthanasia debate is now widening, with more attention being devoted to reducing requests for euthanasia by means of good, compassionate care from the time of diagnosis onwards. Physicians who consider euthanasia a means of last resort, to be carried out only in very exceptional circumstances, agree that a further development of palliative care is imperative in order to decrease the number of cases of euthanasia in the Netherlands (Janssens, 2001). In 1995, there were, apart from the 3,200 cases of euthanasia and the 400 cases of physician-assisted suicide, 900 cases in which patients' lives were terminated without their request. In 14 percent of those cases in which there had been no negotiation with the patient (63% of the 900), the reason for not having negotiated was that the patient was suffering from dementia (Van der Wal & Van der Maas, 1996). It is unclear whether dementia and associated symptoms were the main reason for the life termination or whether concomitant, progressive illnesses were present.

Current differences of opinion on the issue of whether euthanasia can be a part of palliative care indicate that palliative care has been subject to important changes in the last three decades (Wils, 1999). The consensus of the early hospice movement that euthanasia should be rejected can no longer be taken for granted (Jennings, 1997). Furthermore, the connection of palliative care with the hospice movement itself is no longer self-evident (Billings, 1998). In the near future, palliative care will increasingly be formed in the context of a variety of institutions and a variety of medical practices (Clark & Seymour, 1999). In addition to those suffering from cancer (the traditional recipients of palliative care), attention will be shifting to many other groups of patients. Not only persons with AD but also individuals suffering from chronic diseases will be cared for by caregivers who affiliate themselves with palliative care. This also means that palliative care is no longer limited to terminal care. According to many, the scope of palliative care is expanding, back to the moment of diagnosis (Janssens & Willems, 2001). Remarkably, in the context of palliative care for patients with AD, the traditional hospice concept (presupposing at least a certain degree of competency and potentiality for meaningful experiences) may be more relevant in the beginning of the AD process than in the end. Such patients are hardly ever admitted to hospices. The group of patients suffering from advanced malignant disease is still the majority of persons receiving hospice care. And even though care for patients with AD does imply specific burdens—for caregivers and fellow patients, principally—hospice care for these patients and their loved ones is not impossible at all.

Integration of palliative care with the formal health care system thus presents new challenges. The traditional axiology of hospice is now undergoing revision since different patient categories fall under the scope of palliative care. Research in palliative care, underestimated for a long time, will be focused on the establishment of an evidence base, and the care provided must be cost effective and efficient (Clark & Seymour, 1999). While this process of integration has been the goal of many hospice caregivers, it will also lead to increasing ambiguity in the general concept of palliative care. If palliative care forms a part of many medical, even curative, practices, how can we differentiate the concept and practice of palliative care from these medical practices? As indicated above, the moral values underlying palliative care are specific. They differ to a certain extent from the values of curative medicine. That being the case, a demarcation of palliative care from other practices is also an ethical enterprise. Historical, philosophical, and theological analysis of moral notions is necessary to allow new perspectives to emerge, thus providing a richer understanding of the specific morality of palliative care practice.

The paradox is that an ethic of care that does not pretend to have a direct relationship with medical practice is of more practical relevance than a medical ethic that pretends to have an immediate relationship with medical practice. As was indicated above, it is specifically the care for those suffering from AD that can profit from a reorientation of the currently prevailing form of medical ethics. After all, especially in this context, notions such as quality of life, competence, and (in)dependence appear ambiguous. Prevailing dualistic anthropologies, stressing cognitive capacities, appear of little relevance.

Alternatively, the goal of an ethic of care is not so much to solve dilemmas and propose guidelines as to clarify and analyze the articulated experiences of caregivers and patients. The ethics of care has abandoned medical scientific methodology and the dualistic anthropology of medical ethics. Instead, it acknowledges the relevance of philosophical and theological theories. Thus, new, enriching perspectives on palliative care can be anticipated.

REFERENCES

Aristotle. (1961 trans.). *The Nichomachean ethics* (H. Rackham, Trans.). Cambridge: Harvard University Press. The original date of this work is unknown.
Barnard, D. (1995). The promise of intimacy and the fear of our own undoing. *Journal of Palliative Care, 11,* 22–26.

Billings, J. (1998). What is palliative care? *Journal of Palliative Medicine, 1,* 73–81.

Bruntink, R. (1999). Vooral de thuiszorg moet zich gaan ontwikkelen. Interview met G. van den Berg [Home care especially must develop: Interview with G. van den Berg.] *Pallium, 1,* 14–15.

Cella, D. F. (1992). Quality of life: The concept. *Journal of Palliative Care, 8,* 8–13.

Clark, D., & Seymour, J. (1999). *Reflections on palliative care.* Buckingham, UK: Open University Press.

Crul, B. J. P. (1999). *Mens en pijn: Achtergronden en mogelijkheden van pijnbestrijding* [The human being and pain: Foundations and possibilities for pain relief]. Nijmegen, Netherlands: Valkhof Pers.

Desmet, M. (1996). *Dag en nacht: Een spiritualiteit van de medische ervaring* [Day and night: A spirituality of medical experience]. Tielt, Belgium: Lannoo.

Engelhardt, H. T. (1991). *Bioethics and secular humanism: The search for a common morality.* London: Trinity Press International.

Engelhardt, H. T. (2000). *The foundations of Christian bioethics.* Lisse: Swets & Zeitlinger.

Gracia, D. (2002). From conviction to responsibility in palliative care ethics. In H.A.M.J. ten Have & D. Clark (Eds.), *The ethics of palliative care: European perspectives.* Buckingham, UK: Open University Press.

ten Have, H.A.M.J., & Clark, D. (Eds.). (2002). *The ethics of palliative care: European perspectives.* Buckingham, UK: Open University Press.

Hermsen, M. A., & ten Have, H.A.M.J. (2001). Moral problems in palliative care journals. *Palliative Medicine, 15,* 425–431.

Janssens, M.J.P.A. (2001). *Palliative care: Concepts and ethics.* Nijmegen, Netherlands: Nijmegen University Press.

Janssens, M.J.P.A., & ten Have, H.A.M.J. (1999). Medische ethiek en zorgpraktijk: Een diagnose vanuit moraaltheologisch perspectief [Medical ethics and care practice: A diagnosis from the perspective of moral theology]. *Tijdschrift voor Theologie, 39,* 162–177.

Janssens, M.J.P.A., ten Have, H.A.M.J., Clark, D., Broeckaert, B., Gracia, D., Illhardt, F. J., et al. (2000). Palliative care in Europe: Towards a more comprehensive understanding. *European Journal of Palliative Care, 8,* 20–24.

Janssens, M.J.P.A., & Willems, D. L. (2001). *Ethische vragen in de palliatieve zorg* [Ethical questions in palliative care]. Houten, Netherlands: Bohn Stafleu van Loghem.

Jennings, B. (Ed.). (1997). *Ethics in hospice care.* New York: Haworth Press.

Katz, J. (1984). *The silent world of doctor and patient.* New York: Free Press.

Manschot, H., & Verkerk, M. (Eds.). (1994). *Ethiek van de zorg: Een discussie* [Care ethics: A discussion]. Amsterdam: Boom.

Moody, H. (1992). *Ethics in an aging society.* Baltimore: Johns Hopkins University Press.

Pellegrino, E. D., & Thomasma, D. C. (1993). *The virtues in medical practice.* New York: Oxford University Press.

Pijnenburg, M. A. M. (1992). Marginalisering van zieken en zorgbehoevenden [Marginalization of patients and those needing care]. In M. J. Houdijk (Ed.), *Theologie en mar-*

ginalisering: Ethiek en theologie vanuit de marge [Theology and marginalization: Ethics and theology from the margin] (pp. 111–126). Baarn, Netherlands: Gooi en Sticht.

Rothman, D. J. (1991). *Strangers at the bedside: A history of how law and bioethics transformed medical decision making.* New York: Basic Books.

Roy, D. (1997). Palliative care: A fragment towards its philosophy. *Journal of Palliative Care, 13,* 3–4.

Saunders, C., Summers, D., & Teller, N. (1981). *Hospice: The living idea.* Leeds, UK: Edward Arnold.

Schotsmans, P. (1995). Palliatieve zorg als totale zorg aan terminale patiënten [Palliative care as total care of terminal patients]. *Acta Hospitalia, 35,* 5–17.

Sporken, C. P. (1983). *Begeleiding en ethiek: Verantwoordelijkheid en solidariteit van de hulpverlener* [Supportive care and ethics: Responsibility and solidarity of the caregiver]. Baarn, Netherlands: Ambo.

Task Force on Palliative Care, Last Acts Campaign, Robert Wood Johnson Foundation. (1998). Precepts of palliative care. *Journal of Palliative Medicine, 1,* 109–111.

Tronto, J. (1993). *Moral boundaries: A political argument for an ethic of care.* New York: Routledge.

Van den Berg, H. J. (1969). *Medische macht en medische ethiek* [Medical power and medical ethics]. Nijkerk, Netherlands: Callenbach.

Van der Wal, G., & Van der Maas, P. (1996). *Euthanasie en andere medische beslissingen rondom het levenseinde: De praktijk en de meldingsprocedure* [Euthanasia and other medical decisions at the end of life: Practice and notification procedure]. The Hague, Netherlands: SDU.

Van Hooijdonk, A. S. (1999). Van genezen via zorg naar liefdevolle aandacht [From healing via care to loving attention]. *Pallium, 1,* 17.

Van Tongeren, P. J. M. (1988). Ethiek en praktijk [Ethics and practice]. *Filosofie en Praktijk, 9,* 113–127.

Van Willigenburg, T. (1991). *Inside the ethical expert: Problem solving in applied ethics.* Kampen, Netherlands: Kok Pharos.

Widdershoven, G. (2000). *Ethiek in de kliniek* [Ethics in the clinic]. Meppel, Netherlands: Boom.

Wils, J-P. (1999). *Sterben: Eine Ethik der Euthanasie* [Dying: An ethic of euthanasia]. Paderborn, Germany: Schöning.

Zwart, H. A. E. (1995). *Weg met de ethiek? Filosofische beschouwingen over geneeskunde en ethiek* [Getting rid of ethics? Philosophical reflections about medicine and ethics]. Amsterdam: Thesis Publishers.

Part IV / Clinical Ethics Issues

Focus on Patients and Caregivers

The Tendency of Contemporary Decision-making Strategies to Deny the Condition of Alzheimer Disease

Jos V. M. Welie, M.Med.S., J.D., Ph.D.

Even the most cursory review of the contemporary bioethical literature reveals that respect for the autonomy of patients has become the leading bioethical principle, easily trumping more traditional principles such as the principles of nonmaleficence and beneficence. This principle has been operationalized most clearly in the patient's right to grant informed consent to proposed medical interventions. Health care providers may not initiate treatment, including palliative treatment, unless the patient has consented. Except in medical emergencies, informed consent is a necessary condition of treatment.

This means that patients who are mentally incompetent to make decisions about their own health care, and hence legally unable to grant consent, cannot be treated. The classic example is that of the patient suffering from Alzheimer disease (AD). Unlike the patient who is unconscious after an accident, the AD patient will never again regain her capacity to make decisions about her own health care. Unlike the cancer patient who takes high doses of painkillers on most days but can do without on "good days" and be quite lucid, most AD patients do not have "good days." Dementia patients are permanently unable to exercise their right to autonomous decision making.

If patient autonomy is such an important value that it trumps all other values in decision making about health care, how can we treat incompetent patients in an ethically sound manner? If the single most significant vice of health care providers is to treat patients in a paternalistic manner, making health care decisions for patients without involving them in the decision making process and without allowing them the final say in these matters, what should care providers do when their patients have become incompetent? Obviously, it would be wrong to suddenly treat them in a paternalistic manner. The simple fact that a patient has become incompetent cannot possibly change the vice of paternalism into a virtue.

A commonly proposed solution to this problem is the so-called advance directive. Advance directives allow patients to exercise their right to autonomy before they become incompetent. Patients may write down a set of specific instructions about their future health care that is binding for health professionals, called a "living will." Alternatively, patients can grant another person a "power of attorney"; that is, the authority to speak on their behalf once they have become incompetent. The patient can specify how this surrogate should make decisions; or, in the absence of specific instructions, it is commonly believed that the surrogate should step into the shoes of the patient and decide what the patient would have decided had she been competent, a process known as "substituted judgment by a surrogate."

These two decision-making mechanisms—living wills and substituted judgments by a surrogate—are generally contrasted with a third alternative: best-interest judgments. If health care decisions for incompetent patients are based on best-interest judgments, it means that the decision will reflect what is objectively in the patient's best interest. Obviously, a patient's objective best interests may differ from what the patient would have preferred subjectively. Patients—people in general—frequently decide to do what they know not to be in their own best interests. Examples include enjoying unhealthy diets, living sedentary lifestyles, noncompliance with prescribed medications, undergoing dangerous aesthetic surgeries, and the committing of self-sacrificial suicides for the sake of relieving loved family members of their caretaking burden.

Since autonomy allegedly trumps all other values, including the values of well-being, health, and even life, best-interest judgments are abhorred by many bioethicists and health lawyers (though not by all; for a recent example, see Sailors, 2001). Their argument against best-interest judgments may take the form of the following analogy. It is ethically wrong to force a competent patient into undergoing medical treatments that she has refused, even if her refusal will have evident detrimental consequences to her own well-being. By the same token, it would be wrong to impose onto an incompetent patient treatments she has not consented to, even if those treatments are objectively in her best interests. The fact that a patient has become unable to resist and refuse does not suddenly justify the use of unconsented treatments on her.

I argue in this chapter that this line of argumentation and the resulting decision-making strategies for incompetent patients are seriously flawed, particularly when those patients are rendered incompetent because of a chronic, irreversible illness such as Alzheimer dementia. Living wills and substituted judgments can entail severe violations of the patient's intrinsic dignity because these decision-making strategies, unlike best-interest judgments, tend to deny the condition from which the patient is suffering now and for the remainder of his or her life. In doing so, they deny the patient's present personhood. I argue that a best-interest judgment, though by no means perfect, is an ethically more defensible decision-making strategy than either living wills or substituted judgments by surrogates.

✒ Living Wills

Since Alzheimer patients are certain to become legally incompetent to make decisions about their own health care, many bioethicists advocate the use of living wills as a way for the patient to retain control even after she has become incompetent (Vollmann, 2001). A living will is the decision-making strategy of choice because it comes closest to a regular informed consent. Following the logic of "implied consent," "presumed consent," and "parental consent," it might as well have been called an "advance consent."

Given the extremely high value that modern Western societies place on individual choice, leadership, independence, and self-determination, the prospect of being at the mercy of family members, health care professionals, or hospital risk managers once the onslaught of AD has rendered the patient incompetent is a terrifying prospect to many. In that light, the ability to prevent this from happening by making these kinds of decisions in advance of becoming incompetent appears comforting.

In and of itself, the idea of exerting one's autonomy into the future makes a lot of sense. In fact, most people do so routinely, though usually not in written form. The student who embarks on a particular academic study knows that his decision will have a determinative impact on his future, both in terms of what he will be doing for the next couple of years (i.e., studying) and in the more distant future (i.e., his future occupation, work environment, type of colleagues, income, possibly even place of residence). Many people determine their future by entering into marriage, having children, building retirement funds, and even leaving testaments as to what shall be done with their corpse and other worldly goods after they have died.

However, there is an evident difference between all these examples, on the one hand, and a living will, on the other hand. Whereas the former can be revoked at any time during the person's lifetime, the latter cannot. Of course, once the patient has died, a testament cannot be revoked either, but the patient who has fallen prey to AD has not yet died; after a certain point, she has merely become incompetent to exert her autonomy. The student who now is in his last year of study but realizes that he may have chosen the wrong academic discipline still is free to reverse his earlier decision. It will be a costly decision, if only because he has wasted precious years of his life, but he can do so. The woman who realizes after ten years of marriage that she cannot attain true happiness in her marriage, can still break her wedding vows and marry another person. We even allow parents to give their children up for adoption. But the AD patient cannot undo her living will (at least, theoretically she should not be able to do so; some jurisdictions nevertheless allow incompetent patients to revoke a living will).

This aspect of a living will also distinguishes it from a regular informed consent by a competent patient. Such a patient can at any time revoke a previous consent. If the patient's cancer is not responding as was expected to chemotherapy or if the side effects turn out to be more severe and distressing than was initially predicted, the patient can at any moment stop the chemotherapy. The reverse is true as well. Consider the energetic person who had always feared being hooked to life-sustaining technologies. He has a serious car accident and awakes in an intensive care unit hooked up to all possible life-sustaining technology. If he comes to find that there is more to life than the hindrances imposed by such technologies, he is free to consent to the continuation of the technology. But if consent is given or withheld by means of a living will, no such changes are possible once the person has reached a state of incompetence.

Now it is true that the freedom to change one's mind is of limited value. Most people do not cherish that freedom for the sake of simply being able to make changes on the spur of the moment, whenever it appears appealing to do so.

When life becomes a series of free but unrelated and momentary decisions reversing yesterday's decisions only to change them again tomorrow, the freedom to determine one's own course of life becomes a vacuous value. We embark on a study, wed, and conceive children precisely because we want to commit to a particular occupation, marital life, and parenthood. These are important and far-reaching choices. Even though we can still change course down the road, we do not expect that to happen and certainly do not plan for it. And so we prepare well for these choices. We think about them long and hard; we carefully review different academic disciplines before choosing one; we become acquainted with the nature of marital life and date different people before making a final choice in these areas; we are taught in many ways about the portentous task of parenthood in the hope that we take it very seriously.

But this is exactly what does not happen with living wills. Even though a living will is quite literally a matter of life and death, most people issue them without really knowing what they are signing. Many living wills are prepared for patients by attorneys who have never seen an intensive care unit from the inside, who do not know about the success rate of cardiopulmonary resuscitation, or who are unfamiliar with the side effects of drugs. In fact, the people who sign such documents, themselves tend to know little more about these matters. In the best of scenarios, they will discuss the issue with their primary care provider, but it is very difficult to reach a truly informed consent about future treatments for future conditions, neither of which is presently known.

But even if patients consult with their physicians before authoring a living will, serious problems remain. Earlier, it was pointed out that the living will is the extension of the patient's right to informed consent; it is an *advance* informed consent. We know it is not an easy task for either the competent patient or her caregiver to reach a regular informed consent about a particular treatment for a known condition of which the patient is presently suffering. Patients remember few of the facts they are told, and often they have great difficulty comprehending the true nature of their disease and the complexities of the treatments proposed. Consequently, physicians who have to get an informed consent from patients before they can provide treatment, have to be trained in communication skills, learn how to explain jargon and statistics, check that the patient has heard all that has been said, and verify that what is heard is truly understood. And just to be sure, we give patients informative flyers to take home and a written informed consent form to be checked and signed. If all of this has to be done to obtain a regular informed consent, what are the chances that a living will covering many possible illnesses and many possible remedies is truly an advance *informed* consent?

This serious problem is exacerbated by the fact that certain conditions, and particularly AD, are poorly understood conditions. They are poorly understood scientifically, but, more importantly, they are poorly understood existentially. It may be possible, though very difficult, for a healthy person to understand what it means to become paralyzed and dependent on various technologies; it is probably impossible truly to imagine what it means to become an Alzheimer patient. Of course, we may have seen loved ones fall prey to this disease. We may have seen how they have lost their memory, their recognition of family and friends, their ability to sustain a thought, their orientation and decorum. We may have seen them change so much that at times it is hard to acknowledge it is still the same person. We may have seen all of this, and the mere thought that this might happen to us, too, truly terrifies us. But do we really know how it will be for us to become such a patient—how we will experience our own existence once the disease has impacted our nervous system? Precisely the fact the AD appears to have such a radical impact on the victim's personhood—the very fact that terrifies us so much—also renders it impossible to truly understand what it will be like.

It is impossible for a three-year-old child to understand what adulthood is about. And it is equally impossible for an adult to once again experience how it is to be a three-year-old child. Once grown up, we can never again experience ourselves and the world as does a small child. Even though in some regards we are the same person as we were at age three, we cannot go back to that state of being. We have changed too radically. By the same token, it is impossible to imagine what life will be in an advanced state of AD. That state is too different from our own to be truly imaginable. This means that the factual basis of a living will, written by still competent patients diagnosed with AD, is very weak.

To make matters worse, such a living will is founded on a questionable "evaluative" base. It is, as we have seen, very difficult for anybody to predict the facts of one's future as an Alzheimer patient. But it is even more difficult to predict one's evaluation of that future state. Most of us dread severe illness and, even more so, chronic disabilities. We would rather be dead. And yet, most patients who are stricken by severe illness or chronic disabilities do not choose death. Once they have actually fallen ill, their appreciation and evaluation of these conditions change. For that reason, patients have a right always to change their minds about treatments consented to or refused. It is also ethically justifiable for health care providers to bargain with patients who initially refuse treatments, talking them into a trial period, hoping they will develop a new appreciation of those treatments. But all of this is impossible when consent is given or refused by means of a living will. The living will of an AD patient is based on a hypothetical evaluation of a very poorly understood future condition. Yet for most of these patients, it cannot be changed once the idea becomes reality, when the facts materialize and the actual evaluation of the situation develops. For by that time, the patient has become legally incompetent to change the will.

The question thus arises as to why a living will binds on the caregivers of an AD patient. Or, more precisely, why the living will supersedes the judgments of caregivers about the patient's present best interests. As I argue later, to grant priority to the living will is akin to treating the AD patient as a nonperson, as a dead man walking. Irrespective of the undeniable imperfections of best-interest judgments, none can be more serious than to treat a living human being as if she or he had already died. But before I defend this thesis, let us first look at the second favored decision-making strategy, substituted judgments by surrogates.

❧ Substituted Judgment by Surrogate

Many advocates of the patient's right to self-determination prefer living wills as the decision-making mechanism that comes closest to the informed consent of a competent patient. After all, the living will is authored by the patient herself, hopefully based on thoroughly researched data and a careful evaluation by the patient. Substituted judgments by a surrogate are an acceptable secondary option, but cannot possibly reflect the patient's own wishes as authentically as can a living will. Although the surrogate ideally is supposed to step into the patient's own shoes, this is de facto impossible. Hence, there is the inevitable danger of paternalism—that is, reaching decisions that do not in fact reflect the patient's own wishes in the matter but the surrogate's assessment of what is in the patient's best interests.

The fact that the surrogate is a close friend or family member of the patient increases the probability that the surrogate will reach a decision that is in fact in the patient's best interest. But it is not yet a substituted decision proper (i.e., the same decision the patient would have reached had she been competent to make a decision herself). To make such a decision would presume that a surrogate can actually get into a patient's mind and heart and reach the decision the patient would have reached. If this were possible, the surrogate could do so as well while the patient was still competent. In fact, it probably would be easier to do so since the surrogate could interview the patient before reaching her substituted judgment. And yet, we do not allow surrogates to make these kinds of decisions as long as the patient is competent. This shows that we do not believe that substituted judgment can ever be as authentic as the explicit consent by the competent patient herself.

Let us examine how accurate a substituted judgment can be, in particular for an AD patient. To reach a sound substituted judgment, the surrogate will have to do some homework. Typically, the surrogate will collect as many as possible patient "testimonials" and evaluate their reliability in yielding a good impression of what the patient might have decided had she been competent at this moment. The surrogate decision maker will order by rank all available testimonies according to their degree of trustworthiness. First: written notes, letters, old wills, anything that most closely resembles a living will. Second: corroborated oral testimonies from close family members. Third: ideas of a more intuitive nature that can be corroborated by other family members, and so forth.

Clearly, the two problems we have encountered with living wills surface again. First, if the patient is presently suffering from AD, all of these testimonials are factually questionable. None of these sources can tell how the patient is *presently* experiencing her condition. And second, they certainly cannot reveal accurately the patient's own evaluation of her present condition.

It may be countered that the substituted judgment has one advantage over the living will. Whereas the living will was written before the patient was struck by AD, at least the surrogate encounters the patient in her present condition; that is, qua Alzheimer patient. An empathic surrogate will be able to interpret the patient's behavior, expressions, and gestures, and deduce from these how she is feeling. I believe this objection is correct, and will return to it later. However, it cannot support the validity of a substituted judgment. For a substituted judgment is one that the patient would have made had she been competent at this very moment. But it is only possible to assume that the patient is competent by denying the Alzheimer dementia from which she presently suffers. To assume that the patient is suffering from advanced Alzheimer dementia and is at the same time competent is contradictory. Either the surrogate assumes that the patient is competent by denying the effects of the AD (but in that case, her substituted judgment is analogous to the living will written by the patient before she fell prey to AD) or the surrogate accepts the patient's medical condition as a fact, including all the changes brought about by the Alzheimer dementia. But in that case, her judgment is not a substituted judgment proper. Instead, it is a best-interest judgment that takes into account—as all sound best-interest judgments should—the patient's own experience of her condition.

✿ Understanding Alzheimer Disease

The Externalist Model

We thus find that living wills and substituted judgments entail an understanding of Alzheimer disease as being external to the patient. There is the patient, competent to make autonomous decisions about her own health care. And there is the disease. The latter has no constitutive impact on the former. We can bracket the disease, partition it off, and thence reach the competent patient.

In and of itself, this is not an unusual imagery. Not only health care professionals but patients as well often view diseases as something external to their selfhood. Disease is a hindrance to the self, sometimes even a violent enemy of the self. We strive to get rid of diseases much like we get rid of house pests or terrorists. Even if the illness is evidently localized inside of the patients, it is still experienced as something external that is invading them and should be cut out again. AD is no exception. Many caregivers and patient advocates are concerned about Alzheimer patients' being identified with the disease, as if these patients are essentially the disease process, or nothing but the disease process. They insist that patients "have" AD, or are patients "with" AD, instead of "being Alzheimer patients." In other words, the disease becomes a factor external to the patient's personhood or self.

If AD is external to the patient as a person, then it follows logically that the patient is best respected by bracketing the condition of AD, by partitioning it off. In as much as the caregiver can discern the "original" self "under" or "in between" the symptoms of the disease, they should allow the patient to make decisions herself (limited competence). And to the extent that this does not appear possible, they should revert to an older (but presumably identical) version of this "self" who wrote the living will. This former "self" endures, but is in some way hidden inside the prison of AD.

This understanding of diseases as being external to the patient's self is by no means unique to AD: it is an approach commonly adopted toward diseases and handicaps. When the illness concerned disables only a small part of the human body or mind, like an eye infection, a broken wrist, or a phobia for cats, its impact on the existence of the patient is so minor that it seems only reasonable to consider the illness external to the patient. This is ever the more true if the illness is curable or can be contained so well that the patient does not experience any symptoms. We can then afford to view the illness as something external precisely because we know that the patient will be rid of it soon.

But what if the illness or disability will never again leave us? What if we are chronically ill or disabled? What if, moreover, the illness or disability concerns vital organs or its symptoms are so severe that they cannot be bracketed? To consider such a chronic and systemic disease as external to the person is like being permanently locked inside a crumbling and condemned house. Such an externalist view of chronic illnesses and disabilities is likely to engender frantic attempts by both patient and caregivers to restore the house, to patch the leaking roof, to strengthen the foundations, to repaint the walls. These frantic attempts may induce a sense of control and hope, of youth, strength, and health. But in the end, they are doomed to be futile. Precious time and energy is wasted that could have been used to learn how truly to cope with the illness, how to squeeze whatever is positive out of it through palliative instead of curative care efforts and live with all that is negative in a meaningful manner.

The Destructive Model

Even though an externalist understanding of AD is usually adopted for benevolent reasons—we want to give patients hope in the early stages of the illness and make sure that they are not simply identified with their illness once it has progressed—this understanding can easily lead to a very maleficent attitude toward them. Consider again the externalist thesis that somewhere "below" or "in between" the symptoms of the disease there is still the patient's original self. If we next ask what this "self" consists of, an answer is forthcoming. This self is a phantom self, at best, a ghost of old trapped into a body that should have died long ago. Indeed, the logical conclusion seems to be that the patient's selfhood is not simply hidden but actually destroyed by AD. In some sense, the patient as a person has already died. The living will thus becomes analogous to a financial will regulating affairs portmortem. It is the will of a past person. All decisions necessarily are to be based on the patient's "antecedent autonomy" (i.e., anteceding the destruction of her self).

The Constitutive Model

The alternative to the prevailing destructive model requires that we do not understand the person as "having" AD, but as "being" an Alzheimer patient. Alzheimer disease is a constitutive characteristic of this person, not the only constitutive characteristic, but one that cannot simply be disregarded as an external or accidental factor. Race, gender, age—all these are constitutive characteristics. For example, we do not talk about women as persons *with* female gender. They *are* female. Although their womanhood is not their only constitutive factor, it certainly is not external to their being. Neither is one's race or age. The same is true of AD. There is no "other" self that has either been imprisoned or destroyed by AD. Alzheimer disease has impacted, transformed, the person—much like growing old does, or having a sex change or losing one's spouse.

Although this thesis needs further elaboration, one can already see how a constitutive understanding of AD impacts the ethics of health care decision making on their behalf. Consider an eighty-five-year-old gentleman who recently lost his wife after fifty-five years of marriage. If this widower needs health care himself but happens to be incompetent, how should we decide on his behalf? Should we revisit his medical dossier and search for notes about his previous decisions dating from the time that he was still happily married? Should we treat him as if the trauma of losing his wife never befell him—as if his world still includes the presence, support, love, and joy from his wife? Surely, that would be a significant violation of his personhood. Rather, our treatment planning must take into account the loss of his dearly beloved wife. We have to consider the patient's present life goals, needs, and interests. The same should be true for the Alzheimer patient. The fact that the patient is no longer competent to assess, weigh, and describe his own needs and interests in a clear and convincing manner, such that his choice qualifies as a legally binding consent, does not mean that he no longer has new needs and new interests. Since the Alzheimer patient is by no means deceased, he continues to act and respond to the new conditions of his life journey and develop new interests and needs.

We do not expect a competent person to abide by an older living will; he or she is free to change that will at any time; moreover, the patient's present consent overrides any preexisting instructions in a living will. The Alzheimer patient deserves the same respect. In the constitutive model, the living will retains importance as a source of information about the patient, but only to the extent that the will appears relevant to the patient's new condition and appears to facilitate rather than obfuscate the determination of the patient's present needs and best interests.

❧ Best-interest Judgments for Alzheimer Patients

Before we discuss the feasibility of such best-interest judgments, I should make one more comment about the place of the principle of respect for patient autonomy in the care of Alzheimer patients. My plea for the restoration of beneficence does not exclude respect of patient autonomy. In fact, it is perfectly consistent with that principle, provided the latter principle is interpreted in a historically correct manner—that is, as a defensive principle (Welie, 1998).

The right to respect of one's autonomy is, foremost, a political concept that can be invoked to counter the tendency of governments to invade the private sphere of individual citizens. Although medicine and health care do it in a different manner, they invade that same private sphere. Patients hence have the right to resist such an invasion if it is not appreciated, even if the treatment is objectively beneficial to them. In practical terms, caregivers must obtain consent before they can initiate treatment. By withholding consent, the patient de facto refuses the recommended care. But this defensive principle of respect for patient autonomy helps neither patient nor caregivers in determining what *is* a beneficial, recommendable treatment. It is only *after* it has been determined what treatment will benefit the patient that the patient can turn around and refuse it. From this perspective, there cannot be conflicts between the principle of beneficence and the principle of respect for autonomy; or, more precisely, there cannot be conflicts between the principle of benevolence and that of respect for patient autonomy.

We have granted competent patients the right to refuse care that is objectively in their best interests. We have also granted patients the right to extend their autonomy into the time of incompetence by means of advance directives. Whether such advance directives retain their performative force, particularly vis-à-vis AD, remains a point of debate (Welie, 2001). However, an advance directive is not any more likely to invalidate a best-interest judgment than is the refusal of a competent patient. Let us, then, turn to best-interest judgments.

Best-interest judgments for Alzheimer patients are not fundamentally different from those for other categories of patients, including competent patients. The same methods for arriving at such a judgment apply. Without claiming to be exhaustive, I will briefly review three such methods: diagnostics, biography, and perception.

Diagnostics

A patient's best interests are determined in large part by her medical condition. In some cases, patients are unaware that they are or will soon be patients, because their medical condition has not yet resulted in symptoms. Although it is a point of discussion whether all predictive information is beneficial, particularly if no treatment is available, in most cases patients' interests are served by early diagnosis and preventive interventions. But even if the patient is well aware that she is ill, she is unable to bring about relief of her symptoms. The determination of the origins of her symptoms and their future development is necessary in order to establish an effective treatment plan. In short, diagnostics (and, likewise, prognostics) are components of a best-interest judgment.

It is important to emphasize that the results of diagnostics are by no means value-neutral. For example, a diagnosis is normative because it establishes the ways in which this particular patient digresses from certain norms. On the one hand, these norms are never merely statistical, but always axiological as well. On the other hand, the particular patient's digression is judged sufficiently harmful to merit therapeutical intervention.

We should furthermore remember that a good diagnosis is always specific to the particular patient. As long as the patient is *likely* to have a broken rib or *may* have a malignancy, the diagnosis has not been completed. Sometimes, the quest for a perfect diagnosis becomes an obsession and the patient is subjected to ever more diagnostic tests, even though the outcome is already known to have little if any impact on the treatment plan. But this unfortunate obsessiveness also reveals that diagnostics is a prime example of the art of medicine—the ability to attain truthful information about an individual patient.

We conclude, therefore, that the physician who diagnoses a patient with AD has already begun making best-interests judgments on the patient's behalf. By applying the diagnosis, the physician underscores, at least implicitly, that this patient's loss of memory is harmful to her and merits treatment (even if we presently do not have effective treatment). Likewise, her digression from the norms of etiquette and decorum is thought to merit therapy, as do changes in personality, aggression, or depression. The very diagnosis of AD entails a best-interest judgment.

Note, furthermore, that the physician's ability to establish a diagnosis is not markedly affected by the patient's incompetence. His inability to volunteer information and answer questions in a rational and clear manner is an obvious complicating factor when diagnosing any incompetent patient. But in the case of AD, the patient's irrationality paradoxically becomes a significant diagnostic datum. More importantly, some or all of the other diagnostic methods, from physical examination to electronic imaging, are available to the physician, allowing for a careful and reliable diagnosis, both of the Alzheimer disease itself and of accompanying illnesses that may require treatment.

Biography

The diagnosis of the patient's condition entails a best-interest judgment, but only a partial one. This is because the diagnosis cannot provide a complete insight into her condition. The methods of medical diagnostics are designed to uncover the organic origins of the patient's complaints, thus enabling a very targeted therapeutical intervention. These methods are necessarily biased. For example, almost all diagnostic methods are analytical; they are aimed at separating out different structures. Percussion allows the physician to separate lung tissue from liver tissue; auscultation enables an analysis of different intestinal rumblings; X rays reveal different tissue densities; and laboratory analysis separates the many ingredients of human blood into a long list of ingredients. Another peculiar aspect of diagnostics is its focus on the patient's interior milieu. Auscultation, percussion and palpation, X rays, MRIs and sonography, laboratory analysis and pathological microscopy—all aim at discovering what is hidden in the depths of the patient's interior. This is true even of history taking: "Where does it hurt?" "Does it get worse after you have eaten?" "Do you become dizzy when you get up out of bed?"—all are questions aimed at uncovering hidden processes in the depths of the patient's interior.

These biases and reductions are necessary to reach a reliable diagnosis that enables targeted therapeutic interventions. However, it is not the liver that is ill; it is not the blood that needs healing; it is not the brain that has interests. The patient is ill and needs healing. It is the patient's interests that must be assessed and fostered. To assess the needs and interests of the patient as a person, medical diagnostics has relatively little to offer. In fact, the methods of diagnostics have a tendency to obscure from view the patient as a person.

To gain an understanding of the patient as a person, the diagnostic information must be integrated into a biography of the patient. Whereas the primary question of the diagnostician is "*What* is this person?" the biographer asks, "*Who* is this person?" The amount of biographical information that the health care provider needs will differ. But even in cases that appear straightforward diagnostically, such as a fractured collarbone, it must be assessed biographically whether there is, for example, a primary caregiver who can assist the patient with daily chores and whether her line of work will allow for the necessary healing. The more the patient's diagnosed condition affects her existence as a person, the more biographic insight must be attained to reach a best-interest judgment.

There are many sources for obtaining such information. First, there is the patient herself: the patient may be able to volunteer most of what is generally needed. Living wills and, better yet, so-called values histories written in advance of a patient's becoming incompetent, can be important sources of information when the patient has become incapable of providing detailed biographical information. Then there is the care provider's own recollection about the patient—if, that is, the care provider has known her over an extended period of time. Often, there are family members and close friends who can provide valuable information.

Unfortunately, biographical information gathered from different sources is not always consistent and compatible. This problem is not at all peculiar to incompetent patients. A competent patient may describe himself as very health conscious, while his spouse may bemoan his unwillingness to comply with medication regimens or prescribed diets. But the problem does become much more pronounced. The first author of each person's life story is that person herself or himself. When that person continues to write but is no longer able to share the story written, care providers have to rely on the secondary authors, all of whom have their peculiar biases. As most clinical ethicists and members of ethics committees know first-hand, piecing together the patient's story is often very difficult, but also the key to the resolution of the ethical dilemmas.

If the patient is unconscious and unable to share any biographical information, secondary sources are the only ones. However, most Alzheimer patients, even if legally incompetent, still write their life story in a legible manner. It may take readers an additional effort to understand the story as the patient tells it, but as Sabat's many examples show, what may seem nonsensical at first makes a lot more sense on second or third reading (2001).

When interpreting the Alzheimer patient's story, we have to guard carefully against superimposing others onto the patient's own. It is the prerogative of parents of young children that they may write such stories for their children's lives, or at least initiate them. But as children grow up, parents, teachers, friends, colleagues, and spouses have to become secondary authors. No person can ever be the sole author of his own life story, but the essence of respect for the autonomy of others is allowing them to become and remain primary authors of their own stories. Alzheimer patients are no different.

Note that writing a story is not the same as making decisions. All through our lives, others will be making decisions for us. We have to incorporate those decisions into our life stories. Some of these decisions are small, as when the grocery store no longer carries our favorite brand of cereal. Others are major, as when our spouse initiates a divorce and we are forced to relocate. Alzheimer patients may be confronted with similar such decisions, whether it is the menu in the nursing home that is not to their liking or their becoming too big a burden on their spouses, forcing relocation to a clinic. But even in those cases, we can allow patients to retain primary authorship—since they are always writing their own life story, anyway—instead of us superimposing the story we would like to write for them.

The risk of superimposing such a story occurs foremost when proxies are supposed to reach a substituted judgment for Alzheimer patients. As pointed out earlier, such a judgment entails the denial of the patient's present condition, which is an obvious example of superimposing a story that proxies would like to write, but one that is not the patient's own. A similar danger emerges with living wills. Even though, by definition, a living will is written by the patient herself and as such is a chapter in the patient's own life story, it is never the most recent chapter. To treat the Alzheimer patient according to a living will is like superimposing onto the chapter that is presently being written by the patient one that was written a long time ago.

Perception

The third source of information for reaching best-interest judgments is the immediate perception of the patient by the care provider. It is immediate in that it is mediated neither by diagnostic protocols and technologies nor by the grammar and syntax rules of biographical narration. Many contemporary ethicists deny the feasibility of such immediate perception of the patient. As I have argued elsewhere (Welie, 1998), I believe the therapeutic relationship between caregiver and patient is (or can be) characterized by empathy such that caregivers can in fact know what is in their patient's best interest.

Although the information thus gathered cannot be verified or even corroborated in the same way as diagnostic and biographic information can, that does not undermine the veracity of the information. In fact, all of health care and all of biomedical science is based on the perception of other people's suffering and illness. This perception necessarily precedes the use of diagnostic tools because it motivates their employment. Conversely, the reliability of these diagnostic tools can be assessed only in reference to the perceived illness/well-being of patients if a circular argument is to be prevented.

Most assuredly, it is not easy for health care professionals to perceive patients' needs and interests. First, the reliability of such perceptions is directly related to the time spent with the patient, and care providers have ever less time. Second, health care professionals are actually trained to bracket their perceptive understanding of the patient, always distrusting such immediate information and relying instead on mediated data-collection strategies. And third, there is the inevitable anthropological fact that the patient is ill, while the care provider is not. The care provider can never experience what the patient is feeling.

But even if the care provider does not share in the patient's illness, even if he has never experienced the same kind of illness, still it is possible for an empathic care provider to perceive the patient as a person in her own world. As Toombs has shown convincingly, it is possible for a physician to enter the world of the patient stricken by multiple sclerosis (Toombs, 1992). Unfortunately, AD is particularly challenging in this regard. As foreign as multiple sclerosis is to most physicians, dementias such as AD are in a class of their own. They are so much unlike other diseases that it becomes very difficult for caregivers to empathize with the patient, to understand what the new phase in life is all about, to uncover its meaning and place in life, and to relate all of this in a manner authentic to the patient's past. AD appears so foreign to us, almost alien, that it is difficult to make any sense of it. The challenge ahead of us, then, is to develop the hermeneutical frameworks that enable a more insightful interpretation of the Alzheimer patient's life qua Alzheimer patient.

REFERENCES

Sabat, S. R. (2001). *The experience of Alzheimer's disease: Life through a tangled veil.* Malden, MA: Blackwell Publishers.

Sailors, P. R. (2001). Autonomy, benevolence, and Alzheimer's disease. *Cambridge Quarterly of Healthcare Ethics, 10,* 184–193.

Toombs, S. K. (1992). *The meaning of illness: A phenomenological account of the different perspectives of physician and patient.* Dordrecht: Kluwer.

Vollmann, J. (2001). Advance directives in patients with Alzheimer's disease: Ethical and clinical considerations. *Medicine, Health Care and Philosophy, 4* (2), 161–167.

Welie, J. V. M. (1998). *In the face of suffering: The philosophical-anthropological foundations of clinical ethics.* Omaha, NE: Creighton University Press.

Welie, J. V. M. (2001). Living wills and substituted judgments: A critical analysis. *Medicine, Health Care and Philosophy, 4* (2), 169–183.

CHAPTER ELEVEN

Advance Directives and End-of-Life Decision Making in Alzheimer Disease

Practical Challenges

Winifred J. Ellenchild Pinch, R.N., Ed.D.

Practical challenges in palliative care, advance directives, and end-of-life decision making in the context of Alzheimer disease (AD) encompass all individuals in these circumstances: the person who has been diagnosed as well as those who serve as caregivers, both professional and lay persons, and anyone who in turn is in contact with them. As an advocate for family-centered care and joint decision making, I find it is important to understand the perspective of the family, especially when individuals with AD are no longer able to make decisions for themselves. Some of the most salient points are included here in the form of a letter written by a spouse caregiver to her sister. This spouse was intentionally left nameless to emphasize the invisible nature of caregivers, as we have come to expect selfless devotion in this role. The caregiver is the wife of Michael, who was diagnosed with AD several years ago. But that, too, is a role, not her total identity.

Dear Rachel,

I have finally managed to squeeze in some time to write to you—being able to sit down and sort out some of the situations I have been dealing with has not been easy to accomplish. But, it seems like it may work out this afternoon. I wanted to write rather than telephone and simply chat because there have been such serious issues that have arisen lately. If I can organize my thoughts to share them with you, I might be able to think more clearly about them for both Michael and myself.

Your responsiveness to my needs during this very trying time in my life is very important and I want you to know that. Michael's diagnosis with AD was one of the most devastating events in our marriage. Since wives do tend to outlive their husbands, I had this nagging thought in the back of my mind as Michael and I approached retirement, that someday I might be in a position to care for him. As I considered the usual risk factors, I envisioned the possibility of a very serious heart attack that might restrict his activities, or that he might be incapacitated by a stroke. Since my experience with my own mother's diagnosis of Alzheimer's, I guess I really feared my own risk for dementia rather than Michael's developing such a condition.

At first responsibilities were not too difficult—occasional forgetfulness seemed to be an annoyance rather than a problem, looking back on things. Then the forgetfulness became more serious. It wasn't simply forgetting where he put his keys or if he paid the electric bill. He began to forget how to do things, and we eventually got the diagnosis of Alzheimer disease. Obtaining some definitive information was certainly not an easy path to negotiate. Michael's primary care physician was not in tune with my description of events and insisted that I simply needed to adjust to my husband's aging. But I persisted—it took a lot of energy, and of course time. We finally got the appropriate referral but it still took quite some time again before the specialist was able not simply to tell us his diagnosis, but also to talk with us and relay what Alzheimer's would mean in terms of our lives and future plans. They told Michael and me together, since I said I would want to know my own diagnosis under these circumstances, and Michael seemed to take it quite well.

As Michael's needs become more encompassing, I am having more and more difficulty separating when I need to be his caregiver from those times when I want—and need—to be his wife. Perhaps I should just forget about being his wife altogether. It's not that easy, however. I need his love and affection and loss of that emotional piece is exceedingly difficult to adjust to. Mostly I need to be a caregiver, decision maker whenever momentous events rain down upon us—as they now seem to pelt us like a thunderstorm as opposed to the gentle rain of problems we dealt with earlier.

Although you do not get to see us very often, I know I can call on you at any time—good or bad—and you are always there. But more than that, you don't just listen but you hear what I say and have made some invaluable suggestions. The children are here more often than you, but they have a tough time seeing Michael, their dad, as a patient with a deteriorating condition. They resist losing that strong father they have known all of their lives. I wish that they had been able to be here when Michael's physician told us the final verdict. It was very strenuous—telling them the results of the tests myself, but more than that—the changes we would have to expect in the future. Their reluctance to fully acknowledge his need for care could have the potential to be a problem as we face some of the challenges that are coming up for us. I know that I do not need their agreement, but their support is going to be important with some of the decision making I am encountering.

Very basically, I am not sure how much longer I can keep Michael in our home, and I feel so guilty just writing these words. Some days it is just so physically exhausting. I know that he would not want to be a burden—but just the necessary vigilance can be arduous. Also he is larger and stronger than I am. Doing the same tasks of assisting with dressing and grooming for our grandson Toby are far easier than attending to those same tasks for Michael. Toby accepts the need for help; Michael resists.

Then when he disagrees about something I say, or he insists I should know something I do not, he acts out. This seldom occurs, but I am afraid that sometime he might try to hurt me. I don't think he would intend this, but it might occur. More so, I am afraid that he might hurt himself, and I could never forgive myself if he was hurt because I did not care enough. I am taking him to a day care two days a week now. The center comes and gets him, which is helpful in that Michael does not see me drive the car those days. Ending his driving career was so, so difficult. These two days provide me with a break to get some errands accomplished. I wish they had a different name for day care. It is one more reminder of some of the infantile effects of this disease and how different Michael is now from all our earlier—and many—satisfying years of marriage.

Along with decisions about long-term care and the facility we might want to use, we also have to prospectively think about health care decisions as Michael's disease progresses. He is never going to be cured, and eventually I will have to make decisions about what to do or, even more challenging, what not to do. Whether or not we want simply comfort care or more aggressive therapy will help determine where Michael might eventually go. The philosophy of care at a long-term care institution is an important consideration. Some places I have visited admit patients only with the intent to provide comfort care once the Alzheimer's has progressed to a terminal stage. I can understand what comfort care might be for a patient with cancer, since so many of them seem to have problems with pain. Comfort would naturally mean taking away the pain. But Michael doesn't seem uncomfortable with this condition.

Do you remember Bernadette, my neighbor? Her husband did not have Alzheimer's but he did end up in the hospital in a coma due to his diabetes. Well, all she can talk about since he died is how the doctors kept doing more and more treatments when she didn't think anything was doing him any good. When she looks back on it all, Bernadette isn't sure the physicians were ready to let him go, or if they didn't realize that they could stop some of the things they were doing. It can all seem so overwhelming. What if Michael needed to be treated for some other illness? I truly do not know what Michael would want. He always seemed to know what he wanted and he was so resolute once he made up his mind about something.

Michael was very careful about his financial arrangements so we do not have any problems about how he planned his retirement, possible insurance for long-term care, and sources for health care benefits. For some families, the costs thus far would have been prohibitive. I am very lucky. However, Michael did not prepare any advance directives for health care. He never considered that his mind might go before he suffered a debilitating physical illness. I think that the doctors will most likely consult me since Michael cannot make decisions on his own, but I have discovered two things. One, is that the physicians will want to be sure that what I say is likely to be what Michael wanted, and two, when the whole family does not agree—then there can be a problem. I also heard that in some cases, spouses have to go to court in order to have decisions executed.

One day I was looking for information on the Internet and I found two cases where the women's sons went to court after the hospital insisted upon putting in a PEG—that's a feeding tube put directly into the person's stomach, Rachel. One son refused consent while the other son requested that he be made the legal guardian in order to deny the tube. The courts in both cases decided in favor of the sons. In the one, the court agreed with the woman's son, based on statements he said his mother had made. In the second case, the court justified its action based on the woman's incapacity. Then the other day I read about a third case. Here the wife objected to some life-sustaining treatment for her husband and the judge ruled that her testimony about her husband's previous statements did not clearly relate to his current condition, so her petition was denied and he was treated. I wonder if the decision depends upon the person making the appeal, whether or not women might have less credibility in the courtroom than men, or if it depends upon the sex of the patient, and making decisions for a woman is more easily accepted.

Michael is just like most others. They think they will not need to have someone else make health care decisions for them so they don't prepare a living will or make an advance directive, including naming a durable power of attorney for health care decisions. We certainly talked some about such decisions and what we might want, but given the court cases I've read now, it is not certain that our discussions will be adequate evidence. Yet I am clearly the person who best knows Michael. But will my perspective be respected? I may have to make decisions about whether or not to hospitalize him should he become seriously ill—depending upon where he goes to live and his condition at the time. If he should be hospitalized, there may be decisions to make regarding one of those breathing machines, or if he should be revived should his heart stop or he stops breathing, or if he should get antibiotics, or even if he should have food and water. Of course, not food or water in the usual way. But, like I mentioned earlier, through a tube into his stomach or into a blood vessel. It seems to me that food and fluids are somewhat different from the other possible choices, especially when he cannot feed himself. I am sure there are many different ways of thinking about these alternatives. Think about these issues with me, Rachel, and then we can talk sometime. I know that you love Michael as well and that you would not knowingly suggest anything that would not be in his best interests. So, give these future possibilities your considered thought and your perspective. I know that it will be helpful for me.

If Michael went into a coma or did not respond at all—even in an unintelligible way—it would be easier to not do these treatments. But, if he becomes critically ill, and was still responding in some way, then it would seem to be more logical to give him those treatments. Except if his heart stopped. If his heart stopped, perhaps that is the message that he is ready to go and we shouldn't try to start it again. I think that I would need to have some fairly in-depth discussions about these issues should they come up before I could make a decision.

A couple of other questions are on the horizon as well—I think the last two, at least for this letter. I want Michael's quality of life to be as high as possible—no matter where he is and what he is able to do. I already mentioned his acting out and I am not sure, as yet, how any facility will handle this when he is finally admitted elsewhere. I have some difficulty with his wandering, but mostly am able to deal with it by simply accompanying him when locked doors do not easily remind him to stay indoors. His resistance to certain events or his angry objections to what people say has not resulted in an unacceptable level of negative responses as yet—but you already know I fear we are moving on that trajectory. Will restraints have to be used? Restraining people—fellow human beings, especially my husband—seems so primitive to me. But suppose such devices are necessary for Michael's own safety? What will I decide?

Additionally there is, for me, considerations of pain and suffering—his comfort. Since he is not always able to accurately express himself, I wonder about pain. How will we know if he gets sick? You know, Rachel, we all have an ache here, a cramp there, a sore throat, or a headache that might be nothing—but on the other hand may herald something more serious. Do you suppose Michael feels these things? I know he seldom says anything about not feeling well—but of course he never was one to complain about the little things.

The meetings that we have had thus far about Michael's treatment have gone well. I cannot complain about them. The professionals, once he was diagnosed, have been supportive. We seem to have gotten the help that we have needed in order for us to stay together here at home thus far. But I know things are changing as Michael becomes worse and worse. I will need to be making some choices about the next steps in this process.

One final idea about which I know the least at the moment and then I must close this letter. New treatments are always on the horizon. To think that there might be a useful treatment or cure for AD would be just the miracle we needed. I hear that researchers are working on all sorts of ideas and that it might be possible to try some of these things with Michael. Whether or not he should be able to be part of an experiment, however, is somewhat of a scary idea. I am not sure I would like Michael to be a guinea pig. Yet, if the investigators thought that people with Alzheimer's would benefit, and Michael might benefit—how could I say "no."

As I said earlier, think about these things with me. If I have a chance to go over them with you before I talk with the doctors and nurses, I will be in a better frame of mind. I am so grateful that you have been there right by my side. I am thankful, too, that the children are concerned and worried, but they do not think things are as serious as they are. They do not see the day-to-day issues I face, but I hope that once this summer comes and their own schedules are less hectic—they will become more in tune with our situation and come around. Give me a call in a few days.

Love, Your sister

During the course of AD, many decisions are made and such decision making will only increase given the predictions about the incidence and prevalence of this condition (Pollard, 2001). However, decreasing cognitive capacity is a hallmark in the progression of AD to its final stage, as evident in this letter about Michael. Simultaneously, his decision-making ability declined. In U.S. society, great importance has been placed on autonomous decision making, including those decisions related to health care, which are viewed as a patient right. Beginning in the 1960s concurrent with the Civil Rights movement, patient rights became a widely debated topic, resulting in the publication of formal documents such as the American Hospital Association Patient's Bill of Rights (Annas, 1995).

Support for living wills and advance directives flourished as means to direct care when individuals were unable actively to participate in decision making. Eventually, in 1991, the Patient Self-determination Act was passed to add legislative support to the preparation of such documents in the United States (American Hospital Association, 1991). This federal legislation required health care institutions to inform patients about their right to participate in decisions related to their health care, including the right to create and implement instructions such as those in living wills and advance directives. There is some evidence such preparation has occurred (Teno et al., 1997).

✿ Formal Validation for Advanced Decision Making

In chapter 10, Welie raises some serious questions about advance directives. However, I propose that they are essential tools given the state of our understanding of AD and the family's need to involve their loved one as much as possible. In fact, the importance of preparing such documents or the naming of a durable power of attorney for health care (DPA) increases in the case of AD, as the eventual inability to make competent decisions will occur, resulting in the loss of autonomy. The individual with AD is robbed of language, memory, and reason (Pollard, 2001). Michael's wife indicated that he was like most people and did not prepare such advance directives. Not only is it likely that individuals will not have advance directives, living wills, or DPAs, but they may not have adequate knowledge about these options (Hague & Moody, 1993). Although the letter is a fabricated product based on evidence from the literature on AD, the purpose of such a format is to translate those issues from the research and observations of several experts into the practical situation of a family member faced with caregiving responsibilities for the person with AD. The letter included numerous issues, among them defining the information to be shared with the patient, aspects of the dynamics of family functioning, caregiving responsibilities, context for caregiving (residence at home, respite care, or placement in a long-term care facility), financial considerations, and types of health care treatments required or desired for the patient (aggressive versus palliative interventions). These sample issues are influenced by relationships with health professionals and the legal dimensions of health care, especially the legitimacy and authority of surrogate decision makers as the person with AD becomes incompetent in various dimensions of life.

There are some additional features about advance directives that can help us to understand the practical aspect of this issue when we attempt to implement the preparation of such documents in the case of AD. Numerous formats are available for individuals to document their preferences for future health care needs, giving consumers choices about how they go about this process (American Medical Association, 1999; Emanuel & Emanuel, 1989). As already noted, the public generally lacks knowledge about these documents and their use; hence, educational efforts need to continue to inform people (Hague & Moody, 1993). Additionally, systematic efforts need to be organized to inform individuals and then facilitate both the creation of the documents and their preservation in a place where they are available when health care decisions are required. The Education for Physicians on End-of-Life Care program is one endeavor that targets the responsibility of physicians to include discussions about advance directives and other end-of-life issues with their patients before the acute need arises. The Internet is another means to both educate the public and provide examples of possible forms to create their own documentation.

❧ Respecting Individual Choice

Various studies have explored selected individuals' choices about such issues as resuscitation preferences (Carlsen, Pomeroy, & Moldow, 1998; Griffith et al., 1995) and the desirability of advance directives in the event that AD develops (Sehgal et al., 1992). More important practically is not a laundry list of all treatments that one might want, or even those that one might want most to avoid, although the latter type of statement tends to be more helpful (Holzman, 1999). Rather, the fostering of communication among those individuals who will be making the health care decisions should be emphasized (Teno & Lynn, 1996). Families need to set aside opportunities for members to dialogue about life goals and health care preferences.

One problem noted by several investigators relates to their discovery that people change their minds from the time they actually write down choices to the time of the particular circumstance when that choice would be relevant (Lee et al., 1998). Ongoing dialogue could minimize such a problem, if the original document focused on general ideas and included designation of a DPA, instead of the lists of what was wanted or not wanted. Another problem comes from those who question the validity of previously prepared documents after incompetence occurs (Holstein, 1998). Questions arise, such as: Once in an incompetent state, would this now incompetent person continue to have the same perspective as prior to the incompetent state? (Holm, 2001). At the present time, this seems to be an impossible question to answer in the practical sense.

However, whatever the person has become from a psychological or personality perspective, there still remains only one personal history for that individual. Regardless of the radical changes that manifest themselves as a result of the disease, the singular history of an individual is a strong, unifying, usable factor as a basis for decision making. Additionally, although changes occur in every individual for a multiplicity of reasons—aging, new knowledge, fresh experiences— changes wrought by AD are fundamental to pathological processes imposed upon the individual. We simply must work from the information we have about that person and from the knowledge that all caregivers bring to the decision-making process. Perhaps someday we will have patients' stories about their more serious incompetent states when pharmacological agents completely restore memory and they are able to relate such events.

❧ Elements of Advance Directives to Consider

Patterson, Baker, and Maeck (1993) noted some gender differences related to decision making that might inform us. Although the differences were not statistically significant, more women than men rated planning for health care decisions as "very important." Additionally, more women considered themselves to be the primary decision maker about health care, regardless of what the physician said. That is, women viewed the doctor's knowledge and position as informational, but considered themselves to be responsible for the final health care decisions. Women's decisions in this study reflected the fact that they were likely to live longer and have more health care needs than men. They were less likely than married men to name the spouse as a possible surrogate; they named a larger number of potential individuals for this role, and, compared with the men, they were more likely to name an adult child as a surrogate.

Moreover, planning should consider AD as a terminal disease. Decisions about death and dying will eventually become a part of the process even, if those decisions are twenty years in the future, and such decisions may include assisted suicide (Post & Whitehouse, 1995). While assisted suicide is not widely practiced nor strongly supported legally, it is an autonomy-related issue for a number of people. Occasionally, the withdrawal of food and fluids is believed to be a form of assisted suicide since eventually, without sustenance, the individual will die. The concern about nutrition and hydration was noted in the letter by Michael's wife, reflecting increased public awareness of tube feedings as an issue for the AD patient (Grady, 2000). Generally speaking, neither the lay public nor many health professionals have an adequate base of knowledge concerning nutrition and hydration issues, including the various effects of tube feeding. But people especially lack information about the provision of fluids. Family members often view nutrition and hydration from personal experience, with a significant overlay of symbolism associated with celebration, festivities, and the opposite end of a continuum—hunger, thirst, and starvation. People in general require information about the negative effects of providing food and fluids as individuals enter a dying state and bodily systems begin to fail (Zerwekh, 1997).

Other areas that could be included in prospective planning are issues involving research (Dressler, 2001; High, 1992), genetic testing (Post, 1998), and behavior control (Post, 1998; Post & Whitehouse, 1995). Certainly, the need for information and understanding are common themes among all of these areas. There is an obvious need for research related to AD, and persons with AD are vulnerable individuals. The American College of Physicians supports the preparation of an advance directive to indicate a willingness to participate in research in the future should such a possibility arise. Tension exists between the need for research, the caregiver's desire to have improvement, both in the individual and in the circumstances in which they live, and a moral obligation not to use vulnerable individuals for research when they might not personally benefit from the results. Some questions are raised about decision-making capacity and competence when statements about AD and research are included in the advance directive; that is, specific designation of a willingness to participate in research if AD is diagnosed. By the time the diagnosis is made and there is some recognition of the potential to address participation in research, is the individual already beyond a competent stage? Now in the throes of the disease, would they continue to want to participate?

Families may also have an interest in the genetic aspect of AD once a diagnosis is made. Currently, only minimal information is available related to prediction and risk. Caution is advised in this area since susceptibility testing in asymptomatic individuals is not useful (Post, 1998). Here genotyping for patients with symptoms presents problems since the potential for early treatment is at odds with the acquired information that may lead to discrimination for insurance and health care benefits coverage. Then, for the area of behavior control, caregivers, driven to the limits of their patience, can pressure health professionals to prescribe medications for hyperactivity, restlessness, resistiveness, wandering, memory loss, and assaultiveness (Post, 1998). Determining whose needs most require the professional's attention is fraught with problems since the patient with AD is often unaware of what others judge to be unacceptable behavior. Should this individual be treated in order to reduce stress and emotional distress in the caregiver? Women are more frequently the caregiver and, if they are also providing care for children, can be caught in the middle. An especially difficult decision is related to pharmacological agents that might improve memory and behavior, but that will then necessitate the individual's eventual return to undesirable behaviors as progressive stages in the disease must once more be traversed. These areas are possible considerations for advance planning documents or as issues for the surrogate decision maker.

❧ The Milieu of Decision Making

Families come in many sizes and shapes. When decision making occurs it is bound to include variations depending upon the people involved, the context of the decision making, and the history that the individuals as individual and individuals as a family/group bring to the decision-making process. The Alzheimer's Association is an obvious resource for more formal material. One helpful preparatory action for some families is to be informed about how other persons managed similar circumstances. A variety of products are available that provide a translation of relevant issues into a discussion of practical approaches. Personal stories are available (Alzheimer's Disease, 2001; Alzheimer's support, 2001; ALZwell, 2001), some books provide detailed narration (Akin, 2000; Bayley, 1999; Mace & Rabins, 1999; Wright, 1993), and shorter examples as well as interactive discussions can be accessed through the Internet (Hart, 1997). A most engaging version of a woman coping with her mother's AD comes from the gifted Amy Tan. Although not strictly autobiographical, *The Bonesetter's Daughter* incorporates portions of Tan's and her mother's experiences with AD through the fictionalized settings and events of Ruth Young's family in her novel.

The most practical approach to decision making in AD would seem to result in a combination of preparing formal documents such as an advance directive or living will, along with the important appointment of a durable power of attorney (legal representative) for decision making about health care, together with ongoing discussions about preferences and values (Emanuel, 1994). For individuals physically living together, this might occur more regularly than those separated by geographical distances. However, telephone, E-mail, and other communication devices do not preclude sharing important ideas related to care giving and care receiving in chronic disease, especially AD where incompetence will undoubtedly become an issue. Once the diagnosis of AD is made, maximizing the window of opportunity for autonomous decision making by the individual with the disease is imperative (Vollmann, 2001). In the early stages, people are likely to be able to understand the disease and its prognosis as well as to determine their preferred treatment, and select a surrogate decision maker if one has not already been named.

❧ The Relevance of Competency

Caregivers must guard against premature assessments of incompetence based on depression, which could be treated, or other responses that are the result of patients' frustration, rather than the progression of the disease (Sabat, 1998, 2001). Even when language skills deteriorate, Sabat implemented strategies enhancing the person's ability to recover words and expressions. He labeled this communication tactic "the intentional stance." He uses the example of a woman, emphasizing that her interlocutor had to "position as someone who was indeed trying to communicate something intelligible, engage her with a readiness to understand, and provide her with feedback which indicated to her that he was actively involved in conversation" (2001, p. 85). Time consuming though this may be, meaningful communication can slow the downward spiraling of the patient's persona resulting from a cycle of inability to express one's self, impatience by listeners, anger and frustration from a lack of their understanding, and increased anxiety when the next opportunity to speak arises. With the promise of successful communication, alertness and energy are engendered, which decrease anxiety and promote the ability to share ideas and emotions. All of this serves to enable the patient with AD to continue to make known values, preferences, and expectations.

In any case, the incompetence portion of the process is the challenging part. Written documents can offer evidence of some thought on these matters as a starting point when decisions about health care are required. But where to go next? May (1998) examined competency and its relationship to autonomy in order to make a recommendation that fell between a free-rein option to abide by the preferences of the patient regardless of the reason and "objective" standards that may remove decision making from the person's preferences and values. He argued that the quality or the merit of the decision itself should not be a determining factor. Others agree (Vollmann, 2001). Instead, given the unique circumstances of the decision-making process, goals, and limitations under a specific set of circumstances, he recommended viewing each situation in light of the patient's preferences and values. Such an approach would result in a balanced decision between free-rein choices and the use of some objective standard to evaluate an individual's choices. Blustein (1999) seems to agree, but puts the process in the context of "continuing the life story" of the individual who has become incompetent. He places trust and responsibility in the hands of proxy decision makers for those who have lost their narrative capacity. Those who know the self-definition of the person and her or his interests can continue the story by making treatment decisions that cohere with the direction of the life story insofar as this can be ascertained. Post and Whitehouse (1995) would call this respect for choice—respect that is accompanied by a concomitant obligation to examine risks inherent in the choice. One would also need to differentiate clearly between high and low risks related to the available options.

❦ The Significance of Decision-making Theory

If we are to understand health care choices in the context of AD, we also need to address the relevance of theory in the decision-making process. These individuals are not likely to integrate sophisticated, complex ethical theories and philosophical principles in their decision-making process nor use them to defend their judgments. Holmes (1990) disagrees with the strategy of taking isolated principles and theories and attempting to use them objectively to solve ethical dilemmas. In his analysis, when this approach is used, it is often a prop, not a rigorous, nonobjective method of problem solving. Instead he finds that philosophical arguments often are used to support a position already held by its proponent, rather than an individual using theories and principles to solve a dilemma impartially. Holmes also cautions that a theoretical/principled approach often fails to include the broader social, cultural, and historical contexts in which bioethical issues actually reside. These latter aspects must be included because those most affected by the decision must be able to live with the outcome.

Another dimension of decision making to consider as we examine the decisions relative to advance directives affirms the above philosophical critique from a second perspective. Langer (1994) examined decision making as a psychologist. Based on her research, decision making is not objective, regardless of how it might be developed or perceived. At first, options generally appear to be more or less equal when the decision maker is personally faced with a dilemma and the need to make a decision. When this conflict occurs, information must be gathered until one option begins to distinguish itself from all of the others. However, options actually considered by the decision maker are not *all* the possible options, or even more limited, viable options are not *all* possible options. The particular set of options that are initially examined in the decision-making process may only encompass a set of acceptable options for that individual.

For example, Langer tells us that when we walk into an ice-cream store attempting to assuage our need for something sweet, all flavors that are for sale are not viable options—they are not considered within a range of possible outcomes for our decision making. We arrive at the store with a set of options already reduced by personal values and past experiences. For instance, the buyer might never consider sherbets as a choice; or the ice cream may have to contain nuts to be acceptable. As one gathers information about the acceptable flavors for sale that day, one option begins to distinguish itself, to stand out from all the others. When this option becomes sufficiently prominent to the buyer, the decision maker then makes a "cognitive commitment" to the selected flavor. Subsequently, the individual will conduct a cost/profit analysis or a risk/benefit analysis and/or develop a formal rationale for the decision in order to support it. Once the analysis is done or the rationale is identified, then decision making is complete. Both of these commentaries on decision making draw our attention to the importance of those values, beliefs, traditions, experiences, and histories that individuals and families bring to their health care experiences and decisions. Ethically responsive health care professionals acknowledge and respect those elements as they work through the decision-making process with families in the course of caring for the patient with AD.

Health care situations in which AD plays a role will only increase in the future. Both the lay public and health professionals need to prepare prospectively for circumstances in which they will be involved in decision making—either with or for the person with AD—including decisions related to palliative care. Education will play a profound role in this process as evidenced by the caregiver's letter in this chapter as she considered the various decisions she would have to make (see the chapters by Furlong and Scheirton). Understanding by and collaboration with professionals are essential ingredients for the decision-making process, including a deep appreciation for the family's perspective. Such appreciation begins with a recognition of the individuality and needs of the caregivers, who (unlike Michael's wife) in reality are not nameless, invisible creatures, ready and willing to assume around-the-clock responsibility. Decision making must encompass the entire context of the situation, including the caregivers' own lives as they care for those with AD.

REFERENCES

The references are divided into two parts—"Part 1: The Letter" and "Part 2: Discussion." Specific locations for citations to material in the letter are available from the author. Some of the same references are also used later in the chapter. Part 2 of the references consists only of those sources used in addition to the ones listed for part 1.

Part 1: The Letter

Abel, E. K., & Nelson, M. K. (1990). Circles of care: An introductory essay. In E. K. Abel & M. K. Nelson (Eds.), *Circles of care: Work and identity in women's lives* (pp. 4–34). Albany: State University of New York Press.

Ainslie, N., & Beisecker, A. E. (1994). Changes in decisions by elderly persons based on treatment description. *Archives of Internal Medicine, 154* (19), 2225–2233.

Blackhall, L. J., Murphy, S. T., Frank, G., Michel, V., & Azen, S. (1995). Ethnicity and attitudes towards patient autonomy. *Journal of the American Medical Association 274* (10), 820–825.

Bradley, E. H., Peiris, V., & Wetle, T. (1998). Discussions about end-of-life in nursing homes. *Journal of the American Geriatrics Society, 46* (10), 1235–1241.

Connell, C. M., & Gallant, M. P. (1996). Spouse caregivers' attitudes toward obtaining a diagnosis of a dementing illness. *Journal of the American Geriatrics Society, 44* (8), 1003–1009.

Drickamer, M. A., & Lachs, M. S. (1992). Should patients with Alzheimer's disease be told their diagnosis? *New England Journal of Medicine, 326* (14), 947–951.

Drickamer, M. A., & Lachs, M. S. (1993). Telling the diagnosis of Alzheimer's disease [Response to a letter to the editor]. *New England Journal of Medicine, 328* (10), 736.

Freedman, M. L. (1996). Should Alzheimer's disease patients be allowed to drive? A medical, legal, and ethical dilemma. *Journal of the American Geriatrics Society, 44,* 876–877.

Holstein, M. B. (1998). Ethics and Alzheimer's disease: Widening the lens. *Journal of Clinical Ethics, 9* (1), 13–22.

Hurley, A. C., Volicer, L., Rempusheski, V. F., & Fry, S. T. (1995). Reaching consensus: The process of recommending treatment decisions for Alzheimer's patients. *Advances in Nursing Science, 18* (2), 33–43.

In re Christopher. (1998). New York Supplement, 2d series, *675* (21 May), 807–810.

In re Gordy. (1994). Atlantic Reporter, 2d Series. *658* (30 December), 613–619.

In re Martin. (1995). North Western Reporter, 2d Series. *538* (22 August), 399–420.

Maguire, C. P., Kirby, M., Coen, R., Coakley, D., Lawlor, B. A., & O'Neill, D. (1996). Family members' attitudes toward telling the patient with Alzheimer's disease their diagnosis. *British Medical Journal, 313,* 529–530.

Markle, G. B. (1993). Telling the diagnosis of Alzheimer's disease [Letter to the editor]. *New England Journal of Medicine, 328* (10), 736.

Meyers, B. (1997). Telling patients they have Alzheimer's disease. *British Medical Journal, 314,* 321–22.

Mezey, M., Kluger, M., Maislin, G., & Mittelman, M. (1996). Life-sustaining treatment decisions by spouses of patients with Alzheimer's disease. *Journal of the American Geriatrics Society, 44* (2), 144–150.

Miles, S. H., & August, A. (1990). Courts, gender and the "right to die." *Law, Medicine, and Health Care, 18* (1 and 2), 85–95.

Miller, D. L., Jahnigen, D. W., Gorbien, M. J., & Simbartl, L. (1992.) Cardiopulmonary resuscitation: How useful? Attitudes and knowledge of an elderly population. *Archives of Internal Medicine, 152* (3), 578–582.

Pinch, W. J., & Parsons, M. E. (1992). The patient self-determination act: The ethical dimensions. *Nurse Practitioner Forum, 3* (1), 16–22.

Pollard, R. (2001). In pursuit of the unknown: Seeking an answer to Alzheimer's. *Bostonia,* (2), 20–24.

Post, S. G. (1998). The fear of forgetfulness. *Journal of Clinical Ethics, 9* (1), 71–80.

Post, S. G., & Whitehouse, P. J. (1995). Fairhill guidelines on ethics of the care of people with Alzheimer's disease. *Journal of the American Geriatrics Society, 43,* 1423–1429.

Silberfeld, M., Grundstein-Amado, R., Stephens, D., & Deber, R. (1996). Family and physicians' of surrogate decision-making: The roles and how to choose. *International Psychogeriatrics, 8* (4), 589–596.

Solomon, M. Z., O'Donnell, L., Jennings, B., Guilfoy, V., Wolf, S. M., Nolan, K., et al. (1993). Decisions near the end of life: Professional views on life sustaining treatments. *American Journal of Public Health, 83* (1), 14–23.

Part 2: Discussion

Akin, C. A. (2000). *The long road called goodbye: Tracing the course of Alzheimer's.* Omaha, NE: Creighton University Press.

Alzheimer's disease message board. (2001). www.healthboards.com/alzheimer's (retrieved August 17, 2001).

Alzheimer's support community chat. (2001). http://content.communities.msn.com (retrieved August 17, 2001).

ALZwell caregiver stories. (2001). www.alzwell.com/Thisweek.html; 22 June (retrieved August 17, 2001).

American Hospital Association. (1991). Preparing for advanced directives (video broadcast and resource book). Chicago: Author.

American Medical Association. EPEC Project, (1999). *Education for physicians on end-of-life care.* Chicago: Author.

Annas, G. J. (1995). Patients' rights: Origin and nature of patients' rights, In W. T. Reich (Ed.), *Encyclopedia of Bioethics* (pp. 1925–1927). New York: Simon & Schuster Macmillan.

Bayley, J. (1999). *Elegy for Iris.* New York: St. Martin's Press.

Blustein, J. (1999). Choosing for others as continuing a life story: The problem of personal identity revisited. *Journal of Law, Medicine & Ethics, 27,* 20–31.

Carlsen, M. S., Pomeroy, C., & Moldow, D. G. (1998). Optimizing discussion about resuscitation: Development of a guide based on patients' recommendations. *Journal of Clinical Ethics, 9* (3), 263–272.

Dressler, R. (2001). Advance directives in dementia research. *IRB: Ethics & Human Research, 23* (1), 1–6.

Emanuel, L. (1994). Appropriate and inappropriate use of advance directives. *Journal of Clinical Ethics, 5* (4), 357–359.

Emanuel, L. L., & Emanuel, E. J. (1989). The meal directive: A new comprehensive advance care document. *Journal of the American Medical Association, 261,* 3288–3293.

Grady, D. (20 January 2000). Calls growing for stopping tube feeding in dementia. *New York Times* http://query.nytimes.com/gst/abstract.html?res=F30A14FD3E590C7 38EDDA.

Griffith, C. H., Wilson, J. F., Emmett, K. R., Ramsbottom-Lucier, M., & Rich, E. C. (1995). Knowledge and experience with Alzheimer's disease. *Archives of Family Medicine, 4,* 780–784.

Hague, S. B., & Moody, L. E. (1993). A study of the public's knowledge regarding advance directives. *Nursing Economic$, 11* (5), 303–307, 323.

Hart, M. (1997). My journal. Re: Development of Alzheimer's. Claude Hart. www.virtuallawoffice.com/journal.html (retrieved March 22, 2001).

High, D. M. (1992). Research with Alzheimer's disease subjects: Informed consent and proxy decision making. *Journal of the American Geriatrics Society, 40,* 950–957.

Holm, S. (2001). Autonomy, authenticity, or best interest: Everyday decision-making and persons with dementia. *Medicine, Health Care and Philosophy, 4*, 153–159.

Holmes, R. L. (1990). The limited relevance of analytical ethics to the problems of bioethics. *Journal of Medicine and Philosophy, 15* (2), 143–159.

Holzman, I. R. (1999). The horns of the dilemma are sharp. *Cambridge Quarterly of Healthcare Ethics, 8* (4), 480–484.

Langer, E. (1994). The illusion of calculated decisions. In R. C. Schank & E. Langer (Eds.), *Beliefs, reasoning, and decision making: Psycho-logic in honor of Bob Abelson* (pp. 33–53). Hillsdale, NJ: Lawrence Erlbaum.

Lee, M. A., Smith, D. M., Fenn, D. S., & Ganzini L. (1998). Do patients' treatment decisions match advance statements of their preferences? *Journal of Clinical Ethics, 9* (3), 258–262.

Mace, N. L. & Rabins, P. V. (1999). *The 36-hour day: A family guide to persons with Alzheimer disease, related dementing illnesses, and memory loss in later life.* Baltimore: Johns Hopkins University Press.

May, T. (1998). Assessing competency without judging merit. *Journal of Clinical Ethics, 9* (3), 247–257.

Patterson, S. L., Baker, M., & Maeck, J. P. (1993). Durable powers of attorney: Issues of gender and health care decision-making. *Journal of Gerontological Social Work, 21* (1 and 2), 161–177.

Sabat, S. R. (1998). Voices of Alzheimer's disease sufferers: A call for treatment based on personhood. *Journal of Clinical Ethics, 9* (1), 35–48.

Sabat, S. R. (2001). *The experience of Alzheimer's disease: Life through a tangled veil.* Malden, MA: Blackwell.

Sehgal, A., Galbraith, A., Chesney, M., Schoenfeld, P., Charles, G., & Lo, B. (1992). How strictly do dialysis patients want their advance directives followed? *Journal of the American Medical Association, 267* (1), 9–63.

Tan, A. (2001). *The bonesetter's daughter.* New York: G. P. Putman's Sons.

Teno, J. M., Licks, S., Lynn, J., Wenger, N., Connors, A. F., Phillips, R. S., et al. (1997). Do advance directives provide instruction that direct care? *Journal of the American Geriatrics Society, 45* (4), 508–512.

Teno, J. M., & Lynn, J. (1996). Putting advance-care planning into action. *Journal of Clinical Ethics, 7* (3), 205–213.

Vollmann, J. (2001). Advance directives in patients with Alzheimer's disease: Ethical and clinical considerations. *Medicine, Health Care and Philosophy, 4*, 161–167.

Wright, L. K. (1993). *Alzheimer's disease and marriage: An intimate account.* Newbury Park, CA: Sage.

Zerwekh, J. V. (1997). Do dying patients really need IV fluids? *American Journal of Nursing, 97* (3), 26–31.

CHAPTER TWELVE

Saying No to Patients with Alzheimer Disease

Rethinking Relations among Personhood, Autonomy, and World

Franz J. Illhardt, D.D., Ph.D.

During a geriatric symposium at Freiburg University, a visiting theologian introduced his lecture with the remark that he liked to be invited to Freiburg because of the chance to visit his elderly father, who had dementia and lived in a nursing home nearby. These social contacts were highly important for the dignity of his father because a person with dementia has only the dignity we give him in social contact (Ritschl, 1993). We should not forget that dignity is not, or at least not only, a trait of the person as an "object" of care, but a trait of the caregiver as well. By way of comparison, a veterinarian alleviating the pain of a dog acts in accordance with human dignity, not the dog's dignity, because the vet realizes his own human character by relieving the pain. Some argue that the vet's actions should be undertaken to honor the dog's dignity, but I propose that it is for the veterinarian's own dignity that the action should be undertaken. Therefore, the most important issue is not whether we attribute dignity to a patient with Alzheimer disease (AD). When we do not care for these poor persons appropriately, we lose our own dignity (Thomasma, 1986).

These facts present crucial questions for our society in regard to AD: the late onset of AD after fifty years of age; the increasing number of afflicted persons (Larsson, 1993); the average duration of patients' lives (6.1 years for patients at home or in ordinary nursing homes and 8.2 years for those in special care units

(Lynn et al., 1999). The increasing span of life, and contemporaneously the threat of dementia, demands solutions for the maintenance and enhancement of the quality of life. Further, "societies are just beginning to define and deal with the challenges" (Lynn et al., 1999, p. 271); in other words, societies are not yet familiar with solving these problems.

In the first phases (neurological impairment) of AD, communication is, of course, possible, but the worse the dementia becomes the more difficult each kind of controlled action becomes. The word *interaction* suggests that both the patient and the caregiver are acting. Can the interaction of an AD patient and a healthy person be balanced? Interaction means that actions are balanced and part of a network—the one is the precondition of the other. Interaction includes our preferences, value judgements, and priorities; therefore the first step is never to begin with hard and set rules.

A journalist meeting people with dementia for the first time wrote, "I was angry about the inconceivable. I could not cope with that. Until I learned that they laughed when I laughed, that they were pleased when I was pleased, and that their babbling was not shocking, but their last possibility of expression" (Jürgs, 2001, p. 275). Thus, to measure autonomy as an inner characteristic is not the most important task of caring for AD patients; instead, it is to support the interaction that makes their autonomy possible.

✢ Saying No as a Symbol of Setting Limits

Caregivers of patients with AD often face the conflict that they must stop the patient from doing something that appears to be silly, such as knocking, moving around restlessly, and so forth. Professional caregivers would say no only when the strange behavior is a burden to others. The dilemma arises when there is risk for the AD patient herself. For example, a patient with AD trying to leave the chair while the nurse makes up her bed could, without support and control, fall and break legs, arms, or a hip. Should the nurse take this risk or should she set limits? She may decide in the best interest of the patient, but in doing so she is very likely to limit the patient's freedom.

In weighing risks and benefits, the caregiver must recognize that for the AD patient, moving is one of the most important things in the world. The patient will never understand the benefit of this *no* since it limits her expression. Her development will decrease, not increase. Further, the argument that the caregiver's intent to provide care is more valuable than the patient's intent to move about depends on one's perspective, not on a moral discourse, because the patient cannot participate in this discourse. Before saying no, the caregiver must differentiate between important and less important or unimportant actions of the patient. Being trained, ready, and sensitive to question which actions support, rather than limit, a patient's autonomy is a hallmark of professional behavior (Zsolnay-Wildgruber, 1997). It should be a therapeutic principle of nursing homes that injuries for the patient are not as bad as the violation of their freedom (Crabtree, 1994; Schützendorf & Wallrafen-Dreisow, 1998).

Saying no has many repercussions. We know from transaction analysis that the word *no* is not only a cognitive judgment of the facts but also a judgment on the relationship (e.g., that I am right while the other is not). Whatever someone wants to say when saying no, she must be aware that this simple word can include a personal judgment about the other. *No* can refer to the existence of things. It can also refer to how things "ought" not to be. In everyday life, we often muddle the one with the other level (e.g., observe that something is not the case and then derive the norm that it *ought* not to be the case to do something from that). The philosopher David Hume drew attention to this difference of *is* and *ought*. Ethicists call this confusion the "naturalistic fallacy." People with dementia cannot differentiate between these two levels of reality; thus, for them, *no* is never factual—the world of facts is too complicated for them, but always prohibitive and a personal judgement. Gerontological psychiatry gives us some rules to guide communication and action. They describe the special problem in caring for an AD patient who may not understand what we do or say as another patient might. These guidelines are:

1. Differentiate avoidable and unavoidable risks.
2. Help the patient to live in a world that is simple and easy to control.
3. Guarantee constancy in their life and contacts.
4. Avoid simultaneously talking to, touching, and glancing at the patient.
5. Avoid saying no; rather, try to distract the patient's risky ideas and impulses.
6. Try physical gestures rather than words.
7. Allow small competitions between patients, rather than segregating demented and nondemented persons.
8. Restrain the patient as little as possible.

9. Even in advanced phases of dementia, support learning in a setting of calmness and clarity of instruction.

10. Relate new experiences to pleasant sensual and emotional stimuli. (Bruder, 1996)

Some of these rules aim directly at the problem of saying no; others do it indirectly, but refer to it. A major problem of AD is the fact that in "normal" diseases, we can understand the situation of the patient (e.g., we know the biomedical mechanisms—or if not, we state the multifactorial genesis of the disease) and can feel with the patient's problems. Not with AD.

❦ Coherence—Personhood—Dementia

Especially in the treatment of persons with dementia, for caregivers to say yes and to do no creates a feeling of widespread incoherence and confusion. The principle of beneficence requires empathy for the inner situation of an incompetent patient. Coherence in a formally understood fashion (i.e., the correspondence of judgment and reality) does not take into account the challenge of empathy in this type of situation.

What do we mean by coherence on the part of the caregiver? Authenticity is more important than mere consistency. To be authentic means to be a unique, acting person in one's own view as well as in other's. Whatever this coherent person does, she does not do it simply as part of a professional role-expectation, but due to a conviction that has its roots in thoughtfulness rather than in adherence to rules. Naturally, such a person can say and must say no sometimes. But the caregiver's coherence makes her an authentic advocate only as long as she can truly accept the demented patient; otherwise, she is not abiding by the therapeutic covenant. The coherent caregiver never uses the word *no* in circumstances that reject the person. This very difficult task may be a reason for the widespread burnout in nursing homes that serve a high percentage of residents with dementia.

Second, what do we mean by coherence on the part of the people with dementia? It is most useful to understand *coherence* according to A. Antonowsky's theory of salutogenesis. He explains this sense as the basic feeling that all things that happen make sense, have a connection with other events in life, and thus produce health. Patients with AD have difficulty making such sense; nor are they

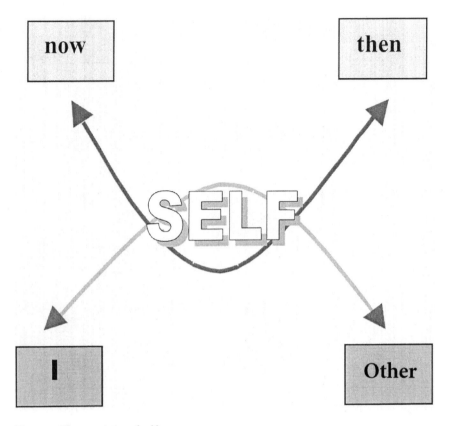

Fig. 12.1. Characteristics of self

healthy in this regard. Because AD patients cannot have this sense, we must pay attention to it and take care that the events that happen to these patients fit together (Antonowsky, 1981).

When Stephen Post differentiates between the "then" self and the "now" self, he requires that we weigh autonomy more for oneself than the other (Binstock, Post, & Whitehouse, 1992). He does seem to suppose a coherence between then and now—at least as a narrative identity referring to events from the patient's life. He pleads for the preference of the then-self over the now-self when a patient's recognition of loved ones declines and aphasia increases. Reflecting on the problem of advance directives, he argues against Dresser & Whitehouse (1994), who hold that the patient's awareness of actual quality of life, however small, has a high value. Post (1995) agrees, of course, but in the case of an absolute lack of communication and participation in the present, he wants to return to the then-self, who "in better times" determined not to enhance the treatment or to prolong the end of life.

Post's conclusion is problematic. As Welie points out in chapter 10, who am I to judge what is more important: the present or the past, the now-self or the then-self? We are never entitled to assess the degree and actuality of autonomy because we cannot quantify quality or measure the unmeasurable. We only are entitled to *support* autonomy and/or create it if it is destroyed or weakened. This approach and this alone can be termed "shared autonomy." Post does not go far enough. We will never succeed in striking an appropriate balance between the two states of the AD patient, the then-state and the now-state, for this assessment would require a superbrain and a neutrality that does not prefer "now" or "then." Either is illusionary. Post's solution disregards three important points:

1. Only a person who lives in the present ("now") can know what he experienced in the past ("then"), but not vice versa. Thus, this differentiation contributes nothing to the solution.

2. Any tourist may find that the most beautiful places in the world can be awful places if the first person he meets is unfriendly and cold. This is also true for AD: reality is not a matter of facts but a matter of relationships.

3. A person's autonomy does not result from a steady state of autonomy, but only from the continuity of different states. In the case of a demented patient, autonomy reflects the coherence of the "then" and the "now," of the ego and of the other.

The configuration of coherence must be taken seriously. The lines overlap and form a center of personal acts that I call self, displayed in figure 12.1.

The difference between my scheme and Post's model is that the self is not a state, bound to one dissolving ego, or replaced by others. The self is displayed by the configuration of coherence. That means a person's self is not "this" or "that" but a network and intersection of the different states and relationships. All involved in this intersection have to care for the self, not assess it. This approach is true especially for the caregivers of patients with AD. They interact in this intersection; the self is a result of interaction. The Czechoslovakian novelist Milan Kundera describes the story of his father:

During the last ten years of his life he lost his faculty of speech step by step. First he only could not remember some words or he replaced them by others, similar ones, and afterwards laughed immediately. But when the end of his life came closer, he could say only a very few words. Things lost their names and were amalgamated into a mere being without distinction. And it was I alone who could change for moments this nameless infinite into a world of named things, when I spoke with him . . . Thus, we spoke about music [Kundera's father was a musicologist], but it was a strange conversation between someone who did not know anything [of music], but knew many words, and one, who knew everything [of music], but actually did not know any words. (Kundera, 1978, p. 217)

The intersecting lines of coherence are the only possible basis of a "communicative ethics" (Moody, 1992). At a fundamental level, communication does not require competence or balance, but mutual respect. This is very similar to the concept of ethics based on "consensual standards" (i.e., a valid decision can never be made in a paternalistic way by one professional alone, but must be a consensual assessment of several persons concerned with the AD patient and the various perspectives involved) (Dresser & Whitehouse, 1994). To consider the ethical challenges of AD without the importance of the social surroundings means to overlook the role of others and to overlook our feelings of being close to someone and "also how we defer from them" (Lynn et al., 1999).

Wicclair interprets this configuration by requiring that decisions of cognitively impaired persons that are "consistent with core preferences and values . . . prior to the onset of mental deterioration" be respected (Wicclair, 1993, p. 143). For these decisions "in character"—in contrast to those that do not fit in the patient's character—we need experience of the patients' preferences and values, their biographic curriculum, their "Sitz im Leben," the ideas of other caregivers, and so forth.

AD challenges the Western understanding of a person and her illness. Subjectivity is the only really decisive criterion of personality. The Christian religion offers, instead of this criterion, belief in, and salvation by, God (i.e., the belief that someone, whatever the status of her competence, is a human being and a person loved by God). Close to this idea is the concept of care ethics of W. T. Reich (Jecker & Reich, 1995).

The same perspective in a surprising turn is expressed in what the South

American poet Gabriel García Márquez has the Roman Catholic cardinal say to the earl whose daughter has been bitten by a rabid dog. The cardinal suspects that the girl is possessed and calls for the father. The father confesses his difficulties with faith, and the cardinal replies: "Así que lo esencial no es que tú no creas, sino que Dios siga creyendo en tí" ("What is essential is not that you do not believe, but that God continues believing in you") (1994, p. 67). Thus it is not the activity of the ego that matters but the trust of others in the disabled ego. Not only do I create the world but the world also creates me—a perspective that the bioethical contributions to the AD problem lack.

Especially in eastern parts of the world, but also in European medieval times, a human being is/was a person because of his place in the social environment— because a human being is only a person within the family, the clan, the tradition, the Christian community and so forth. "Place in the social environment" is totally different from the Darwinist pattern of "social utility," because the latter thinks in terms of cost-benefit, the former in terms of the person's living with others. Thus, we have a problem treating an AD patient as a "person" when understanding a personhood only through individuality, subjectivity, and so forth, as does the European Enlightenment of the eighteenth century. But personhood can be explained differently.

The French philosopher Maurice Merleau-Ponty (1973, 1945) holds the following criteria for being a person: (1) bodily extension that can be perceived; (2) being perceived by others; and (3) being self-conscious about both of these. This existence transcends the body and views the body *être-au-monde*. It is a body with a living soul that is perceiving as well as being perceived. Personhood can be realized only through relationships, thus interaction is essential.

Those who live with AD patients can observe that the patients lose the opportunity to have fun and lose interest when they cannot anticipate any valuable or meaningful activity. Recall the book later made into a film of the neurologist Oliver Sacks, *Awakenings* (1990). A young doctor has found that the drug L-dopa works with the demented inhabitants of a New York nursing home who have been diagnosed "state after meningitis." This doctor observes an old man catching a ball that threatened to hit him or an old lady catching her falling glasses, whereas, for the most part, they sit apathetically. The doctor comments to his medical colleagues that the patients may borrow their will (their autonomy) from the object. The colleagues leave the room because they have never heard such a medicine-free explanation in medicine. If we transfer this case to AD, we can ask, "Isn't it possible that AD patients borrow their personhood from the people around them?"

❧ The Crisis of Autonomy

What do we mean by autonomy? Someone who determines not to be autonomous is autonomous, but someone who is autonomous without having others recognize it is not autonomous. Thus, the *differentia specifica* is the recognition. Thomasma lays out a more differentiated autonomy:

1. Freedom from obstacles
2. Freedom as knowing one's options
3. Freedom as choosing
4. Freedom as acting
5. Freedom as creating new options (Crabtree, 1994, p. 184).

These five freedoms of autonomy may be assessed differently according to the state of dementia, whether limited to neurological or expanded to further central or peripheral bodily and psychological functions. Thus, nobody can assess clearly what autonomy does mean for a patient with AD, but we know that autonomy is more than a check list of psychological skills. Rather, it is (1) relationship; (2) interest in the surrounding world of things and of persons; and (3) the ability to contact them. The caregiver's problem is not to assess whether there are symptoms of autonomy. The caregiver's task is to assist the patient by relating to her, to foster her interest in the surrounding world of things and persons and her readiness to contact them. Thus, assisted autonomy means

1. protection by "appropriate democratic governance of a nursing home"
2. "facilitation of a better understanding" of patient's rights and freedoms
3. "fostering of a supportive environment" for persons with dementia (Crabtree, 1994, p. 185)

Some years ago, the psychiatrist J. Bauer shocked his German colleagues with the hypothesis that vascular dementias as well as the dementia of Alzheimer type have their origin in a crisis of autonomy. The vascular dementias stem from the loss of control over the world around oneself (e.g., children leave the house; loss of a spouse; retirement; etc.). In other words, in the case of AD, because of steadily being humiliated or experiencing flops and failures, there is the loss of feeling that oneself is a valuable and important person (Bauer, Qualmann, & Bauer, 1995). This study has been criticized because it was a pilot, not followed by a major study. But beyond what causes dementia, the question is raised as to whether (to use Crabtree's words) we foster an environment that supports autonomy or render living autonomously more difficult. We know that autonomy can be corrupted in many events of our lives, but we fail to consider the problems of autonomy in the parent-child relationship, in friendship, in marriage, in relationship to working colleagues, and so forth. The education for and refinement of everyday autonomy seems a marginal theme in public life. The price is an increasing number of people who must fade from a world that is not theirs.

The crisis of control is a very important feature of autonomy. One can define control as "the perception that one can take charge of what happens in one's life" (Lachman, Ziff, & Spiro, 1994, p. 216). The problem for the patient of hearing *no* is because the ability to control is so essential. Control provides an opportunity for internal mastery that should not be separated from types of social supports that are provided by others (Lachman, Ziff, & Spiro, 1994). It embraces the consciousness of which things are connected to one's life and one's reaction to this understanding. It does not mean adequacy as judged by others. Communication in this context is most significant because autonomy as human dignity is not a trait. It is, rather, a result of interaction. I give an example: Some years ago, I visited an elderly couple in a nursing home and talked with the wife. Her husband, an AD patient, sat to one side and played with her jewelry box, which was standing on the table. During our conversation, she looked at him and protested now and then, saying, "Josef, stop it." She didn't succeed in stopping him. So, I repeated loudly, distinctly, and a little bit more sharply, "Josef, stop it." I, too, did not succeed. This behavior seemed to me to be a protest as if he were saying, "Be aware that I am also here, what you are saying does not reach me." When I was considering this episode later, I understood my reaction as supportive of the wife—but was it supportive of the husband? His aggressive reaction seemed undoubtedly to show that he was not interested in my presence and conversation. The social correctness of persons who do not have AD prohibits the straightforward conduct of patients and makes communication a struggle of social power,

TABLE 12.1. Characteristics of Persons with and without Alzheimer Disease

Expected Characteristics of Persons with AD	Expected Characteristics of Persons without AD
Divided (then-now / I-other) state of the patient	Structure of the "multiple personality" (everybody varies in roles and states of self)
Special vulnerability of impaired persons	As a healthy structure, largely invulnerable
Overwhelmed by social stress, failure, disappointment, etc.	Masters situations of social stress, failure, disappointment, etc.
Inappropriate behavior (sexual, aggressive, disturbing, and other actions in public) expected	Sudden inappropriate emotions are controlled
Unpredictability of patient's reaction	Expected to behave predictably according to good boy / nice girl patterns

rather than an opportunity for honesty and the real need to be genuinely included.

A further aspect of this story is that the husband was a good and hardworking craftsman who twice tried, but failed, to establish his own company. His wife told me that he suffered from her being intellectually superior to him. She was proud of it. It is easy to understand his becoming aggressive when he saw me (an intellectual) talking and interacting with his (intellectual) wife, not with him. He did not have this insight at the cortical level, but felt it at the level of Post's "then-self."

Some informational materials coming from centers for those concerned with dementia or their burned-out relatives are focused on shaping smooth communication and preventing "negative" reactions. Saying no can be such a dangerous communication. "Use only affirmative sentences" (Alzheimer Europe, 1999, p. 16) is a variation of this advice. Existence needs affirmation. Nonetheless, coexistence requires limits—and, somehow ridiculously, limits against other people (the other as an enemy) because of their so-called right to their privacy. Dealing with AD means rather to deal with a world in which smooth communication and affirmation, which flow from empathy, are expected.

❧ "Time Deferred": A Dichotomy of Worlds

Diachronic (from the Greek for "time deferred") means that the care for AD patients begins with the dichotomy of the caregiver's and the patient's worlds. From this dichotomy follows the necessity to act from one's own world into the strange one of the patient. Each bioethical guideline has to reflect this difference. Some of the guidelines mentioned above (e.g., those covering the process of learning) are less important in the last phases of AD, such as the terminal phase. These guidelines must consider the differences between the caregiver world and patient world if they are to be meaningful in this concrete situation.

Saying no can mean, as for instance with young people, that someone takes them very seriously; they experience limits in their contact with others and become sensitive to respecting their privacy. To the incompetent demented person, *no* signifies a divergence, a gap. We must take into account that persons with AD do not share the world with others (e.g., their caregivers act in one world and the patient shrinks ever further into a more cryptic world).

For example, a seventy-nine-year-old patient with AD in a nursing home fell and fractured his femur. In the hospital, the necessary surgery was performed. His son was appointed guardian, according to German law. In order to include his father in this strange world and to take away possible angry feelings, the son explained in very simple words to his father what had happened and what the physicians planned to do. The son knew that a dementia patient, in contrast to those who are depressed, are overwhelmed by new surroundings. The father, a soldier in World War II, replied to his son, "Yes, I have reported already." Obviously, the father lived in the military world of about fifty years ago, when he was young, healthy, well-oriented in a steadily changing surroundings, in a world of duty, superiors, law and order, unavoidable fear and suffering.

Why are we fixed on the perspective that the patient is distorted from the correct view of the world? There is no need to defend the one (right) against the other (wrong) perspective. It is not "our" ethos that is questioned, but our ability to meet the reality of the patient. Since bioethics requires caregivers to "meet patients as moral strangers" (Engelhardt, 1996, p. 80), and medicine becomes "stranger medicine," closeness appears to be beyond ethics and medicine. The AD diagnosis causes embarrassed and stony silence, but sometimes ignores the challenge of bridging the gap between the diseased person and the caregiver.

On November 5, 1994, the former U.S. president Ronald Reagan, an AD patient, wrote a letter to Americans. The last paragraph read: "I now begin the journey that will lead me into the sunset of my life. I know that for America, there will always be a bright dawn ahead" (Merki and Krämer, 2001, p. 47). Reagan's world and that of his countrymen are diachronic—the one going down, the other rising. Words from the one to the other must bridge this gap, but the word *no* mostly cannot succeed in bridging; instead, it sets new limits—more divergence.

❧ Reframing the Caregiver

There are basically two possibilities of how to react to the AD patient in her diachronic world: The first is to correct her or to express one's own confusion. Unquestionably, the patient cannot understand the correction that in her view comes from a strange world. Her disorder and angry feelings increase; the second possibility is to stay in the patient's world. At first glance, that seemingly can mean to admit lies and/or distortion of reality. Caregivers may feel as if they are accepting something that they consider wrong. To show the difference, consider that a lie gets its moral quality from the intention to put someone on the wrong track and to deceive her. The intention of the gerontopsychiatric caregivers is different. They intend to put the patient on the right track and accept the only way she can understand with good feelings.

To hold the idea of AD patients as inadequate and a symptom of a damaged brain is too simplistic even if one can find such concepts in some bioethical writing. Psychotherapy (Eckstein, 1997) as well as linguistics (Lincoln, 1997) offer helpful approaches in solving the distortion problem. An AD patient tells a story that seems strange and disoriented. We must acknowledge that reality is not only factual but also is constructed by people through their experiences, social surroundings, culture (including their spirituality), and so forth. We need to discuss theories of philosophic constructivism, but we should acknowledge the social and spiritual influence on the perception of reality.

This influence is also valid for AD. "Distorted" reality is also reality. But perhaps those who do not understand the strange uttering of the patient also suffer some distortion. Who is in prison—the gorilla in the zoo that is prevented from coming out or the visitors who are prevented from entering the enclosure? The answer depends on the perspective; it is not a question of reality. In the psychotherapeutic technique of "reframing," a therapist offers a new perspective to an irritable woman who suffers from the idea of having a dirty carpet: "Every footprint that appeared on the carpet was a sign that her loved ones were near, and that she was with her family" (Eckstein, 1997, p. 421). The psychotherapist did not convince her that her observation was wrong; instead, she supported the patient with ideas of closeness and warm feelings. The AD patient does not confront us with dirty carpets, but does present us with very similar problems.

The patient confronts us with a "symptom [that] has an existing function for the individual person," at least the function of understanding the world and feeling a part of it. The difference between the "normal" client of psychotherapy and the AD patient is the AD patient's failing memory, ability to learn, to plan, and to feel success. Whatever the neurological state of a feeling may be, the point is that every human being must have the chance to realize her potential. "The same is valid for deviant behavior whose ecological benefit is confirmed at first and thereafter may be replaced by attitudes used in a differentiated manner" (Margraf, 2000, p. 438).

To illustrate this, I will go back to the story of the patient who fractured his femur: The son supported his father's interpretation of the strange situation and pain through withdrawing to his fifty-year-old military world. The son did not correct his father by putting him on the "right" track of the "normal" world. His father would not have understood this correction, and his confusion would have increased. Of course, he did not say to his father, "Yes, Sir, stand down." One must not, after all, play theater, but should not send the patient into a situation that he can neither understand nor control (Lachman, Ziff, & Spiro, 1994). Consider the question of whether a mother who lies does so to comfort her baby, "Be quiet, it's all okay" (Berger & Luckmann, 1966). Newspapers tell us everyday that little is okay.

Why can saying no be a catastrophe for the dying AD patient? Saying no to the patient can become a catastrophe since it

1. limits the patient's autonomy
2. confuses the patient's place in the social world
3. rejects *the person* of the patient with AD

To prohibit the word *no* seems at first glance to be the sediment of "antiauthoritarian education." At second glance, we see the difference. The theory of education tried to set no limits on a child, but believed that the child will find and decide its own way and limits. The caregivers of the AD patient can be never sure which state of the self (then, now, I, other) the word *no* will address. Not knowing the consequence obliges caregivers to avoid saying no. Does this requirement tie the hands of caregivers? No, it demands that they explore the world of dementia patients—first of all, to make a value assessment (Sass, 1998; Thomsen et al., 1998; Illhardt, 2000). They need not discuss the issue of whether an AD patient's now-self is of greater value than her then-self or whether her I-self is more important than her other-self. No judgment facilitates the treatment decision, but observing the following steps may be helpful:

1. Gather all information on the different possible self-states of the person.
2. Be alert to the coherence of this information and avoid preference of one type of information over the other.
3. Explore whether the patient is giving any sign about which self-state she is in at any one moment. If there is a sign, act in accordance with its message.
4. Only in cases of emergency or unsolvable dilemmas can one decide as a surrogate and advocate of the person in the "best interest of the patient." (Kayser-Jones, 1993, p. 95)

Why must the dying AD patient be autonomous? Nobody should be hindered in becoming what she could be. Although "healthy" persons might think that they must decide for the patient, relieving her from all responsibility, this is not so. Claiming that the AD patient has no mental resources at her disposal would constitute prejudice and superficiality instead of careful scrutiny and thought. Rather than a substantial concept, autonomy is, in Merleau-Ponty's words, an être-au-monde.

Saying no is a symbol of communication. In the process of coping with patients with AD it always has the impact of being a prohibitive and personal judgment. One must analyze the world of AD patients as well as the state of one's own self. It is rather simplistic to state that the demented patient has lost the cortical functions that make rational communication possible. Communication is a mutual endeavor, and thus embraces states of now, then, I, and others. Basing caregivers' decisions on a process that excludes communication supports prejudices and superficial experience, instead of scrutinizing the experience. Autonomy is not a substantial concept; rather, it is an être-au-monde.

The integration of the dying AD patient into the network of communication and human solidarity is doubly problematic and meets double resistance: The dying person is beyond communication and a shared world of values, duties, empathy, and symbols. The AD patient appears to be an incompetent partner for communication. Autonomy is very important to patients in the last phases of the disease. At the first glance, it seems to be impossible for the caregiver to ease this phase while complying with the standards of palliative care (e.g., to act according to patient's wishes). Autonomy is "shared autonomy" based on sharing and understanding common worlds, symbols, values, and competence. This sharing applies to the so-called normal persons as well as to those with dementia. Thus, autonomy presents a chance also for the dying AD patient.

REFERENCES

Alzheimer Europe. (1999). *Handbuch der Betreuung und Pflege von Alzheimer-Patienten* [Manual for care and nursing of patients with Alzheimer's disease]. Stuttgart: G. Thieme. www.alzheimer-europe.org.

Antonovsky, A. (1987). *Unrevealing the mystery of health* (1st ed.). San Francisco: Jossey-Bass.

Bauer, J., Qualmann, J., & Bauer, H. (1995). Psychosomatische Aspekte bei der Alzheimer Demenz und bei vaskulären Demenzformen [Psychosomatic aspects of Alzheimer's disease and of vascular dementias]. In G. Heuft, A. Kruse, H. G. Nehen, & H. Radebold (Eds.), *Interdisziplinäre Gerontopsychosomatik* (pp. 214–228). München: MMV, Medizin-Verlag.

Berger, P. L., & Luckmann, T. (1966). *The social construction of reality: A treatise in the sociology of knowledge.* Garden City, NY: Doubleday.

Binstock, R. H., Post, S. G., & Whitehouse, P. J. (1992). The challenges of dementia. In R. H. Binstock, S. G. Post, & P. J. Whitehouse (Eds.), *Dementia and aging: Ethics, values, and policy choices* (pp. 1–17). Baltimore: Johns Hopkins University Press.

Bruder, J. (1996). Vergessen und Traurigkeit: Psychische Veränderungen im Alter [Forgetting and sadness: Psychological changes in aging]. In G. Naegele & A. Niederfranke (Eds.), *Funkkolleg Altern.* Studieneinheit 8. Tübingen: Deutsches Institut für Fernstudienforschung an der Universität Tübingen.

Crabtree, J. L. (1994). Autonomy of the elderly living in nursing homes. In J. F. Monagle & D. C. Thomasma (Eds.), *Health care ethics: Critical issues* (pp. 179–187). Gaithersburg, MD: Aspen.

Dresser, R., & Whitehouse, P. J. (1994). The incompetent patient on the slippery slope. *Hastings Center Report, 24* (4), 6–12.

Eckstein, D. (1997). Reframing as a specific interpretative counseling technique. *Individual Psychology, 53,* 418–428.

Engelhardt, H. T. (1996). *The foundations of bioethics* (2nd ed.). New York: Oxford University Press.

García Marquez, G. (1994). *Del amor y otros demonios* [On love and other demons]. Barcelona: Mondadori.

Illhardt, F. J. (2000). Grenzen therapeutischer und rehabilitativer Maβnahmen [Limits of therapeutic and rehabilitative interventions]. In T. Nikolaus (Ed.), *Klinische Geriatrie* (pp. 772–775). Heidelberg: Springer.

Jecker, N. S., & Reich, W. T. (1995). Contemporary ethics of care. In W. T. Reich (Ed.), *Encyclopedia of bioethics* (Rev. ed. Vol. 5) (pp. 336–344). New York: Macmillan / Simon & Schuster.

Jürgs, M. (2001). *Alzheimer: Spurensuche im Niemandsland* [Alzheimer: Searching for tracks in no man's land]. Munich: Econ/Ullstein/List.

Kayser-Jones, J. (1993). Surrogate decisions for nursing home residents. In G. R. Winslow & J. W. Walters (Eds.), *Ethics and health care for the elderly* (pp. 96–99). Boulder, CO: Westview Press.

Kundera, M. (1978). *Das Buch vom Lachen und Vergessen* [Book on laughing and forgetting]. *Roman*. (S. Roth, Trans.) Munich: Deutscher Taschenbuch Verlag.

Lachman, M. E., Ziff, M. A., & Spiro, A., III. (1994). Maintaining a sense of control in later life. In R. P. Abeles, H. C. Gift, & M. G. Ory (Eds.), *Aging and quality of life* (pp. 216–232). New York: Springer.

Larsson, E. B. (1993). Illnesses causing dementia in the very elderly. *New England Journal of Medicine, 328*, 203–205.

Lincoln, Y. S. (1997). Self, subject, audience, text: Living at the edge, writing in the margins. In W. G. Tierney & Y. S. Lincoln (Eds.), *Representation and the text: Re-framing the narrative voice* (pp. 37–55). New York: SUNY Press.

Lynn, J., Teno, J., Dresser, R., Brock, D., Nelson, H. L., Nelson, J. L., et al. (1999). Dementia and advance-care planning: Perspectives from three countries on ethics and epidemiology. *Journal of Clinical Ethics, 10*, 271–285.

Magraf, J. (2000). *Lehrbuch der Verhaltenstherapie* [Textbook of behavior therapy]. Vol. 1. Heidelberg: Springer.

Merki, K.-E., & Krämer, G. (2001): *Rückwärts! Und alles vergessen: Anna und Otto Nauer: Mit Alzheimer leben* [Backwards! And forgetting everything: Anna and Otto Nauer: Living with Alzheimer's disease]. Munich: Econ/Ullstein/List.

Merleau-Ponty, M. (1945). *Phénoménologie de la perception* [Phenomenology of perception]. Paris: Gallimard.

Merleau-Ponty, M. (1973). *L'oeil et l'esprit* [The eye and the mind]. Paris: Gallimard.

Moody, H. R. (1992). A critical view of ethical dilemmas in dementia. In R. H. Binstock, S. G. Post, & P. J. Whitehouse (Eds.), *Dementia and aging: Ethics, values, and policy choices* (pp. 86–100). Baltimore: Johns Hopkins University Press.

Post, S. G. (1995). Alzheimer disease and the "then" self. *Kennedy Institute of Ethics Journal, 5*, 307–321.

Ritschl, D. (1993). Alter und Gesellschaft [Aging and society]. In H. W. Heiss (Ed.), *Das Geriatrische Zentrum im Spannungsfeld der Vernetzungsaufgaben* (pp. 8–28). Freiburg: Zentrum für Geriatrie und Gerontologie der Albert-Ludwigs-Universität Freiburg.

Sacks, O. (1990). *Awakenings*. New York: Vintage.

Sass, H. M. (1998). Images of killing and letting die, of self-determination and beneficence: The ethical debate on advance directives and surrogate decision making in Germany. In H. M. Sass, R. M. Veatch, & R. Kimura (Eds.), *Advance directives and surrogate decision making in health care* (pp. 137–172). Baltimore: Johns Hopkins University Press.

Schützendorf, E., & Wallrafen-Dreisow, H. (1998). *In Ruhe verrückt werden dürfen: Für ein anderes Denken in der Altenpflege* [Be allowed to go crazy in peace: Towards an alternative approach to the care of elderly persons] (8th ed.). Frankfurt: Fischer.

Skoog, I., Nilsson, L., Palmertz, B., Andreasson, L.-A., & Swanborg, A. (1993). A population-based study of dementia in 85-year-olds. *New England Journal of Medicine, 328*, 153–158.

Thomasma, D. C. (1986). Philosophical reflections on a rational treatment plan. *Journal of Medicine and Philosophy, 11*, 157–165.

Thomasma, D. C., & Pellegrino, E. D. (1988). *For the patient's good: The restoration of beneficence in health care.* New York: Oxford University Press.

Thomsen, A., Illhardt, F. J., Dornberg, M., & Heiss, H. W. (1998). Erweiterung des geriatrischen Assessment durch ein Ethik-Assessment: Auswertung eines Pilotprojektes zu medizinethischen Fragestellungen im geriatrischen Assessment [Expansion of the geriatric assessment through an ethics assessment: Evaluation of a pilot project on bioethical issues in geriatric assessment]. *Geriatrische Forschung, 8*, 193–201.

Wicclair, M. R. (1993). *Ethics and the elderly.* New York: Oxford University Press.

Zsolnay-Wildgruber, H. (1997). Alzheimer-Kranke und ihr primäres Bezugssystem: Grundlegende Untersuchungen für ein Kommunikationstraining pflegender Angehöriger [Patients with Alzheimer disease and their primary frame of reference. Foundational investigations concerning communication training of family care givers]. Freiburg: Lambertus.

CHAPTER THIRTEEN

The Ethical Challenge of Treating Pain in Alzheimer Disease

A Dental Case

Gunilla Nordenram, D.D.S., Ph.D.

Dementia may be defined as an acquired global impairment of intellect, memory, and personality, but without impairment of consciousness. Many types of dementia disorders exist, of which Alzheimer disease (AD) is the most common. AD involves serious communication problems, speech being limited to a few words or incomprehensible sounds. If behavioral and psychological symptoms in dementia occur, aggression, shouting, anxiety, and hallucination become particular problems. It has been shown, however, that persons in a severe stage of the disease can still react to various stimuli and experience uncomfortable sensations (Asplund et al., 1991). This latter aspect of their situation has been an important motivation for this book, which explores various types of palliation or comfort care that should be provided to such patients.

Although cognition and social behavior in moderate and severe dementia are impaired, the afflicted patients have a rich and powerful emotional life. Loss of intellect is not loss of personhood (Bernat, 1996). Decisions regarding treatment needs and the management of treatment must attempt to maximize the patient's quality of life and improve safety. An often overlooked area is oral care.

The oral region is a "private" zone of the body. Entrance to the mouth is restricted to persons who are near and dear to us and to certain professionals (e.g., dentists, dental hygienists, speech therapists, and physicians). Personal space in terms of the oral region varies from person to person—whether a friend, an acquaintance, or a stranger, and in this hierarchical scale, enemies are far away. Elias Canetti (1960) talks about teeth as an instrument of power or a weapon, not just a biological part of the body, and asserts that the teeth are the armed guardians of the mouth.

For a newborn baby, the sucking reflex is vital for its survival, notwithstanding that nowadays we can feed a baby artificially through a tube. When we touch the cheek of a newborn, the baby turns its head toward the touched side—the orienting reflex. For a tiny infant, feeding also means close contact with the caregiver and the first opportunity to establish confidence and nonverbal communication. In the late stage of dementia, the sucking reflex and the orienting reflex have returned, and the oral zone may be as significant for the severely demented person as it is for the newborn baby.

When persons suddenly become afraid, they often put their hands in front of their faces, instinctively and immediately guarding their mouths. The aggressive behavior of persons with AD in oral care situations may be an expression of fear caused by a lack of understanding of what is going on and of why people want to look into their mouth. They feel that the private oral zone has been invaded, arousing emotions that the patient can no longer interpret or verbalize. The most natural reaction in this situation is to hide the mouth or forcefully reject any attempt to enter it.

However, refusal behavior in dental care can also mean something else. As an illustration, I describe one of my patients, Cathy, whom I met in about 1990. When I first met her in the hospital, she was aggressive, restless, and agitated. She screamed, bit, and fought whenever anyone tried to open her mouth.

Cathy's life is a living illustration of modern European history. She was born in Saint Petersburg, Russia, at the beginning of the last century, into a wealthy family. She was brought up by a private governess, learning several languages and how to play various music instruments, to embroider, to manage a household—all the things that a fine young lady needed to know at that time.

She married young. In her thirties, her husband was executed by the Stalin regime. She managed to leave the Soviet Union and settled down in France. After World War II, she remarried, taking as husband a French diplomat. They lived in various parts of the world and her knowledge of languages was very convenient. Her husband's last post was at the French embassy in Stockholm, and when he retired they remained in Stockholm, living in a large apartment in the city center, in a district where such accommodation is now very expensive.

Cathy's husband died a few years after his retirement, and Cathy had been a widow for more than twenty years. She had no children and gradually reached a situation where she was quite alone. She had no relatives or friends left and no social contacts. Only rarely did she let anybody into her flat. An exception was one of the neighbors, who enjoyed her confidence and used to help her in emergencies (e.g., by changing her lock after she had lost her keys). In fact, this had happened quite often lately.

In May 1990, Cathy's neighbor contacted the district nurse about this elderly lady. He thought something was wrong with her: she was behaving strangely from time to time. Recently, she had gotten into the habit of walking around the city at night with 100,000 Swedish crowns (US$ 10,000) in her handbag and carrying all her antique and expensive jewels in a plastic bag. She could easily have been robbed, but she was lucky. She was unable to find her way home. Even in dark city streets, she stood out from the crowd—the police had learned who she was and they drove her back to her flat on several occasions.

After the call from the neighbor, the district nurse and a geriatrician visited her. That day she was in a good mood and let them in. The flat was rather untidy. There was a smell, especially from the kitchen. But one does not go into people's homes in order to inspect them, so the visitors simply took note of all this and wondered how Cathy coped when it came to eating.

Cathy seemed to spend her time looking at old photos and drawings from Saint Petersburg. The old lady still gave off an appearance of high class; she was mobile and seemed in good health. She denied having problems with her memory or any other problems. At that time, she spoke Russian fluently, French, and rather good Swedish. The only thing she complained about was her neighbor who used to help her. In a whisper, she insisted that he was a secret agent, presumably a KGB officer. She obviously suffered from paranoid delusions. She was offered help from the municipal care for the elderly, but she was not interested.

A few months later, her neighbor heard screams coming from her flat.

She was found lying in the floor with a femoral neck fracture and was taken to the hospital for surgery. She was examined and tested for dementia and the assessments indicated severe AD. In addition, she was no longer able to walk and sat in a wheelchair. She was completely uncooperative, angry, agitated, and rather aggressive. It was considered necessary to place her in a unit for the demented and she was put on continuous heavy medication with neuroleptic drugs. She was admitted to a hospital for long-term care, where I was the hospital dentist at the time.

By now she had lost her Swedish and her French. With the assistance of a Russian interpreter, the nurses tried to find out what she was saying with the few words she used, often in a screaming voice. The interpreter said they were better off not knowing what Cathy was screaming, because it consisted only of swearwords and abuse. She was very uncooperative, and dependent in all her daily activities, apart from eating, when she used her hands, instead of utensils: she had totally lost her table manners. Despite heavy sedation, she still showed aggressive and hostile behavior, and the ward staff found it difficult to take care of her. Naturally, she did not allow anyone to brush her teeth. She bit and screamed and forcefully rejected every attempt to approach her face.

Cathy seemed to have healthy teeth as far as the staff were able to judge. I was asked to examine her teeth, and it was not easy—I was able to take only a brief look. There seemed to be a lot of caries, and some molar teeth had fractured crowns with sharp edges. Her oral hygiene had been rather neglected. A second treatment attempt with heavy sedation and an interpreter present also failed.

We (the ward nurses, the doctor, and myself, the dentist) concluded that the patient could be in pain from her teeth. However, an assessment, including an X ray, determined that dental treatment could be carried out only under general anesthesia. The patient had no relatives, only a guardian—a bank clerk who took care of her finances. As far as her dental treatment was concerned, he said that we could do whatever was needed, money was not a problem. So the treatment decision was discussed and made with the consensus of the physician, the ward staff, and me. We thought it was neither fair nor beneficial for her to have toothaches, and that this could affect her quality of life. The dental treatment should be in accordance with "science and approved experience" as supported in the Swedish Act of Supervision. The treatment was aimed at making the patient feel as comfortable as possible.

One month later, the oral treatment was performed under general anesthesia. In the meantime, Cathy had fractured the crowns of her upper central incisors, and suddenly she lost the appearance of a person with healthy teeth even when viewed from a distance. The X rays, taken when the patient was asleep, revealed a large amount of infection. The only possible treatment was extraction of all teeth and roots.

Some days later, I was contacted by the doctor, who was rather upset that all of Cathy's teeth had been extracted. Cathy was also quite black and blue after the extractions, although it looked worse than it was. After the doctor had looked at the X rays, she understood the treatment decision and accepted it as the only course of action. Healing was normal.

Three months later, the doctor asked me to make dentures for Cathy. I considered such treatment to be quite useless, but the doctor insisted, and I agreed to try. Cathy now seemed to be calm, but I was unable to get a response from her. I decided to start with an upper denture to see if it was possible. The patient was not exactly in a cooperative mood, but she was not actively refusing treatment. The ward staff wanted Cathy to have new teeth to make her look prettier: they really cared for her.

However, when the denture was ready and in place in her mouth, initially she was not at all interested in looking at her face in the mirror. According to the nurses, Cathy became really pretty with her new teeth, but after eventually looking into the mirror for a long time, she took out the denture and placed it on the table in front of her. She did not want it. We were the ones who wanted her to have new teeth. If her attention was distracted, she seemed to forget her new denture and could wear it for several hours, but from time to time she would remove it from her mouth. She did not want to use it.

Oral pain and discomfort were the cause of the refusal behavior in this AD patient. She felt pain but could not interpret the signals and need for adequate treatment. Her reaction was aggressive, with screaming and biting whenever anyone tried to look into her mouth or feed her with warm or cold food. After the healing of the lesions following the tooth extractions, her heavy medication with neuroleptic drugs had been totally discontinued. Her aggression and irritability had completely disappeared. Of course, she was still severely demented, but she looked and behaved as though she was satisfied—and she got her good table manners back. She was much easier to care for, and the ward staff were happy.

❧ Ethical Considerations

We find Cathy's accusing her neighbor of being a secret agent and her going out at night with her jewels and money to be curious and irrational. Considering Cathy's earlier life, she and her former husband had undoubtedly encountered spying, and she had escaped from Russia with some of her belongings in a bag. Her behavior was rational in that context, but not in her then-current life situation.

As the AD progressed, she gradually lost her acquired languages and reverted to her mother tongue, which is common in persons with dementia. Living as an immigrant or in a foreign country, as Cathy was, a person with dementia becomes even more confused when verbal communication fails, due to the cognitive impairment suffered.

Cathy was brought up as a fine lady and was taught good table manners as a child. When she got rid of her oral pain, she was able to behave properly in mealtime situations. The importance of this for Cathy is impossible to know, but with her background it might well have been a dimension of dignity for her to eat with instruments as she was used to that helped her to remain integrated and as active as possible.

The ethical dilemmas facing the people who cared for Cathy were paternalism, beneficence, autonomy, and informed consent. Balancing her individual autonomy with the caregivers' desires to protect cognitively impaired persons from harm and provide optimum treatment is difficult. It is an obligation to choose the alternative that best satisfies the patient's need for integrity and dignity.

Informed consent is the formalized process of protecting patient autonomy, and the person is supposed to understand the burdens and the benefits of the treatment. Caring for patients with cognitive impairment requires evaluation of the patient's ability to participate in the treatment decision. Several other chapters in this book address aspects of this challenge, notably those by Welie, Pinch, and Illhardt. If the dementia patient has a diminished decisional capacity or is not competent to reach rational decisions, in Sweden the care requires the involvement of a proxy decision maker. "Living wills" are rare in Sweden, and not legally binding within the Swedish context (Sandman, 2001). The advocate for a patient with AD in a dental treatment situation may be a relative, the hospital staff, and the dentist, working in consensus. The treatment philosophy must be tempered by considerations of burdens and benefits of the treatment for patients—that is, acting in the patients' best interests. (Niessen, Wetle, & Wirthman, 1966; Nordenram & Norberg, 1998; McNally & Kenny, 1999). Human dignity must be respected, and care must be beneficial and of good quality.

Chemical or physical restraints, even general anesthesia, as in Cathy's case, may be necessary. This burden, including a possible postoperative period of confusion, must be weighed against the benefit provided by the treatment. In Cathy's case, the benefits of the tooth extractions turned out to be relevant, although the new denture was of no use to her. This treatment was too much, even though it brought minor harm to her.

The strain experienced by the dentist in coping with patients with AD is similar to that experienced by nurses and informal caregivers such as relatives. Dentists, like other providers of care, must understand and perceive their dementia patients as unique and valuable human beings, including the patient's premorbid life and current situation.

The assessment of treatment need for patients with severe dementia must take into account not only such factors as autonomy, benefit, and relief of pain, but also include the caregivers' insight into the person behind the diagnosis (Nordenram & Norberg, 1998). Cooperation between a number of categories of caregivers—both the various professionals and the nonprofessional caregivers such as family members and friends—is necessary.

Fair and proper oral care for patients with dementia is resource demanding, and this becomes especially obvious in times of constraints on public funding. Justified and respectful care for older people requires careful consideration of care needs in clinical situations and in policy (McNally & Kenny, 1999). In the face of health and welfare cutbacks in the public sector, it is a challenge to argue for adequate resources for irrational patients such as cognitively impaired people. Care is a moral project, and the challenge is based on a belief in mankind and the concept of intrinsic human dignity. In our diversified world, with rapid changes in technology and economic situations, shifts in contemporary biomedical ethics are evident (Pellegrino, 1993). An ongoing dialogue of biomedical ethics is therefore essential. It should be based on actual practice with authentic cases that augment and extend the notion of good and bad, right and wrong, within the professions as well as within society as a whole.

REFERENCES

Asplund, K., Norberg, A., Adolfsson, R., & Waxman, H. (1991). Facial expressions in severely demented patients: A stimulus-response study of four patients with dementia of the Alzheimer type. *International Journal of Geriatric Psychiatry, 6,* 559–606.

Bernat, J. L. (1996). Ethical issues in the management of demented patients: The American Academy of Neurology Ethics and Humanities Subcommittee. *Neurology, 46,* 1180–1183.

Canetti, E. (1960). *Masse und Macht* [Crowds and power]. Düsseldorf: Claassen Verlag.

McNally, M., & Kenny, N. (1999). Ethics in an aging society: Challenges for oral health care. *Journal of the Canadian Dental Association, 65,* 623–626.

Niessen, L. C., Wetle, T., & Wirthman, G. P. (1966). Clinical management of the cognitively impaired older adult. In P. Holm-Pedersen & H. Loe (Eds.), *Textbook of geriatric dentistry* (pp. 248–257). Copenhagen: Munksgaard.

Nordenram, G., & Norberg, A. (1998). Ethical issues in dental management of patients with severe dementia: Ethical reasoning by hospital dentists: A narrative study. *Swedish Dental Journal, 22,* 61–76.

Pellegrino, E. D. (1993). The metamorphosis of medical ethics. A 30-year retrospective. *Journal of the American Medical Association, 269,* 1158–1162.

Sandman L. (2001). Palliative care in Sweden. In H.A.M.J. ten Have & R. Janssens (Eds.), *Palliative care in Europe* (pp. 60–82). Amsterdam: IOS Press.

CHAPTER FOURTEEN

Alzheimer Disease and Euthanasia

Bert Gordijn, Ph.D.

Alzheimer disease (AD) is the most common form of irreversible dementia. It is a progressive, irreversible brain disorder. There is still a lot to learn about the causes of the disease and a cure has yet to be developed. Among the symptoms are memory loss, confusion, impaired judgment, personality changes, disorientation, and loss of language skills. Although AD starts with relatively mild symptoms, it finally results in a severe loss of mental function and makes patients completely dependent on other people for their everyday care. Thus, loss of control and increasing dependency on others are pivotal traits of the life of a person with AD. At the same time, empirical research has demonstrated that fear of dependence on others and the prospect of loss of control are important reasons to ask for euthanasia. Hence, the dreadful prospect of progressive dementia may drive persons with AD to request euthanasia. Moreover, there are different developments that will most likely cause the phenomenon of persons with AD requesting euthanasia to become more significant in the decades to come.

First, in several countries policies concerning euthanasia are on the brink of becoming more liberal. In the Netherlands, for example, a new law came into force in April 2002 that legally embodied grounds for exemption from punishment for physicians who conduct euthanasia and comply with certain requirements (Law on certification of life termination on request and physician assisted suicide, 2001). Thus, the new law transforms the practice of pragmatic tolerance into a legally codified practice of euthanasia, making the Netherlands the first country in the world to legally allow euthanasia under specific circumstances (Gordijn, 2001; Gordijn & Janssens, 2001). In May 2002, a new euthanasia law was also adopted in Belgium, making this country the second, after the Netherlands, to allow doctors to terminate the life of their patients under specific circumstances. Similar, though generally less radical, developments and tendencies to decriminalize and liberalize euthanasia can be seen in other countries (e.g., France, Switzerland, Australia, Japan).

Second, through a further development of palliative care, the treatment of distressing symptoms that can play a role in the causal pathway leading to a request for euthanasia (e.g., pain, clinical depression, dyspnea, vomiting, fatigue, anorexia, constipation, bladder disturbances, bedsores) will most probably be ameliorated. Loss of control and dependency, however, do not seem to be readily amenable by a program of palliative care. Hence, through a further development of palliative medicine, the relative importance of fear of dependency on others and the prospect of loss of control as reasons to ask for euthanasia will increase.

Third, against the backdrop of increasing life expectancy and demographic changes, the number of persons with AD will significantly increase worldwide in the decades to come. For these reasons, the topic of persons with AD requesting euthanasia will increasingly present itself as an ethical problem that will have to be discussed.

In this chapter, I analyze the question of whether it can be ethically justified to perform euthanasia on persons with AD. First, however, I will clarify the concept of euthanasia, sketch the main characteristics of AD, and review some of the research done on reasons to ask for euthanasia. Moreover, I distinguish three different scenarios: (1) an incompetent person with AD asks for euthanasia; (2) an incompetent person with AD has an advance directive in which he asks for euthanasia; and (3) a competent person with AD asks for euthanasia. Presented in this order, the case for euthanasia becomes stronger with each successive scenario. Nevertheless, it will be argued that the arguments against performing euthanasia are stronger even in the last scenario.

❧ The Concept of Euthanasia

The word *euthanasia* comes from the Greek. Taken literally, it signifies a good (happy and painless) death. Nowadays, however, the concept of euthanasia signifies different forms of medically induced death. In the international discussion on the ethical aspects of euthanasia, three different distinctions are made. First, passive euthanasia and active euthanasia are distinguished. Passive euthanasia means letting die by foregoing or withdrawing life-sustaining treatment, for example by removing life-support equipment (e.g., turning off a respirator) or not delivering cardiopulmonary resuscitation and allowing a person, whose heart has stopped, to die. Active euthanasia, on the other hand, means causing the death of the patient by giving a certain life-shortening treatment, mostly by injecting controlled substances into the patient, thus causing death. Second, there is the distinction between direct euthanasia and indirect euthanasia. The latter means inducing the death of the patient as a foreseen but unintended side effect of treatment of pain or other symptoms, whereas the former involves bringing about the death of the patient as the intended effect of the treatment. Finally, voluntary euthanasia, involuntary euthanasia, and nonvoluntary euthanasia are distinguished. This last distinction assumes that euthanasia can either be an object of the will of the patient or not (nonvoluntary euthanasia). Moreover, if it is an object of the will, it can be adverse to the patient's will (involuntary euthanasia) or conforming to the patient's will (voluntary euthanasia).

The analysis in this chapter focuses on patients asking for active, direct euthanasia (ADE). From a moral point of view, this is the most interesting form of euthanasia. As to passive euthanasia, there is a widespread consensus that there are circumstances that justify foregoing or withdrawing life-sustaining treatment. The same goes for indirect euthanasia, which is often defended using the principle of double effect (Boyle, 1980). With regard to involuntary and nonvoluntary euthanasia, on the other hand, the *communis opinio* holds that they are clearly immoral. With regard to voluntary ADE, however, moral standpoints differ. For example, there are many authors who state that if a terminally ill person asks a physician for assistance in dying, the physician is morally justified to offer it, provided the request is made autonomously. Others, however, state that voluntary ADE is immoral on principle.

❧ Alzheimer Disease

Alzheimer disease is an irreversible, progressive brain disorder. It is the most common cause of dementia among people over sixty-five years of age. On average, persons with AD live for eight to ten years after they are diagnosed, though the disease can last for up to twenty years. In years to come, as O'Brien, Brumback, and Bennahum state in part I of this book, we will witness a growing incidence of AD in almost all modern societies. After all, the risk of developing AD increases with age, and there is an increasing life expectancy. As a result, the disease will become very common.

An essential trait of having AD is loss of control. Initially, people with AD tend to have less vigor and impulsiveness. Moreover, they are slow to learn and react and show signs of minor memory loss and mood swings. They tend to forget the names of familiar people and common objects. Moreover, thinking becomes fuzzier. Consequently, persons with AD prefer the familiar and start to shy away from anything novel. They will then be increasingly confused; they will get lost easily and exercise poor judgment. Through all these changes, job performance will be affected.

In later stages of the disease, all cognitive faculties, such as speech, memory, and understanding, will further deteriorate. Advancing AD affects the person's ability to comprehend where he is, the day and the time. Becoming aware of this loss of control may result in depression and irritation. As the person's mind continues to slip away, eventually, he will lose all reasoning ability. Somehow the very cognitive essence of the person seems to vanish. Memory will become very poor, and no one will be recognizable anymore. Finally, persons with AD lose the ability to chew and swallow. In addition, bowel and bladder control are lost. They become vulnerable to pneumonia, infection, and other illnesses. Respiratory problems worsen, particularly when the patient becomes bedridden. This terminal stage eventually leads to death (American Health Assistance Foundation [AHAF], 2002).

The loss of control of persons with AD results in a growing dependency on other persons for everyday care. Many spouses, relatives, and friends take care of people with AD. During their years of caregiving, these families and friends experience different forms of stress (e.g., emotional, physical, and financial). After all, their loved ones become increasingly absent minded, discouraged, puzzled, and dependent. Eventually, they may not even recognize their nearest and dearest relatives and friends anymore. Since persons with AD become totally dependent on others for their daily care as the disease runs its course, family members often face difficult decisions about long-term care. Often, they have no choice but to place their relative in a nursing home.

❧ Reasons for Requests for Euthanasia

In the last decade, empirical research has been done as to why people want to die and why they ask for ADE (Van der Maas, Pijnenborg, & Delden, 1991; Chochinov et al., 1995; Seale & Addington-Hall, 1995; Van der Wal & Van der Maas, 1996; Back, Wallace, Starks, & Pearlman, 1996). One of the interesting results of these studies is the finding that pain is not the most important reason for patients to request ADE. In fact, there seem to be many different reasons why people ask for ADE.

Van der Maas et al. (1991) report that considerations concerning the prevention of degeneration or decay were more important than pain. In their 1996 study, Van der Wal and Van der Maas show that the most important reasons for asking for ADE have to do with suffering in a broad sense. In addition, the prevention of degeneration or decay again appears to be more important than pain. It is not clear to what extent other physical symptoms, such as dyspnea, vomiting, fatigue, anorexia, constipation, bladder disturbances, bedsores, and so on play a role in the causal pathway leading to a request for ADE. However, it can probably be safely assumed that these symptoms significantly contribute to the suffering of patients.

Chochinov et al. (1995) argue that the desire for death is correlated with ratings of pain and low family support, but most significantly with measures of clinical depression—a potentially treatable condition. They conclude that this could indicate that depression is the most important cause for developing a desire for death. Pain and lack of family support may exert more indirect influences (Chochinov et al., 1995). In Chochinov's study, clinical depression appears to be the most significant factor in developing a wish to die. Of course, the wish to die is not identical to the desire to die through ADE, the first being a necessary condition for the latter, but not a sufficient condition for it. Nevertheless, it seems reasonable to assume that clinical depression can also play a significant role in developing a wish to die through ADE.

In other studies, fear of loss of independence and personal control are mentioned as being very important determinants of developing a request for ADE. For example, Seale & Addington-Hall (1995) regard the fear of losing independence as an important determinant of the desire for euthanasia. Another study concerning ADE and physician assisted suicide (PAS) in Washington State confirms the hypothesis that the loss of personal control and independence are very important determinants of the desire for euthanasia (Back et al., 1996, p. 922).

In recent times, a lot has been written on palliative care as a means to prevent requests for ADE (Aulbert, Klaschik, & Pichlmaier, 1998; Gordijn & Janssens, 2000; Husebø & Klaschik, 1998; Zylicz & van Dijk, 1995). After all, quality of life being one of its most important moral notions, relief of suffering is a pivotal goal of palliative care (Janssens, 2001; Janssens et al., 2002). It can be safely assumed that a better treatment of pain and other physical symptoms, as well as clinical depression, will ensue from the further development of palliative care. To the extent that these factors play a substantial role as motives for requesting ADE, adequately addressing them by means of palliative care can probably take away a significant number of these requests (Gordijn & Janssens, 2000).

However, fear of loss of control and fear of dependency seem not to be readily amenable by a program of palliative care (Seale & Addington-Hall, 1995). Even the best palliative care does not seem to be able fully to prevent the dependency and loss of control that are inherently connected with dying from chronic disease (Gordijn & Janssens, 2000; Zylicz & Janssens, 1998). After all, dying from chronic illness fundamentally involves some form of loss of control and dependency. Thus, being-in-control and enjoying-independence having become the culturally idealized icons of our time, future palliative care will at this point probably reach some kind of frontier. Therefore, it can be expected that these two determinants will become more important as future reasons for ADE requests, whereas the relative importance of pain, other physical symptoms, and clinical depression in the causal pathway of the development of the wish for ADE will probably decrease.

❧ Alzheimer Disease and Euthanasia

The relative importance of fear of loss of control and fear of dependency as reasons for requesting euthanasia will grow in the years to come. Moreover, the incidence of AD will significantly rise. At the same time, loss of control and increasing dependency on others are pivotal traits of the life of a person with AD. Therefore, it is to be expected that the phenomenon of persons with AD seeking medical assistance in dying will increasingly present an ethical topic of concern. Not only will the absolute number of persons with AD asking for ADE increase, but also the group of persons with AD asking for ADE (understood as a percentage of all people who ask for ADE) will grow.

As noted above, it is important to distinguish three different scenarios: (1) an incompetent person with AD asks for ADE; (2) an incompetent person with AD has an advance directive in which he asks for ADE; and (3) a competent person with AD asks for ADE. Presented in this order, in each scenario more arguments can be brought forward in favor of performing ADE. In order to be able to justify the performance of ADE on persons with AD, however, the pro arguments will have to be stronger than the contra arguments. For this analysis, I focus on two arguments against ADE: (1) the argument of respect for life and (2) the slippery-slope argument.

Life has an intrinsic value. The norm that actively intentionally terminating the life of an innocent human being is wrong is one of the most universally accepted norms of humanity. In almost all socially and legally accepted exceptions to this norm—for example, in self-defense, war, capital punishment—the victim is not innocent. Only with regard to abortion does legislation of many modern countries allow for the killing of innocent human life. However, if these abortions could be prevented somehow, this would be morally preferable. It seems that, in general, in situations in which killing of innocent human life can be prevented, it is morally better not to kill than to kill. Likewise, in those cases in which patients request ADE, it would be morally preferable not to terminate their lives but instead to help these patients by other means.

The slippery-slope argument states that in a society in which physicians are permitted to conduct ADE on patients who ask for euthanasia, situations could arise that clearly are morally undesirable. For example, in such a society, palliative care would not be developed or would be developed only insufficiently. In the end, killing would be the only solution that medicine would have to offer in situations of extreme suffering. Thereby, the freedom of terminal patients to choose between different models of dying would be severely restricted. Also, increasing cost pressures, as well as greed, laziness, insensitivity, and other factors affecting physicians and their institutions could lead to situations in which extremely suffering patients would be more easily killed nonvoluntarily or even against their will. This would involve a suppression of personal choices and individual rights; for example, the right to die in a natural way. This, again, could undermine the patient's trust in the physician. Of course, these predictions are all a bit speculative, and a sound basis cannot easily be demonstrated for them. However, all predictions with regard to future developments on a societal level have an aspect of uncertainty on principle. Societal processes are too complex and too indeterminate to be predicted with certainty. Therefore, arguments stating that a medical practice in which physicians are permitted to conduct ADE on patients who have developed the desire for euthanasia will not lead to morally undesirable consequences are speculative as well. Therefore, it is better to be prudent and to take no risks.

❧ The Incompetent Person with AD

In the first scenario, an incompetent person with AD asks for ADE. Can it ever be ethically justified to comply with such a wish? The only argument that comes to mind as a candidate that could speak in favor of such a deed is the argument of beneficence. Considerations relating to beneficence play a central role in the debate on euthanasia (van den Berg, 1969). Many discussions on this can be found in the literature (Overberg, 1993; Prouse, 2000; Wilkinson, 1990). The traditional argument of beneficence states that no person should have to endure pointless terminal suffering. If the physician is unable to relieve the patient's suffering in other ways and terminating the life of the patient is the only way to bring the torment to a close, then the physician should be allowed to bring about the death of the patient. This line of argument presupposes two premises: (1) the patient is suffering; and (2) the relief of the patient's suffering cannot be brought about in ways other than by putting an end to the patient's life. With respect to the incompetent person with AD asking for ADE, it is difficult to establish the truth of these conditions.

First, the argument presupposes that the patient is genuinely suffering. How can the physician be sure that this condition is really a given? The patient clearly being incompetent and having lost substantial mental capacities cannot be regarded as a good source to indicate the level of his own suffering. Moreover, since suffering is a subjective, conscious state, it will be difficult to assess the level of suffering of the person with AD from an external, third-person point of view.

Second, the argument presupposes that there are conditions in which relief of the patient's suffering cannot be brought about in ways other than by termination of life. Are there really situations in which relief of suffering cannot be brought about in other ways than by death? Could not even in extreme cases terminal sedation always bring about the same relief of suffering without any direct termination of the life of the patient? Supposing that specialists have done everything in their power to relieve the distress of a patient and nothing has worked, complete sedation still seems to be an option of coping with the otherwise untreatable agony. Complete sedation implies total obtundation. Accordingly, a completely sedated patient cannot suffer anymore. Therefore, terminal sedation can be regarded as a last resort when nothing else works.

Since the two conditions of the argument of beneficence are not givens in the case of incompetent patients asking for ADE, the argument has no force in this scenario. Hence, the only argument in favor of complying with the incompetent AD patient's wish for ADE is disqualified. Therefore, against the backdrop of the argument of respect for life and the slippery-slope argument, performing ADE in this scenario cannot be morally justified.

✌ The Incompetent AD Patient with an Advance Directive

In the Netherlands, the new law on ADE provides a legal basis for the written advance directive. This development brings up the question of whether ADE based on an advance directive of an incompetent person with AD can be justified. The argument of beneficence is equally weak in this scenario as in the case of an incompetent person with AD without an advance directive. Consequently, the main ethical argument for complying with the wishes expressed in an advance directive is respect for autonomy. In general, advance directives are problematic (Health Council of The Netherlands, 2002). First, the physician can often not be sure whether the patient was competent and well-informed at the time he wrote down the directive. Second, after having written down the directive, the patient can have changed his will without having changed the written document. Third, the directive can be too vague; for example, if it does not specify the medical conditions and the wanted or unwanted medical measures in sufficient detail. Therefore, respect for autonomy urges that interpretation of an advance directive be made against the backdrop of all other available information concerning the patient. The physician should never become a technical executor of advance directives.

In addition, there is a specific problem with advance directives in the case of persons with AD. An advance directive is a written instruction about the future medical care of a person, in the event that the person becomes unable to speak for himself. This regulation is based on the assumption that the advance directive is in line with the person's will. As such, it presumes some sort of personal identity or continuity of the person. However, this continuity may very well have disappeared in the course of AD. Many persons with AD may appear to be quite happy with their lives, even if they carry a written advance directive stating that they want ADE to be performed when they have reached an advanced state of AD. The current will of such patients does clearly not correspond to their will at the time of writing the advance directive (Willems, 1999).

Overall, the problems connected with advance directives requesting ADE in the case of incompetent persons with AD are so serious that they disqualify the thesis that an ethically justified ADE of an incompetent person with AD could be based on the person's advance directive.

The Competent Person with AD

In the last scenario, a competent person with AD asks for ADE. The number of persons who have been diagnosed as having AD and who are still competent may now be fairly limited. However, as the diagnosis of AD improves, making earlier diagnoses possible, this could change (HCN, 2002). Supposing that the patient is really suffering and fully informed about her situation, the arguments of beneficence and respect for autonomy present themselves as considerations in favor of complying with the patient's wish.

A competent person with AD can indicate the main causes of his suffering. Probably the prospect of losing all control and becoming completely dependent on others is one of the main factors. Considerations of beneficence demand that attempts should be made to reduce the suffering. Does beneficence also imply that the life of a patient should be terminated if nothing else can be done to help him?

Normally, we presume that a genuine relief of suffering consists of reducing the amount of distress or agony, after which the subject of suffering will be able to feel relieved. Essential for the phenomenon of feeling relieved of suffering is the capacity for noticing the reduced level of torment. In the case of ADE, however, the suffering is brought to an end by annihilating the subject of the suffering. Here, the means to achieve the end consist of an irreversible elimination of the subject of all conscious experience. Accordingly, the reduced level of suffering is never really experienced by the suffering subject itself. This objection, however, could also be brought forward against terminal sedation. After all, in terminal sedation all conscious experience is eliminated. However, here the elimination is not as definitive and irreversible as in ADE. In principle, the sedation could be reversed were there good reasons to do so.

This last scenario also puts forward the question of whether respect for autonomy demands that the physician terminate the life of an autonomous person with AD if he is asked to do so. The answer is not easy, because it is far from evident what is meant by the norm that demands that autonomy should be respected. On the one hand, there is the problem of what are the defining properties of autonomy. On the other hand, there is the question of what respect for autonomy involves. With regard to the defining properties of autonomy, there are different theories (ten Have, Ter Meulen, & Van de Maas, 1998). Many theories seem to agree that three conditions are essential to autonomy: first, some kind of independence from controlling influences; second, the capacity for intentional action; and finally, true information and understanding (Beauchamp & Childress, 1994).

With regard to the question of what respect for autonomy involves, again different opinions exist. Immanuel Kant (1724–1804) and John Stuart Mill (1806–1873) have been the most influential thinkers in this regard. According to Kant, respect for autonomy requires that autonomous persons should never be treated merely as means. Since autonomous persons are ends in themselves, each having the capacity to determine their own destiny, it is morally forbidden to regard them exclusively as a function of the goals of other persons (Kant, 1985).

According to Mill, on the other hand, respect for autonomy implies a ban on interfering with the choices and actions of autonomous persons, provided that the latter, in their turn, do not conflict with the freedom of other autonomous persons. Sometimes, however, when other persons act on erroneous beliefs, interference by way of persuasion is morally allowed. Hence, according to Mill's theory, respect for autonomy involves two different duties. First, there is the negative duty of not interfering with the decisions and actions based on the considerations, beliefs, and values of an autonomous person. Autonomous persons' liberty and freedom to act and think ought not to be restricted arbitrarily. Second, respect for autonomy implies the positive obligation to interfere in order to enhance or restore the autonomy of persons who have a reduced level of autonomy (Mill, 1977).

Returning to euthanasia, it can be doubted whether a patient's requests for euthanasia in situations in which the only alternative is extreme suffering can be regarded as optimally autonomous (Zylicz, 2000). It could be argued that in a situation in which extreme suffering compels a patient to ask for euthanasia, the patient's autonomy is limited—that is to say, there seems to be no independence from controlling influences. The extreme suffering can be regarded as an influence that controls and takes over the will of the patient, thereby effectively reducing the autonomy of the will. But even if we suppose that a patient's request for euthanasia is substantially or even fully autonomous, respect for autonomy would still not demand that euthanasia be conducted. As stated above, respect for autonomy implies two different duties: a negative duty of not interfering with the freedom of autonomous persons; and a positive obligation to interfere in order to enhance or restore the autonomy of persons. Hence, respect for autonomy clearly does not involve an obligation to do whatever an autonomous person asks of one. In the case of a request for euthanasia, a patient asks the physician to interfere with his life. However, a positive obligation to interfere is present only if through this interference enhancement or restoration of the autonomy of a person is possible. Killing a patient would not enhance or restore his autonomy; what is more, it would bring about the annihilation of his autonomy. After all, by taking away the life of the patient, the physician would at the same time destroy the necessary condition for the patient's autonomy. Therefore, a moral obligation for the physician to put an end to a patient's life cannot be founded on respect for autonomy, even if the patient's desire to be killed is fully autonomous.

It is to be expected that in the next few decades the ideal of a choreographed death on command will urge an increasing number of persons with AD to ask for euthanasia. In this chapter, the ethical aspects of performing euthanasia on AD patients have been analyzed. Three scenarios in which increasingly strong arguments in favor of performing euthanasia can be presented have been distinguished: (1) an incompetent person with AD asks for euthanasia; (2) an incompetent person with AD has an advance directive in which he asks for euthanasia; and (3) a competent person with AD asks for euthanasia. However, it has been demonstrated that, even in the last scenario, the case in favor of euthanasia is overruled by the contra arguments. Thus, euthanasia cannot be convincingly ethically justified in the treatment of persons with AD.

REFERENCES

American Health Assistance Foundation. (AHAF). (2002) What are the stages of Alzheimer's disease? www.ahaf.org/alzdis/about/adfaq.htm (accessed January 2002).

Aulbert, E., Klaschik, E., & Pichlmaier, H. (Eds.). (1998). *Palliativmedizin—die Alternative zur aktiven Sterbehilfe: Zur Euthanasie-Diskussion in Deutschland* [Palliative medicine—the alternative to active assistance in dying: The euthanasia discussion in Germany]. Stuttgart: Schattauer.

Back, A. L., Wallace, J. I., Starks, H. E., & Pearlman, R. A. (1996). Physician-assisted suicide and euthanasia in Washington State. Patient request and physician responses. *Journal of the American Medical Association, 275* (12), 919–925.

Beauchamp, T. L., & Childress, J. F. (1994). *Principles of biomedical ethics* (4th ed.). New York: Oxford University Press.

Boyle, J. M. (1980). Toward understanding the principle of double effect. *Ethics, 90,* 527–538.

Chochinov, H. M., Wilson, K. G., Enns, M., Mowchun, N., Lander, S., Levitt, M., et al. (1995). Desire for death in the terminally ill. *American Journal of Psychiatry, 152,* 1185–1191.

Gordijn, B. (2001). Regulating moral dissent in an open society: The Dutch experience with pragmatic tolerance. *Journal of Medicine and Philosophy, 26* (3), 225–244.

Gordijn, B., & Janssens, R. (2000). The prevention of euthanasia through palliative care: New developments in the Netherlands. *Patient Education and Counseling, 41* (1), 35–46.

Gordijn, B., & Janssens, R. (2001). New developments in Dutch legislation concerning euthanasia and physician-assisted suicide. *Journal of Medicine and Philosophy, 26* (3) 299–310.

ten Have, H.A.M.J., Ter Meulen, R., & Van Leeuwen, E. (1998). *Medische ethiek* [Medical ethics]. Houten/Diegem: Bohn Stafleu Van Lochum.

Health Council of the Netherlands. (2002). *Dementia.* The Hague: Health Council of the Netherlands (pub. no. 2002/04).

Husebø, S., & Klaschik, E. (1998). *Palliativmedizin: Praktische Einführung in Schmerztherapie, Ethik, und Kommunikation* [Palliative medicine: A practical introduction in pain treatment, ethics, and communication]. Heidelberg: Springer.

Janssens, R. (2001). *Palliative care: Concepts and ethics.* Nijmegen: University Press Nijmegen.

Janssens, R., ten Have, H.A.M.J., Broeckaert, B., Clark, D., Gracia, D., Illhardt, F. J., et al. (2002). Moral values in palliative care: A European comparison. In H.A.M.J. ten Have & D. Clark (Eds.), *The ethics of palliative care: European perspectives* (pp. 72–86). Buckingham, UK: Open University Press.

Kant, I. (1985). Kritik der praktischen Vernunft [Critique of practical reason.]. In K. Vorländer (Ed.), *Philosophische Bibliothek,* Vol. 38 (9th ed.). Hamburg: Felix Meiner.

Law on certification of life termination on request and physician assisted suicide. (2001). [Wet toetsing levensbeëindiging op verzoek en hulp bij zelfdoding]. Eerste Kamer vergaderjaar 2000–2001, 26691, n. 137.

Mill, J. S. (1977). On liberty. In J. M. Robson (Ed.), *Collected works of John Stuart Mill,* Vol. 18. Toronto: University of Toronto Press.

Overberg, K. R. (Ed.). (1993). *Mercy or murder? Euthanasia, morality, and public policy.* Kansas City, Mo.: Sheed & Ward.

Prouse, M. (2000). Euthanasia: slippery slope or mercy killing? In P. Webb (Ed.), *Ethical issues in palliative care: Reflections and considerations* (pp. 101–125). Manchester, UK: Hochland & Hochland.

Seale, C., & Addington-Hall, J. (1995). Euthanasia: The role of good care. *Social Science and Medicine, 40,* 581–587.

Van den Berg, J. H. (1969). *Medische macht en medische ethiek* [Medical power and medical ethics]. Nijkerk, Netherlands: G. F. Callenbach.

Van der Maas, P. J., Pijnenborg, L., & Delden, J. (1991). *Medische beslissingen rond het levenseinde: Commissie onderzoek medische praktijk inzake euthanasie* [Medical decisions at the end of life: Investigative Committee on the Medical Practice of Euthanasia]. The Hague: Sdu Uitgevers.

Van der Wal, G., & Van der Maas, P. J. (1996). *Euthanasie en andere medische beslissingen rond het levenseinde: De praktijk en de meldingsprocedure* [Euthanasia and other medical decisions at the end of life: Practice and notification procedure]. The Hague: Sdu Uitgevers.

Wilkinson, J. (1990). The ethics of euthanasia. *Palliative Medicine, 4* (2), 81–86.

Willems, D. L. (1999). Hoe steil en hoe glad is het hellend vlak? Levensbeëindiging bij dementie en de grenzen van het willen [How steep and how slick is the slippery slope? Termination of life among persons with dementia and the limits to wanting]. *Tijdschrift voor Gerontologie en Geriatrie, 30,* 147–148.

Zylicz, Z. (2000). Ethical considerations in the treatment of pain in a hospice environment. *Patient Education and Counseling, 4* (1), 47–53.

Zylicz, Z., & van Dijk, L. (1995). Palliatieve zorgverlening en de vraag naar euthanasie [Palliative care and the request for euthanasia]. *Pro Vita Humana, 6,* 161–168.

Zylicz, Z., & Janssens, M.J.P.A. (1998). Options in palliative care: Dealing with those who want to die. In M. Zenz (Ed.), Cancer pain. *Bailliere Clinics of Anaesthesiology, 12,* 121–131.

Part V / Organizational Ethics Issues

Educational Initiatives, Laws, and Allocation Decisions

The Role of Nurses and Nursing Education in the Palliative Care of Patients and Their Families

Elizabeth Furlong, R.N., Ph.D., J.D.

A hospice program is one ethical model of delivering palliative care to patients with Alzheimer disease (AD) in the terminal stages. This chapter, while addressing the role of nurses in promoting a palliative model of hospice care, also provides insight into nursing education challenges in this area. I begin with a description of a hospice model of care and clinical research on this model, and then describe ethical conflicts. I then focus directly on the nurse's role in promoting a palliative model of hospice care. The hospice model of palliative care for patients with AD can meet the conflicting demands among the four ethical principles of nonmaleficence, beneficence, autonomy, and justice and it also integrates with the nursing ethics model of care (Post, 1998). Because of AD's effect on individuals, families, and society, it is recognized as a major public health problem in the world. Because it is a major public health problem, it is imperative to address the ethical aspect of palliative care for this population.

❧ A Hospice Model of Care and Clinical Research

Nurses who wish to promote a palliative model of hospice care must first gain a clear understanding of the premises and limits of this model. Hospice is a "philosophy of care emphasizing comfort and quality of life in contrast to life prolongation except as a side-effect of palliative treatments" (Post, 1997, p. 649). Post distinguishes hospice as a philosophy from a locus of care since there can be many sites—home, hospice, nursing home, hospital, and so forth. Some writers advocate its use in the terminal stage of AD (Zerzan, Stearns, & Hanson, 2000; Post, 1997). Besides being an advocate for hospice for patients with end-stage AD, for the earlier stages Post also recommends routinized treatment limitations, according to advance directives and family entrustment (1997).

In 1986, Volicer et al. described a hospice model of care for patients with advanced AD that had five levels of care. Patients were assigned to the five levels during interdisciplinary team meetings with family members. Level 1 included an aggressive diagnostic workup, treatment of co-morbid conditions, cardiopulmonary resuscitation (CPR), tube feedings, and transfer to an acute medical unit if needed. Level 2 included the same level of care as in level 1, but excluding CPR. Level 3 care also excluded CPR. In addition, it excluded a transfer to an acute medical unit, thereby eliminating the use of respirators, cardiovascular support, and so forth. Level 4 care excluded CPR and mandated no transfer to an acute care unit, no aggressive diagnostic workup, and no antibiotic treatment of life-threatening infections (pneumonia, urinary tract, etc.). Patient comfort needs were met with analgesics and antipyretics. In level 5 care, strategies such as cardiopulmonary resuscitation, transfers to acute medical facilities, diagnostic workups, antibiotics, and tube feedings were not done. Patient comfort care and supportive care were continued. This research is fifteen years old, and changes in practice are acknowledged; for example, nursing homes are sites now for the delivery of care that once only took place in hospitals (ventilators and so forth); percutaneous endoscopic gastrostomy (PEG) tubes have frequently replaced nasogastric feeding tubes; evidence-based outcomes have changed treatment regimes. However, this model of hospice approach continues and research has been done on the decision-making model to decide which level of care to utilize (Hurley et al., 1995). This qualitative study reinforced the ethical nursing model of care in which staff did not separate potential patient outcomes from potential family outcomes (i.e., they viewed the context of the situation). Further, another indicator of nurses' contextual understanding of the situation was their integration of clinical and ethical judgments about proposed patient care.

Luchins, Hanrahan, and Murphy (1997) researched the criteria for enrolling patients with dementia into a hospice program. They note that this model of care delivery is optimal for patients with end-stage dementia both because their prognosis is terminal and because their care is best met by palliative care. Further, others believe aggressive medical care is neither wanted nor ethical (Zerzan, Stearns, & Hanson, 2000). Palliative care will facilitate the individual's comfort, relieve symptoms, and control pain. Several pilot hospice programs for these patients have proven to be both feasible and ethical (1997). Even though Volicer's research was done nearly two decades ago, data show a nonawareness of the hospice model for care of patients with dementia. For example, a 1993 survey showed that only 13 percent of family and professional caregivers of patients with dementia were aware of this hospice care delivery model (Luchins & Hanrahan, 1993). In contrast, 87 percent of these same caregivers were aware of hospice services for patients with cancer. Further, this survey demonstrated that 90 percent of them viewed the hospice care model as appropriate for the end stage of dementia.

Another research study shows families and health providers who care for patients with AD prefer the use of hospice when the individuals are in the end stage of the disease. Of families associated with an Alzheimer's Association, 71 percent wanted this kind of care, as did 61 percent of physicians associated with the American Geriatric Society (Post & Whitehouse, 1995).

However, there are barriers and challenges to using this hospice model. Only 1 percent of patients in hospice have a primary diagnosis of dementia (Luchins, Hanrahan, & Murphy, 1997). Major barriers in many settings include funding policy, an inability to predict survival time for patients with dementia, lack of knowledge about hospice care for patients with dementia, and lack of available services (Zerzan, Stearns, & Hanson, 2000; Rousseau, 1998). The next section describes some challenges to the United States regarding funding policy. Medicare and Medicaid are examples.

❧ Medicare and Hospice

While the modern hospice movement began in the United States in 1974, it did not become a Medicare benefit until 1982 (Rousseau, 1998). Individuals with Medicare Part A can receive hospice care in a Medicare-certified hospice if they have a terminal illness and are predicted to die within six months or less. The first two barriers are intertwined—the Medicare hospice benefit is for patients with a six-month survival time. These barriers present a problem, but it is one that could be solved in a variety of ways. One solution is to change policy to make access to palliative care more available and to not apply a historical, cancer-disease trajectory onto a type of illness that follows a different natural history of disease pathogenesis (Lundy & Janes, 2001; Hospice: Core and Cornerstone, 2000). Thus, a better approach would be to adopt policy and funding changes that are not limited by the current six-month standard. Another way to solve the problem is to accept the policy as status quo and to do clinical research that provides better predictive tools for the six-month survival time in hospice for patients with dementia. Such is the research by Luchins, Hanrahan, and Murphy (1997), who have developed criteria for enrollment of patients with dementia into hospice programs. They were able to identify a group of patients who had a median survival time of four months and a mean survival time of 6.9 months. They conclude: "When the admission guideline concerning a 6-months survival time was initially adopted for Medicare hospice benefit, most hospice patients were dying of cancer. The use of this guideline for the new groups of patients that hospices have begun to serve—notably, dementia patients and AIDS patients—may not be appropriate" (p. 1058). Policy changes could include the elimination of the six-months rule, less rigorous admission criteria, and financial structures reflecting changed public health problems, disease trajectories, patient and family wishes for palliative care, and best ethical practices.

The impetus for recent research by Marsh et al. (2000) was the above-mentioned barriers and the desire to have the most sensitive screening tool for disease severity to maximize the Medicare hospice benefit when admitting patients to a hospice. The tool, the Alzheimer's Hospice Placement Evaluation Scale (AHOPE), was used with a sample of 112 patients with AD and was supported with reliability and predictive validity. Response in Colorado (where the tool was developed) has been significant since publication of this research: (1) long-term care institutions and hospices have instituted the use of this tool; and (2) there has been a sharp increase in the number of admissions of patients with Alzheimer disease to hospices (a 198% increase). Again, the question arises—should policy be changed or should there be an attempt to find a predictive clinical tool that meets status quo policy?

Post writes of a possible new Medicare model for policy: if there is a probability of a patient dying within six months following the onset of a fever and if this probability was utilized with other clinical judgment, then the patient with AD could be admitted to the Medicare hospice benefit (Post, 1997).

Research by Wilson, Kovach, and Stearns (1996) reports on a model that changes worksite policy and facilitates a hospice model in a long-term care setting with no expectation of meeting the Medicare guideline of death within six months. They noted some differences between care of patients with end-stage dementia and those with cancer: Patients with AD require less pharmacologic and more psychosocial and environmental modalities; they also require careful assessment for discomforts because of their loss of ability to communicate. These researchers found "hospice concepts can be effectively modified and incorporated into the care of persons with end-stage dementia" (p. 10) and that this could be accomplished with minimal additional cost to the facility. However, they stressed the importance of staff education about the hospice philosophy.

❧ Medicaid and Hospice

There is concern with Medicaid policy, too. For example, attorneys from the AARP Foundation Litigation and Maryland's Legal Aid Bureau are advocating for a woman with severe dementia where Medicaid policy is not meeting her needs (Personal correspondence, Dr. Rosalie Yeaworth, May 28, 2001). The attorneys argue that Maryland's Medicaid Older Adult Waiver Program is too restrictive in not admitting her to a nursing facility and paying her expenses. She meets the financial, but not the medical, criteria. They argue, further, that the restrictions conflict with U.S. federal law and discriminate against individuals with AD. This patient is currently at home, but her physician refuses to order certain medications unless she has twenty-four-hour supervision in a facility. Thus, she could receive palliative care in a nursing home, but Maryland Medicaid policy prevents it. This is one current anecdotal legal case that reflects state Medicaid policy concerns in the care of patients with AD. Another legal example is attempted legislation in 2001 in Nebraska to improve the availability of registered nurses for assessment of patients with AD in assisted care living facilities so that the patients may receive better care.

❧ Ethical Conflicts

In articulating an ethical analysis of using a model of palliative care for patients with Alzheimer disease, one can anticipate tensions between and among several key ethical principles that will confront nurses. First, there is conflict between autonomy and nonmaleficence that several authors in this book—notably

Welie, Pinch, Illhardt, and Nordenram—have addressed from various perspectives. Does the nurse follow the wishes of the patient and/or family member? or are patient/family wishes analyzed as harmful, and, therefore, one should not respect patient/family autonomy? Second, there is tension between autonomy and distributive justice: if every person/family wanted aggressive medical treatment, might some family members, health providers, ethicists, and policymakers invoke the principle of distributive justice because there is a lack of financial resources for everyone? Post (1998) argues against the hegemonic emphasis on the principle of autonomy. However, Bosek and Shaw (2001, p. 47) identify autonomy as "the primary ethical principle to be promoted and protected during health care decision-making in Western society." Other authors have written of the dominance of autonomy: "[Alzheimer disease] erodes what lies at the very heart of medical ethics—the principle of preserving patient autonomy" (Lynn et al., 1996, p. 44). Third, there is a conflict between nonmaleficence and beneficence: patients, family members, and health providers can have honest, genuine differences on what characterizes treatment to meet these ethical concepts. For example, an individual with severe dementia could interpret aggressive medical treatment as torture. Nordenram's chapter addresses her attempts to provide oral care and the patient resistance she encountered, as well as the nurse's role in helping the patient overcome the resistance. Is this treatment harmful or beneficial? (Post, 1997). Fourth, there can be tension between distributive justice and the continuum of nonmaleficence and beneficence. Treatment modalities (whether they are viewed as harmful or helpful) can be seen as antithetical to the need for societal distributive justice.

From a nursing ethics analysis standpoint, the importance of context and relationships also must be acknowledged. Post's ethical analysis is consistent with nursing and feminist theorists on nursing ethics (i.e., an ethic of care). He advocates that as the AD progresses, the ethic of care should become paramount (Post, 1998). In this model, one considers (1) the context of the situation, (2) others who are involved and how they are related, and (3) decision making that promotes and maintains relationships. This model understands patients as being "in relationship" versus there being an emphasis on individual autonomy. In this model, "being with" the patient is imperative, and it transmits moral hope—to the patient, the family, and other health providers. However, "the medicalized 'doing to' is sometimes easier than the more appropriate 'being with'" (Post & Whitehouse, 1995, p. 1427).

Boyd and Vernon (1998) raise questions about the clinical and ethical challenges of the important interplay between the patient and the family caregivers. This, too, is consistent with the nursing ethic model of care. Will treatment of comorbid conditions, with a goal of comfort, "create symptoms that compound the patient's discomfort in dying? . . . [what effect] will [continuation or] discontinuation of a medication have on the caregivers; that is, will symptoms appear that increase caregiver stress or burden?" Boyd and Vernon state, "A balance between the legitimate needs of caregivers to control troublesome behaviors and the concerns for humanistic care and damaging polypharmacy needs to be carefully considered by the PCP [primary care provider]" (pp. 74–75).

An ethic of care does not preclude giving attention to principles. Nurses have been taught to avoid harm to patients and to practice the principle of beneficence (Code of Ethics for Nurses, June 30, 2001). Bosek (2001, p. 31) advocates that nonmaleficence should be the "primary guiding ethical principle in every action a nurse does." In specific clinical situations, the nurse should ask: Is a certain treatment causing more harm than benefit, or vice versa?

Studies of nurses and physicians have shown they have been compelled against their conscience by prolonging overly burdensome treatments (Baggs & Schmitt, 1995; Solomon, O'Donnell, & Jennings, 1993). This historical tension of differentiation between the two ethical principles of nonmaleficence and beneficence will be modulated in the future by research studies on evidence-based outcomes. As there is increasing scientific clinical evidence for what constitutes beneficial treatment, it may be less ethically burdensome to make treatment decisions. For example, there is increased clinical evidence that forgoing fluids and nutrition in end-stage illness does not cause suffering, whereas artificial nutrition frequently causes aspiration pneumonia and bloating (Post & Whitehouse, 1995). Fabiszewski, Volicer, and Volicer (1990) reported on patients with advanced AD that treatment of fever with antibiotics does not alter the outcome of fever.

Another perspective on beneficence (from an ethical analysis, not clinical research) is that offered by Post (1995), who argues against the societal value that Americans put on the "hyper-cognitive" self. He stresses, instead, the positive value of several indicators of well-being in individuals with severe dementia— for example, the assertion of will (generally in the form of dissent), expression of a range of emotions, initiation of social contact, and affectional warmth. Post also argues against the personhood theory of self for patients with AD: "Used as an engine of *exclusion,* personhood theory easily leads to insensitivity, if not to great wickedness" (1998, p. 72). Thus, if a health provider is to practice beneficence, a palliative care model may be the best model because it recognizes the whole patient and does not put full value only on the cognitive aspect of an individual. It also provides an environment in which emotional, relational, aesthetic, and spiritual needs can be met. However, a caveat is that individuals and family members want certain treatments implemented or withheld based on their strong value system—regardless of what scientific evidence or ethical analysis indicates.

There is also tension between the nonmaleficence/beneficence principle and the principle of justice. Nurses must be sensitive to the fact that a society ought to allocate finite resources wisely. Such allocations are based on the society's values and recognition of futility or nonfutility of treatments. Again, evidence-based outcomes in health care are important guides. For example, Karlawish, Quill, and Meier (1999) report on five studies conducted between 1992 and 1998 in which enteral feeding (1) did not significantly reduce and may have increased the risk of aspiration pneumonia, (2) did not prevent weight loss or the progression of decubitus, and (3) was associated with a substantial one-year mortality rate. In the United States, end-of-life care costs 10–12 percent of the total health care budget and uses 27 percent of the Medicare budget (Emanuel, 1996). Data from the SUPPORT study found a correlation between a family's economic hardship and a patient's preference for palliative care versus life-extending treatments (Tilden, 1999). Palliative care, whether for patients with AD or with other diseases, can be cost effective and meet the principle of justice by wise utilization of resources. Data from the Oregon Hospice Association (OHA) and Medicare demonstrate the economic aspects of such use of financial resources: OHA showed two days of hospital care were equivalent financially to thirty days of hospice care. Medicare data reflects Medicare nonhospice patients spend twenty of their last fifty days in a hospital, whereas Medicare hospice patients spend eight of their last fifty days in a hospital. Because patients with AD are sometimes admitted to hospitals for co-morbid problems, these statistics have implications for models of health care delivery for these latter patients. A hospice model of palliative care for patients with AD can meet the ethical principle of justice.

Oregon is an exemplar case study to analyze because many indicators of palliative care reform occurred after proposed legislation on physician-assisted suicide in that state (Tilden, 1999; Tilden et al., 1996; Gordon & Singer, 1995). For example, Oregon differs from many other states in the following ways: (1) only 33 percent of Oregonians die in hospitals, whereas the majority of Americans die in acute-care hospitals; one-third of Oregonians die in nursing homes, and one-third die in hospices or at home; (2) 90 percent of elderly nursing home residents in Oregon have advance directives; the converse is true for the rest of the nation-about 80 percent of nursing home residents do not have such directives; (3) 33 percent of Oregonians have hospice support, compared with 17 percent of the national population; (4) the state leads the country in the use of medical morphine; (5) their advance directive law is liberal (i.e., "permitting the refusal of any medical treatment and authorizing surrogates to make decisions for patients who are terminally ill or who have dementia and can no longer speak for themselves"); and (6) an Oregon law *requires* that when life-sustaining treatments are withheld or withdrawn, medication to relieve pain and suffering *must* be provided (Tilden, 1999, p. 165).

While ethicists, health professionals, and policymakers discuss and debate ethical approaches to palliative care for patients with AD, another approach taken by Post and Whitehouse (1995) has been "discourse ethics." They held focus groups of family caregivers and individuals with mild dementia and asked them to discuss the issues facing them. "Discourse ethics" is a "shift toward socially deliberated moral consensus and away from heavy reliance on ethical theory and solitary reflection . . . and returns ethics to the affected public world" (p. 1423).

A major ethical question may be: What is the extent to which interested individuals (patients, family members, health providers, ethicists, policymakers, and citizens) are community and political actors to facilitate change in worksite, community, and public policy? Are interested individuals enacting change to facilitate the availability and accessibility to hospice care for patients with AD? Are they changing current Medicare hospice benefit policy and state Medicaid policy?

❧ Nursing Role

The nurse's role in care of patients with AD (as in caring for other patients) includes (1) educating patients on the use of advance directives, (2) facilitating families in making end-of-life decisions, (3) monitoring the compliance of staff to patient preferences, (4) revalidating with patients and family members the treatment plans being followed, (5) facilitating communication among the patient, family, and health providers, (6) involvement in policy making, (7) involvement in the implementation of both life-extending and palliative care interventions, and (8) being culturally competent in the delivery of care (Tilden, 1999).

Nurses educate patients on the use of advance directives in many patient settings. Many individuals, valuing autonomy, decision making, and control over their future lives, will have completed advance directives, including both a living will and a form for durable power of attorney. However, many other patients have not completed such legal documents. Even though the federal Patient Self-Determination Act of 1990 has resulted in more individuals and families having discussions on end-of-life care, studies have shown that 80 percent of nursing home residents do not have such documents (Bradley, Peiris, & Wetle, 1998; Suri et al., 1999). Only 10 to 20 percent of all Americans have advance directives (Robinson & Kennedy-Schwarz, 2001). It is important that nurses educate patients on advance directives when the patients are not in acute illness episodes.

The second role of nurses is to facilitate families in making end-of-life decisions. Norton and Talerico's (2000) research specifically contributes to nurses' (and other health care providers') knowledge base of how to facilitate end-of-life decision making for individuals and families. This study integrates with use of the hospice model discussed above. The following behaviors were considered of prime importance by family members: (1) the health care provider was experienced in the care of the dying, and (2) the health care provider was comfortable in discussing end-of-life decision making. This latter behavior of being comfortable was expressed by the professional caregiver's taking over the initiative and being willing to engage patient or family in end-of-life discussions. "Comfortable" professional caregivers initiated this conversation early in the patient's disease trajectory so that important symptom management could be decided. This has specific implications for nurses caring for patients with AD and their families. The other listed behavior—being experienced—has implications for those who work in hospices: family members appreciate their loved ones being cared for by providers who are experienced.

To return to the overall list of nursing roles, the third and fourth—facilitating patient preferences and staff compliance in meeting patient needs—can be done in several ways. A behavioral standard for nurses is to have knowledge of research on how families make decisions. For example, for end-of-life decision making, the three most important aspects to families are their realization of futility, their understanding of the patient's preferences, and their perception of the patient's suffering (Tilden, 1999). Therefore, nurses must have knowledge of evidence-based outcomes of different treatment plans for the patient with AD with co-morbidities and to be able to explain whether or not this is a futile or nonfutile treatment. Further, it is important to explain patient behaviors to the family. The nurse may educate on patient suffering that is not visible to the family member. Nurses should be bold in utilizing mediators when the occasion calls for it. Such professionals may be of valuable assistance in conflict resolution and healing when there are different preferences among family members and/or health providers regarding treatment regimes. This resource, now being increasingly used with success in several legal areas (divorce, parenting plans, probate, guardianship, conservatorship, etc.), could be a potential resource for ethical conflict resolution for family members making decisions about treatment options for patients with AD. This is a resource in addition to the ethics committees of health institutions.

Tilden's fifth listing is facilitation of communication. Some authors emphasize the importance of language sensitivity when discussing palliative care with individuals and family members. When there is a shift from cure or aggressive treatment to palliative or active comfort care, one should avoid the implication that "nothing can be done" (Robinson & Kennedy-Schwarz, 2001, p. 76). Norton and Talerico stressed "being willing, being clear, and clarifying prognosis and goals of treatment" in communication between health providers and family (2000, pp. 9–10). "Being clear" meant avoiding phrases such as "there is nothing more we can do" and "there isn't any hope." They noted that experienced health providers were able to implement many adequate and appropriate symptom management interventions and that there was always something to hope for. Language sensitivity is an important clinical competence and ethical standard for providers to implement when shifting from aggressive treatment to palliative care.

Nurses also have their policy making role. In facilitating more hospice models of care delivery for patients with AD, nurses are important actors. For example, they could initiate such a change at their worksite, be a part of a community group advocating for such services, and be legislative advocates to facilitate policy and funding decisions that would make this type of care more available and accessible (Rushton & Sabatier, 2001). Besides changing legislation, nurses could advocate for changes in state policy and nursing home regulation to ensure nursing home inspectors and regulators are knowledgeable about the issues described in this chapter. Perhaps, for the patient with dementia, the nursing home inspector could be less concerned with weight measurements and more concerned with palliative care and the ethics of caring for such patients (Post & Whitehouse, 1995). To meet this public health need, nurses will have to stay educated and competent in a variety of ways to best meet the needs of this population. For example, different parts of this chapter emphasize the need for the nurse to know the literature on (1) evidence-based outcomes, (2) increased educational opportunities for health-provider students and practitioners in end-of-life care, (3) ethical analysis, and (4) policy aspects.

The seventh role, that of implementing palliative care interventions, is based on the nurse's knowledge of nursing care and research in this specialty area. Nurses can take initiative in home, community, and long-term care settings by recommending the use of the AHOPE tool when they note deteriorating conditions in patients. If the patient meets the criteria of this screening tool, this may mean beginning hospice care for that patient (Marsh et al., 2000). The researchers do not recommend use of this predictive tool when the patient is hospitalized, because of the negative effects of short-term disorientation in the hospital. In addition, one should be knowledgeable of these specific clinical nursing interventions, including the use of art, music, individualized care planning for wandering, adequate pain management, attention to interventions that enhance emotional and relational well-being, aesthetic and spiritual well-being, and so forth (Post, 1998).

There are numerous implications from the work by Miller, Nelson, and Mezey (2000) on appropriate pain assessment and management. Nurses should (1) know the barriers for these patients to adequate pain management; (2) administer analgesics on a regular versus on an as-needed schedule; (3) use opioid analgesics when needed; (4) be attentive to the relationship of behavioral symptoms with pain (e.g., aggressiveness, agitation, growls); (5) educate other team members—professional and nonprofessional—in this area of care.

❧ Cultural Competence of Nurses

Tilden's final role for nurses is that they be culturally competent in their care of patients. Cultural differences exist in a variety of end-of-life issues. For example, problem solving of treatment regimes for patients with Alzheimer disease could range from aggressive medical treatment to hospice palliative care to physician-assisted suicide and euthanasia (Post, 1997). In 1998, the German Medical Association released new principles about palliative care. They firmly rejected euthanasia and said that physician-assisted suicide violated professional medical rules (Sahm, 2000). Further, they stated that palliative care should include satisfying hunger and thirst subjective needs versus maintaining physiological parameters. This guideline is similar to the American Alzheimer's Disease and Related Disorders Association: "If such a patient is unable to receive food and water by mouth, it is ethically permissible to choose to withhold nutrition and hydration artificially administered by vein or gastric tube" (Post, 1998, pp. 75–76).

Use of advance directives is another way that cross-cultural differences exist. The advance directive may work better in a culture such as the United States, which puts a high degree of value on individual autonomy. However, in cultures that support a family-centered model rather than individual decision making, use of such forms is not commonplace. For example, Korean Americans, Mexican Americans, and Native Americans would have conflicts with these directives (Post, 1998; Lynn et al., 1996). In an increasingly culturally diverse American society, nurses will have to be knowledgeable of these differences and recognize that the dominant American value of autonomy does not apply to all families. Lack of such discussion and/or directives could contribute to inadequate or unauthorized aggressive symptom management. For example, African American and Hispanic patients want more aggressive life-prolonging treatment and are less likely to have advance directives (Tilden, 1999). In countries with (1) national health systems, (2) a strong emphasis on primary care, and (3) health and social systems where there is a longer, more enduring relationship among the patient, family, and the physician, advance directives are viewed negatively (Solomon, 2000). Besides the cultural trait of emphasis (or nonemphasis) on individual autonomy, another cultural difference is related to truth telling. Some Americans would perceive an apparent lack of truth telling by health providers in Italy, Spain, and Russia (Solomon, 2000).

Dementia is also viewed differently in various cultures. Americans highly value independence and economic productivity that necessitates the importance of intellect, memory, and self-control (Post, 1998). These underlying values then shape the clinical and ethical discussions Americans have about treatment for patients with AD. For example, an earlier section of this chapter noted writers who emphasized autonomy as the dominant medical ethical principle in the United States: this springs from basic American value systems. In contrast, research in China shows less dread there about the diagnosis of dementia (Post, 1998). To Chinese family members, an individual with dementia is still "there" and is not "gone," neither a shell nor a husk—metaphors that one might hear in the United States (Post, 1998, p. 72; Post, 1995). In the Japanese culture some find dementia to be "a release from the fetters of everyday cares and occupations" (Post, 1998, p. 72).

Cross-national research shows differences in physician decision making on treatment decisions for patients with advanced AD. For example, in one study, American physicians, compared with Australian physicians, chose more aggressive medical treatment. The Australians were more likely to choose supportive care (Post, 1997).

Family members and health providers may approach ethical decision making from different perspectives. For example, a Jewish perspective of caring for an incompetent parent may be duty-based (Weisensee & Kjervik, 2001).

Different countries have different histories of palliative care approaches. Palliative care—for all patients—is in beginning stages in Poland. While palliative nursing care is an outgrowth of the hospice movement, which started in 1981 (i.e., the Society of Friends to the Terminally Ill), there is much improvement that could be done in their nursing curriculums (Wronska & Gozdek, 1994). This was a finding of a research study of baccalaureate nursing students. The researchers were concerned that for a palliative model of care to succeed in the transformed Polish society of the past decade, there must also be an appreciation of the value of palliative care by health professionals. Hospice care is new to Russia—it began in 1990 (Cooke, 1995). The economic situation in Russia has been one factor that has influenced the use of alternative therapies in their hospices (i.e., imagery, hypnosis, massage). Of particular interest to this writer was the management of bells as practiced by European monks as a pain-management strategy (Cooke, 1995; Nelson, 1995). Nelson observed the following while visiting an impoverished area of Russia:

> As a result of the limited pain control options, they have had to become resourceful with the alternative ways to manage pain, even resorting to bells. Bells? It was related to us that the European monks used bells when they were sick, not to alarm but to appeal to those that needed help. Dr. Andrei Gnezditov showed us a room with excellent acoustics where there were suspended from a rack a number of irregular-shaped, homemade bells ranging in size from gigantic to large. Dr. Gnezditov struck the bells with a soft headed mallet. The mixture of size and vibration was quite incredible and difficult to describe. We could feel the vibration through our bodies and it was a very pleasant sensation. Many patients in pain find great relief from this bell therapy, the modality of which has yet to be investigated and explained. (1995, 7)

Such an example could have positive clinical and financial implications for nurses' and others' care of patients in other countries.

To summarize, this chapter defends a hospice model of care delivery for patients with end-stage dementia because palliative care can relieve symptoms, control pain, and contribute to a better dying process. Research on hospice projects has demonstrated both the feasibility of this kind of care delivery and the barriers to such delivery. Other research has shown that family and professional caregivers perceive this model as appropriate. Arguments have been made that this is an ethical model of care delivery. The greater ethical question may be, "Is enough being done to foster and promote this kind of palliative care?" This chapter has emphasized the eight roles of the nurse in promoting this model of care delivery.

Centuries ago, Jonathan Swift (1945 version, pp. 214–216) wrote in *Gulliver's Travels* about demented "struldbrugs" who had "no remembrance of anything but what they learned and observed in their youth and middle age, and even that is very imperfect . . . and they were despised and hated by all sorts of people." Can a palliative model of care delivery prevent patients with AD from being despised as struldbrugs? Can a palliative model of care enhance the moral significance of such patients, temper the threat of existentiality that accompanies forgetfulness, and decrease the use of metaphors such as shell, husk, "gone," and "not there" that often accompanies the description of individuals with Alzheimer disease? The answer should be yes.

REFERENCES

Baggs, J., & Schmitt, M. (1995). Intensive care decisions about level of aggressiveness of care. *Research Nursing Health, 18,* 345–355.

Bosek, M. (2001). Reaffirming a primary commitment to nonmaleficence. *Journal of Nursing Administration: Healthcare Law, Ethics, and Regulation, 3,* 31–34.

Bosek, M., & Shaw, L. (2001). When surrogate decision-making is not straightforward. *Journal of Nursing Administration: Healthcare Law, Ethics, and Regulation, 3,* 47–57.

Boyd, C., & Vernon, G. (1998). Primary care of the older adult with end-stage Alzheimer's disease. *Nurse Practitioner, 23,* 63–83.

Bradley, I., Peiris, V., & Wetle, T. (1998). Discussions about end-of-life care in nursing homes. *Journal of the American Geriatrics Society, 46,* 1235–1241.

Code of Ethics for Nurses. Available at the official American Nurses Association website, www.nursingworld.org/ethics/chcode.htm (accessed September 2001).

Cooke, M. (1995). The Russian way of hospice. *American Journal of Hospice & Palliative Care, 9–17.*

Emanuel, E. (1996). Cost savings at the end of life: What do the data show? *Journal of the American Medical Association, 275,* 1907–1914.

Fabiszewski, K., Volicer, B., & Volicer, L. (1990). Effect of antibiotic treatment on outcome of fevers in institutionalized Alzheimer patients. *Journal of the American Medical Association, 263,* 3168–3172.

Gordon, M., & Singer, P. (1995). Decisions and care at the end of life. *Lancet, 346,* 163–166.

Hospice: Core and cornerstone of the end-of-life movement. (2000). *Caring, 19* (9), 46–49.

Hurley, A., Volicer, L., Rempusheski, V., & Fry, S. (1995). Reaching consensus: The process of recommending treatment decisions for Alzheimer's patients. *Advances in Nursing Science, 18,* 33–43.

Karlawish, J., Quill, T., & Meier, D. (1999). A consensus-based approach to providing palliative care to patients who lack decision-making capacity. *Annals of Internal Medicine, 130,* 835–840.

Luchins, D., & Hanrahan, P. (1993). What is the appropriate level of health care for end-stage dementia patients? *Journal of the American Geriatrics Society, 41,* 25–30.

Luchins, D., Hanrahan, P., & Murphy, K. (1997). Criteria for enrolling dementia patients in hospice. *Journal of the American Geriatrics Society, 45,* 1054–1059.

Lundy, K., & Janes, S. (2001). *Community health nursing.* Sudbury, MA: Jones & Bartlett.

Lynn, J., Marson, D. C., Odenheimer, G. L., & Post, S. G. (1996). Legal and ethical dilemmas in Alzheimer's care. *Patient Care,* 44–61.

Marsh, G. W., Prochoda, K. P., Pritchett, E., & Vojir, C. P. (2000). Predicting hospice appropriateness for patients with dementia of the Alzheimer's type. *Applied Nursing Research, 13* (4), 187–196.

Miller, L. L., Nelson, L. L., & Mezey, M. (2000). Comfort and pain relief in dementia. *Journal of Gerontological Nursing, 33*–56.

Nelson, F. (1995). Citizen ambassador program of people to people international's hospice delegation to Russia and Poland. *American Journal of Hospice & Palliative Care,* 6–8.

Norton, S., & Talerico, K. A. (2000). Facilitating end-of-life decision-making: Strategies for communicating and assessing. *Journal of Gerontological Nursing, 26*, 6–13.

Post, S. (1995). Alzheimer disease and the "then" self. *Kennedy Institute of Ethics Journal, 5,* 307–321.

Post, S. (1997). Physician-assisted suicide in Alzheimer's disease. *Journal of the American Geriatrics Society, 45,* 647–651.

Post, S. (1998). The fear of forgetfulness: A grassroots approach to an ethics of Alzheimer's disease. *Journal of Clinical Ethics, 9,* 71–80.

Post, S., & Whitehouse, P. (1995). Fairhill guidelines on ethics of the care of people with Alzheimer's Disease: A clinical summary. *Journal of the American Geriatrics Society, 43,* 1423–1429.

Robinson, E. M., & Kennedy-Schwarz, J. (2001). Caring for incompetent patients and their surrogates. *American Journal of Nursing, 101,* 75–76.

Rousseau, P. (1998). Palliative care in managed Medicare: Reasons for hope—and for concern. *Geriatrics, 53,* 59–66.

Rushton, C., & Sabatier, K. (2001). The nursing leadership consortium on end-of-life care: The response of the nursing profession to the need for improvement in palliative care. *Nursing Outlook, 49,* 58–60.

Sahm, S. (2000). Palliative care versus euthanasia: The German position: The German general medical council's principles for medical care of the terminally ill. *Journal of Medicine and Philosophy, 25,* 195–219.

Solomon, M. (2000). Innovations in end-of-life care. *Education Development Center Annual Report,* 23–25.

Solomon, M., O'Donnell, L., Jennings, B., Guilfoy, V., Wolf, S. M., Nolan, K., et al. (1993). Decisions near the end of life: Professional views on life-sustaining treatments. *American Journal of Public Health, 83,* 14–25.

Suri, D., Egleston, B., Brody, J., & Rudberg, M. (1999). Nursing home residents use of care directives. *Journal of Gerontology, 54,* M225–M229.

Swift, J. (1945 version). *Gulliver's travels.* Garden City, NY: Doubleday. Originally published 1726.

Tilden, V. (1999). Ethics perspectives on end-of-life care. *Nursing Outlook, 47,* 162–167.

Tilden, V., Tolle, S., Lee, M., & Nelson, C. (1996). Oregon's physician-assisted suicide vote: Its effect on palliative care. *Nursing Outlook, 44,* 80–83.

Volicer, L., Rheaume, Y., Brown, J., Fabiszewski, K., & Brady, R. (1986). Hospice approach to the treatment of patients with advanced dementia of the Alzheimer type. *Journal of the American Medical Association, 256,* 2210–2213.

Weisensee, M., & Kjervik, D. (2001). Assessment of cognitively impaired elderly: A challenge for public policy in an aging society. *Journal of Nursing Law, 8,* 33–47.

Wilson, S., Kovach, C., & Stearns, S. (1996). Hospice concepts in the care for end-stage dementia. *Geriatric Nursing, 17,* 6–10.

Wronska, I., & Gozdek, N. (1994). Aims and ethics of palliative care-the views of a selected group of Polish nursing students. *Scandinavian Journal of Caring Science, 8,* 25–27.

Yeaworth, R. (2001, May 28). Personal communication.

Zerzan, J., Stearns, S., & Hanson, L. (2000). Access to palliative care and hospice in nursing homes. *Journal of the American Medical Association, 284,* 2489–2494.

CHAPTER SIXTEEN

Ethical Dimensions of Alzheimer Disease Decision Making

The Need for Early Patient and Family Education

Linda S. Scheirton, Ph.D.

She had been with us for one month. She seemed somewhat detached or depressed, perhaps. She stood in the kitchen at dusk, with the last vestiges of light coming through the window illuminating her frail figure as she moved among the shadows. You could see the individual strands of grey hair recklessly uplifted in slight disarray, as the stream of remaining light gave her head an almost angelic appearance. As her son-in-law walked into the room, she politely asked, "Would you like some coffee, honey?" "No, thank you, I usually don't drink coffee this late in the day," he answered. "I was just making some coffee," she replied. All of a sudden it seemed to dawn on her. She appeared to be perplexed. The furrowed brow accentuating the deep wrinkles in her once-beautiful face provided clear evidence of her confused state of mind. She held on to the edge of the counter as if to stabilize herself before walking around to where I was standing. Her faded blue eyes peered deeply into my mine and she asked, "Linda, is this morning or evening?" "It is evening, Mom," I said softly.

Alzheimer disease (AD) begins insidiously with a gradual but progressive deterioration. As chronicled in the preceding vignette, disorientation of time and place as well as changes in mood and behaviors are just a few of the warning signs of AD. Although the course of the disease is generally prolonged and a reasonable quality of life can often be enjoyed during much of that time, in the end the disease erodes all cognitive and functional abilities of the patient and leads to total dependence on caregivers (Ham, 1997). Indeed, AD patients rarely suffer alone because the disease also takes its toll on their family and friends. But if diagnosed in the early stages, patients often retain the ability to guide medical and domestic decisions to be made during later stages of the disease process, thereby fostering the quality of their own care as well as mitigating the burdens of caregivers.

Health consumer education ideally is initiated at this point of early AD, before problems encountered with the disease escalate into crises. Education can empower the patient and give him the tools to successfully navigate through each stage of the disease. What most recently diagnosed Alzheimer's patients need to know is how to live with the disease, what to expect, how to get care and treatment, how to deal with disease-related problems when they arise, and how to ensure that their wishes are honored. Hence, educational programs should provide clear and concise information regarding diagnosis procedures, treatment options, the effects of the disease, and ethical treatment guidelines (Alzheimer Society of Canada, 1995). In addition to these health care related issues, patients and their families will benefit from education about estate planning, living wills, powers of attorney, and choices for guardian or conservatorship.

A wealth of educational resources, training modules, and references for Alzheimer disease (AD) patients related to current research, diagnostic testing, activities of daily living, social services, home health aides, nursing homes, hospices, and support groups is easily accessible via local, regional, national, and international health organizations, universities, and on the web. Explicit instructions on how to access these resources are necessary to enable a person to navigate through the wealth of educational materials available.

This chapter presents an educational agenda, utilizing the following ethical guidelines and principles for Alzheimer care: truthfulness in disclosing the diagnosis of AD; availability of comprehensive information about the progression of the disease; respect for individual choice by facilitation of voluntary transfers of decision making; enhancement of quality of life; prevention of harm to self and others; voluntary participation in genetic testing and research; and justice for caregivers.

❧ Truthful Communication of the Diagnosis

The educational process begins with an early and accurate diagnosis. A proper diagnosis is important for four reasons. First, patient or family concern can be eliminated if it is unwarranted. Second, non-Alzheimer conditions that are treatable can be identified, as emphasized in chapter 3. Thirdly, the earlier that AD is diagnosed, the more likely some symptoms may respond to and benefit from existing treatments. Fourth, early diagnosis allows the patient and family to plan for the future, including making therapeutic strategies (Fox et al., 2001).

While researchers have made major progress in developing diagnostic tests and techniques, there is no one, simple test with which to make a diagnosis of AD. The standard workup includes a health history, physical examination, blood work, radiology, and neuropsychological testing (Geldmacher & Whitehouse, 1997). A health history is taken from the patient and relative or friend. Neuropsychological testing is used to assess a patient's level of cognitive functioning and, when deficits are present, to quantify the severity and scope of existing cognitive impairment. Neuropsychological testing should be carried out as part of the standard medical workup, although many practitioners fail to do so. Standardized assessment instruments can provide information on the patient's capacity for self-care and independent living. During the assessment, a combination of questions, simple tasks, and observation is used to evaluate patients and determine the kinds of skills a person has lost or that have been retained. A baseline assessment of functional abilities is important to track and document disease progression. One of the most common nonneuropsychological tests for assessing and documenting mental status is the Mini-Mental State Examination (MMSE), a brief test of mental status and cognitive functioning (Folstein, Folstein, & McHugh, 1975) (included in chapter 2). The screening tool and its scoring system can be used to chart progress over time.

Individuals with AD must be able to trust that information on their disease will be forthcoming from others. In September 1999, Alzheimer's Disease International (ADI) developed a charter of basic principles considered fundamental to the provision of care for people with dementia. This charter is a working document and is reviewed periodically, most recently in October 2002. The fourth of these core principles stipulates that "people with dementia require up to date information." The fifth principle emphasizes that "people with dementia should as far as possible participate in decisions affecting their daily life and future care." Both of these principles cannot be adhered to unless truthful and full disclosure of the diagnosis takes place.

Occasionally, family members or friends will object to having the diagnosis disclosed to the patient. They may argue that the patient has limited capacity to understand; subjecting the patient to full disclosure could lead the patient to hopelessness, depression, or suicide. Since the diagnosis is imperfect, the prognosis uncertain, and treatment options limited, nondisclosure seems more humane. Although controversy over disclosure continues among ethicists, it is generally assumed that all patients, including AD patients, have either the right to receive truthful information about their own diagnosis or to waive that right (Post, 2000; Meyers, 1997). The main objective should be sensitive disclosure in order to avoid unnecessary despair. Most clinicians agree that the patient will need emotional support when the diagnosis is communicated (Post & Whitehouse, 1995). Therefore, there should be a joint meeting that will include both the diagnosed individual and family members or friends.

❧ Comprehensive Information about Disease Progression

For the recently diagnosed individual, learning more about AD prevalence and progression takes on a new significance, and education becomes more crucial. Educational interventions can assist the patient and future family caregiver to (1) find answers to questions about AD; (2) get information about recent research findings on the disease; (3) learn about new treatment modalities; (4) subscribe to publications about the disease, and (5) locate helpful resources via the Internet and through Alzheimer organizations or governmental health agencies.

The disclosure should begin with the facts of the disease. The individual should be aware that even though the disease is irreversible and progressive, some of its effects can be treated. Since the nature and symptoms of the disease vary significantly among patients, it is important to tailor information to the patient's unique situation and to guard against making undue generalizations. Expectations for the future should be discussed early in the process since the disease's progression may preclude such discussions down the road.

Disease progression is classified in three stages: *early* (mild), *middle* (moderate), and *late* (severe). Symptoms at the time of diagnosis vary from individual to individual, and the disease advances at different rates. There are also very variable ranges of functioning within each stage of the disease; hence, there is always a significant risk that educational programs unduly generalize. Nevertheless, some general patterns can be discerned.

In the early stage of AD, the individual consciously experiences loss of mental faculties and as a result can become depressed. Short-term memory loss, mild aphasia, and disorientation and confusion lead to problems with routine tasks. The individual seeks familiar places and avoids unfamiliar places. Work or social activities are somewhat impaired, but the capacity for independent living remains during this stage. Reminders with some activities of daily living are needed.

As the disease progresses, the symptoms become more noticeable and start clearly to interfere with daily living such as the ability to work, handle finances, or to drive an automobile. Individuals in the middle stage with moderate dementia are sometimes capable of independent living, but require significant assistance with daily tasks. Disorientation, anxiety, panic, paranoia, hallucinations, aggression, and hostility are sometimes exhibited by the individual. The ability to recognize people, to understand the spoken and written word, to speak and write, increasingly impedes communication. The individual loses sense of time, and thus sleeping rhythms become disrupted; the distinction between day and night loses its significance. The individual no longer recognizes familiar places; judgment is decreased; wandering/roaming can be triggered; and the individual becomes fearful, lost, and at risk for serious harm. Creating a safe environment at this stage becomes of paramount importance.

The late stage of AD is marked by severe dementia. Constant supervision, care, and assistance are needed. Individuals lose the ability to understand or use language. There is greater incidence of mood and behavior disturbances. Individuals lose track of their own person and sense of personal history. Physiologic decline such as total incontinence, ability to walk unaided, and difficulty chewing and swallowing occurs. The individual is more prone to pneumonia and bedsores. Finally, an unresponsive state may occur that leads to death. Despite the hopelessness and severity of the symptoms at this late stage, the individual still responds well to touch and familiar, soft voices.

✦ Respect for Patient Choices about Treatment and Care

A diagnosis of Alzheimer disease does not mean that an individual is immediately unable to make decisions on his or her own behalf. Throughout most of the course of the disease, some decisional abilities remain. Whenever a patient appears able to make choices, in principle these choices should be respected. If at all possible, a care plan should be discussed and agreed upon while the individual is still decisionally capable.

A good care plan requires that personal values are discussed. One way to determine those values and preferences is to complete a Values History Form (Doukas & Gorenflo, 1993; Ross et al., 1993). For times when decisions must be made, the form has a series of "questions about preferences in specific medical circumstances, general values, medical values, relationships with family, friends and health care providers, religious views, financial preferences, and other issues likely to be useful" (Lambert, Gibson, & Nathanson, 1990, pp. 204–208). The Values History Form recognizes that the health care decisions we make for ourselves are based on those beliefs, preferences, and values that matter most to us. It allows individuals to think and document these ahead of time. Once the Alzheimer patient is unable to make health care decisions, the patient's thoughts as expressed on this form can help others (family, friends, health care providers, lawyer, clergy, etc.) to make a decision for the patient in accordance with what the patient would have chosen, thus preserving the patient's individual autonomy. Finally, the values history can be utilized as a precursor for (1) executing advance directives (trusts, living wills, durable powers of attorney, durable powers of attorney for health care, etc.); or (2) deciding whether consent should be given to participate as a human subject in a research study.

✦ Future Planning: Estate, Advance Directives, Powers of Attorney, Wills

A variety of legal mechanisms are available to assist in the management of assets and health care when a person becomes incompetent. As one AD researcher has eloquently said, "the precedent self that is fully intact before the clinical manifestation of dementia has the legal right and authority to dictate levels of medical care for the severely demented self" (Post, 2000, p. 52). Advance directives are written instructions that communicate an individual's preferences and wishes about care and treatment that he or she would want to receive if a point was reached where the individual could not speak for him or herself (Reilly, Teasdale, & McCullough, 1994). These instructions could address use of physical restraints, for example, or artificial nutrition and hydration, or other end-of-life care issues. A durable power of attorney for health care authorizes someone such as a relative, spouse, or friend to make health care decisions when the individual is no longer capable of doing so. Educating the patient and family caregivers regarding these mechanisms will hopefully assure that the patient's wishes are later fully honored.

As time passes and the disease progresses, more and more decisions will involve others—family members, caregivers, knowledgeable health care providers. It is important that an ongoing dialogue include the individual with AD. It should remain a core principle that "people with dementia should as far as possible participate in decisions affecting their daily lives and future care" (Alzheimer Disease International, 2002, principle 5). Decisions can vary on a continuum from simple expressions of desire to complex issues requiring specific experience and personal judgment. The Alzheimer Society of Canada (2001) suggests that all decisions should be based on (1) the wishes of the individual with AD; (2) the weighing of risks and benefits of the decision to the diseased individual as well as the caregiver; (3) the effect on the physical as well as emotional well-being of the individual; and (4) the effect on the individual's and caregiver's quality of life.

To help the AD patient plan for the future, a certain knowledge base concerning the disease must be attained while the patient is competent to do so. Therefore, "adequate resources should be available and promoted to support people with dementia and their caregivers throughout the course of dementia" (Alzheimer Disease International, 2002, principle 7). This is a core principle that must be given priority if patient autonomy and self-determination is to be maximized. Alzheimer organizations have developed brochures on planning for the future, steps to understanding financial and legal issues, and where resources can be accessed. These organizations, via their Internet websites, list online resources that include brochures, fact sheets, books, tapes (video and audio modular training packages), values histories, advance directive documents, and other references to where legal and financial assistance can be found. Many local organizations, hospital education departments, health care providers, social workers, and lay volunteers staff telephone help lines, chat rooms, and list serves in an effort to assist the AD patient in advance planning.

In addition to advance directives, estate planning, execution of wills, and guardianship, it is also important for the patient and family to perform an asset and expense assessment. This will give the patient and family caregiver the necessary information to determine if they qualify for governmental or state resources.

Deciding on types of residential care is another major planning topic— choosing among group homes, retirement communities, assisted living facilities, continuing care retirement communities, nursing homes, and hospice or dementia special care units. Again, a wealth of Internet information is available from the major Alzheimer organizations, with links to regional and local resources. Although care at home can be managed in the later stage of the disease, it requires someone to be responsible for providing twenty-four-hour supervision. Late-stage care of Alzheimer patients is often performed in long-term care facilities. Planning placement in a long-term care facility before it becomes an urgent need can ease the transition for both the patient and the caregiver. With assistance from others, the person with AD can gather facts about different facilities, visit the facilities and compare, and weigh pros and cons of each. It can be agreed upon in advance that when observations chronicling decline to the point that possible harm may occur, transition from home to long-term care will occur.

Additional education is needed for management of affairs in the later stages of the disease. Difficult moral choices at the end-of-life should be discussed as early in the disease process as possible. Once the meaning and substance of human life have deteriorated, and certain thresholds—determined by the patient—have been met, the decision not to use life-prolonging technologies is acceptable (Post & Whitehouse, 1995). It should be understood that unnecessary treatment or procedures that will not benefit the patient need not be carried out. Respect for treatment refusal is needed at this point. Comfort care and emotional well-being should be the most important objective. Directives as to the use of life-prolonging technologies, foregoing tube feedings, hydration, and treatment of infection, as well as alternatives to assisted suicide and euthanasia, should be executed (de Wachter, 1992; Post, 1997; Ham, 1997; Boyd & Vernon, 1998; Volicer, 2001).

❧ Enhancement of Quality of Life

Each individual has a personal standard of what is valued and what determines quality of life. Quality of life is partly contingent on the creation of a supportive environment to enhance the individual's well-being (Lawton, 1994). "A person with dementia continues to be a person of worth and dignity, and deserving the same respect as any other human being" (Alzheimer Disease International, 2002, principle 2). This core principle should be a guide when helping to maintain an AD patient's dignity. It is not always easy, even for the most caring and concerned caregivers, to realize and sustain this guiding principle. Family caregivers should themselves seek out educational opportunities in an effort to understand and manage the aspects of the disease. The caregiver should encourage the AD patient to participate in support groups whose goals are to assist the patient in adjusting to and coping with the disease (Yale, 1999). Support groups often provide helpful informational sessions, for example on the use of memory aids that can make life less difficult for the AD patient during the early stage of disease. As routine loss of memory continues, family members and caregivers can assist the individual by giving frequent and simple reminders. What others say and do can be disturbing to the patient. But the patient's comprehension may in fact be better preserved than is apparent, and caregivers should guard against discussing the patient's condition in his or her presence, as though the patient is not there. Conversely, repetition, consistency, and reassurance can help reduce anxiety, agitation, and verbal outbursts (Wilen, Harman, & Alexander-Israel, 1997). Routine is very important in establishing order and structure for the daily life of the individual with AD. Keeping things as normal as possible may come to represent a real sense of security for the individual.

As time goes on and the disease progresses, assessments are necessary to determine which activities of daily living are still possible. Whether a person can dress, eat, handle finances, drive an automobile, use a telephone, tell time from a clock, or travel alone will determine the amount of progressive deterioration and whether there is the ability to survive independently.

While there is currently no cure for AD, quality of life can be extended by the use of certain medications (see chapter 21). Medications are available for people with mild disease. Extensive research is being carried out by pharmaceutical companies on drugs that might slow down the progression of the disease or improve symptoms such as memory loss. However, since AD has an irreversible progression, temporary improvement in cognition can create ethical issues. It has been noted that patients and caregivers who have previously navigated cognitive decline may have to repeat the process after these drugs are taken. "The individual who has lost cognitive insight into his or her losses may regain insight, along with renewed anxiety" (Post, 2000, pp. 63–64). This "intrusion" may not necessarily enhance quality of life; it actually may be more malevolent than benevolent in nature. Therefore, the efficacy of these drugs must be based on long-term studies and not preliminary evidence. It is a pity that after more than twenty years of research, little discernable help has come from medicine or pharmacy to alleviate AD symptoms. It therefore behooves the patient and caregiver to educate themselves thoroughly, seek health care provider information, review drug studies, and remain informed of new drug developments that will alleviate AD symptoms. Medications can play a vital role in assisting a patient to sleep or control agitation or depression. However, AD patients can be susceptible to overmedication, side effects, or reactions from combinations of prescription and over-the-counter drugs. Careful monitoring is necessary in order to avoid harm.

Fortunately, not every patient has every symptom or problem that is associated with the disease, and in fact the agony that many patients with AD feel in the early stage of the disease can often resolve when cognition declines (Ham, 1997). However, in the later stages of the disease, the patient loses the ability to understand or use language, to walk, to sit, to smile, or to eat. This is the stage where the patient and caregivers will receive the most benefit from previous educational interventions and Alzheimer support groups. Constant supervision is clearly necessary at this stage. Preferred environmental and psychosocial interventions often do not work at this stage of the disease, and pharmacologic solutions or physical restraints may be the only alternative. While safety is important, it rarely justifies involuntary restraint and the indignity of being tied down, immobilized. In this situation, it is difficult to determine "a balance between the legitimate needs of the caregivers to control troublesome behaviors and the concerns for humanistic care" (Boyd & Vernon, 1998, p. 75). This creates a true ethical dilemma. A difficult challenge such as this can often significantly and irreparably tax the caregiver's coping skills. This is the point where the patient may be placed in a long-term care facility because the caregiver is no longer capable of caring for the AD patient. Finally, hospice care may be an option for the end stage of AD (Boyd & Vernon, 1998). The cornerstone of hospice philosophy is in the palliation of suffering, the providing of comfort care, and the enhancement of a humanistically attended death.

✤ Prevention of Harm to Self and Others

"People with dementia need a physically safe living environment and protection from exploitation and abuse of person and property" (Alzheimer Disease International, 2002, principle 3). This core principle of nonmaleficence acknowledges the duty not to inflict harm, but to prevent it. It also underscores the need for early intervention and continued concern for the patient's safety. Early patient and caregiver education and advanced planning can facilitate later modification of the environment to promote safety and cooperation of the patient and family when privileges are curtailed for the purpose of protection of the patient and others.

Alzheimer organizations have developed checklists and educational brochures to inform cognitively aware patients and caregivers of ways to make the environment safe for the AD patient. A few of these suggestions for the prevention of injury include installation of gates near stairs, grab bars in bathrooms, removal of internal door locks, and clearing of clutter and dangerous devices such as sharp and flammable objects (Wilen, Harman, & Alexander-Israel, 1997). In the United States, the Alzheimer's Association's Safe Return Program provides twenty-four-hour, toll-free telephone access and maintains an extensive database. It is the only nationwide system that helps to identify, locate, and safely return individuals with AD who have wandered and become lost. Identification products such as bracelets, necklaces, clothing labels, and wallet identification cards are used to alert others that the individual is memory-impaired and needs assistance. The Safe Return crisis number is affixed to the identification product.

There are also forms available on the Internet for chronicling unsafe incidents. For example, unsafe incidents worth recording include wandering outside and getting lost, getting lost inside a building, burning food on the stove resulting in excessive smoke or fire, paranoid delusions involving threats or violence against others, mismanagement of funds, and self-neglect of nutritional, medical, and personal care needs. Written observations chronicling the events leading to a decision to move the patient to a safer setting can alleviate the stress of making and executing such difficult decisions. Based upon the chronicling of incidents, limitations on freedom can occur in the interest of preventing harm to self and others and promoting safety. Automobile driving is a good example. Excellent materials are available on many Alzheimer organization web-sites that educate individuals on balancing independence and safety. Tips and warning signs are listed for caregivers and individuals with AD. One strategy suggested is the use of formal agreements regarding warning-sign observation and evidential support for cessation of driving. This allows the person with AD to continue to drive until presented with proof that safety is now compromised. Other areas of harm identification include patient risk of abuse or neglect from caregivers. Fortunately, agencies have been established to protect frail, vulnerable, elderly persons from abuse and neglect.

❧ Voluntary Participation in Genetic Testing and Research

Several areas where protecting patients and promoting autonomy takes on moral significance is in the area of genetic testing and prospective consent for participation in human subject research. Each one of these areas requires extensive knowledge and education in order to justify participation.

In the area of genetic diagnostics, a number of articles and philosophical treatises are available that define arguments for and against testing. Genetic diagnostics for AD are still in their infancy. While research is proving hopeful, at this time in genetic diagnostics development, it is inadvisable for people to rely on this mechanism fully. There are two types of testing: predictive genetic testing and genetic risk assessment. In predictive genetic testing, only about 5 percent of all families exhibit a specific inheritance pattern for AD, and this is easily identified in families in which early onset clearly passes from one generation to another. But even if there is a genetic link, this does not prove that a person has the disease, or even that he or she might. In genetic risk assessment, the disease can be absent in those people who possess the genetic risk factors. The test predicts only higher or lower risk, not who will get the disease. Apolipoprotein E allele typing is currently recommended only to help support a diagnosis of AD and not to predict disease risk among family members (Mayeux et al., 1998; Post et al., 1997). As research continues, genetic tests could become important. However, for the time being, testing carries the risk of unduly alarming or harming a person.

Since the predictive value is still in question, the test results can also provide a false sense of security.

In the area of research involving advance directives, the most controversial category is the one that exposes people who lack decisional capacity to significant psychological and physical risks without reasonable prospect of direct health benefit. This kind of burdensome research can expose a vulnerable group (e.g., AD patients) to harm purely to promote the interests of others (Dresser, 2001). Allowing such patients prospectively to consent to future research participation after they have lost decisional capacity may not advance their best interests because most dementia studies are designed for the benefit of future patients. While altruism is often a consideration, caution is necessary as well.

❧ Justice toward Caregivers

As pointed out earlier, patients with AD seldom suffer alone. Family members and other caregivers accompany the patient along this taxing, stressful, and painful journey (Grand et al., 1999). On top of this emotional burden comes the burden of daily care giving, often for years and years—a point made in chapter 11 and other chapters. Since many problems associated with the disease are behavioral, not medical, the solutions, too, often are behavioral and entail changes for the patient's family (Gray-Davidson, 1999).

Major caregiver stressors involve (1) the time commitment needed; (2) the psychological loss of a close, cherished relationship; (3) physical exertion and fatigue when assisting with bathing, dressing, and other personal care activities; (4) the financial cost of home care, assisted-living, or long-term care; and (5) role changes and role strains as career, personal, family, health promotion, and leisure routines are disrupted or restricted in order to take into account the growing needs of the person with AD. Sometimes these stressors can lead to emotional distress, poor physical health, family conflict, and even social isolation. Hence, an ADI core principle for the care of people with dementia involves the caregivers: "The family caregivers of a person with dementia should have their needs relating to the care assessed and provided for and should be enabled to take an active role in this process" (Alzheimer Disease International, 2002, principle 6).

Many AD patient caregivers are female. Often these women are "sandwiched" in the middle—that is, they find themselves in the role of caregiving daughter while also fulfilling obligations to children and working for an income (Brody, 1981; Mace & Rabins, 1999). A balance must be struck between the needs of patient and caregiver in order not to risk harm to either (Cohen, 1994). The caregiver must learn to accept help in the care of the AD patient.

A vast network of community, national, and international Alzheimer disease support groups and resources is available to provide information, referral, and educational services to patients and their caregivers. In addition, some nonprofit religious and community organizations offer a range of services to patients and caregivers on a voluntary basis. Getting outside help can range from having someone come into the home to help with patient care, such as a homemaker, home health aid, or personal care aide, to adult day care, day hospitals, or short-stay residential care. These support groups and the services they provide allow patients and caregivers the opportunity to acquire education, counseling or psychotherapy, respite time, and crisis intervention (Teitel, 2001). Certainly, with proper, sustained support, the negative outcomes associated with caregiving can result in positive outcomes such as a sense of purpose, sense of loyalty and fulfillment of commitment, renewal of religious faith, and closer personal ties, with strengthening of the relationship with the patient.

Education is an essential component of care for patients with AD. Many Alzheimer organizations worldwide offer educational services and support patients, families, and caregivers. An extensive network of educational programs offer a comprehensive range of didactic, practical, psychological, and supportive interventions to assist the patient and the family caregivers. For example, as mentioned earlier in this chapter, Alzheimer organizations worldwide have worked diligently to develop multilingual education materials and communication mechanisms in an effort to improve the lives of people with AD.

However, empirical data regarding education and support programs are lacking. A few studies in the 1980s described the effectiveness of information or supportive interventions (Zarit & Zarit, 1982; Lipkin & Faule, 1987; Gray, 1983). More recent studies and reports lead only to a modest increase in disease knowledge, and there is no effect on disease severity or patient outcomes, but they are well liked by family caregivers and offer them greater confidence. The modest outcomes found should not deter these activities (Brodaty, Roberts, & Peters, 1994; Chiverton & Caine, 1989; Doody et al., 2001). Even modest help to patients and their caregivers is worth the effort. "Understanding the experience of living with dementia, especially from the perspectives of persons with dementia and of their carers, is vital to providing effective advocacy, quality care and meaningful rehabilitation. Information, education and training on dementia, its effects and how to provide care must be available to all those involved in the assistance of people with dementia" (Alzheimer Disease International, 2002, principle 8).

REFERENCES

Alzheimer Disease International. (2002) Charter of principles for the care of people with dementia and their carers. October 2002. www.alz.co.uk/adi/charter.html.

Alzheimer Society of Canada. (1995). Alzheimer Care Ethical Guidelines. Task Force on Ethics. www.alzheimer.ca/english/care/ethics-intro.html.

Boyd, C. O., & Vernon, G. M. (1998). Primary care of the older adult with end-stage Alzheimer's disease. *Nurse Practitioner, 23* (4), 63–79.

Brodaty, H., Roberts, K., & Peters, K. (1994). Quasi-experimental evaluation of an educational model for dementia caregivers. *International Journal of Geriatric Psychiatry, 9,* 195–204.

Brody, E. M. (1981). "Women in the middle" and family help to older people. *Gerontologist, 21* (5), 471–480.

Chiverton, P., & Caine, E. D. (1989). Education to assist spouses in coping with Alzheimer's disease: A controlled trial. *Journal of the American Geriatrics Society, 37,* 593–598.

Cohen, D. (1994). A primary care checklist for effective family management. *Medical Clinics of North America: Alzheimer's and Related Dementias, 78* (4), 795–809.

de Wachter, M. A. M. (1992). Euthanasia in the Netherlands. *Hastings Center Report, 22,* 23–30.

Doody, R. S., Stevens, J. C., Beck, C., Dubinsky, R. M., Kaye, J. A., Gwyther, L., et al. (2001). Practice parameter: Management of dementia (an evidence-based review): A report of the quality standards subcommittee of the American Academy of Neurology. *Neurology, 56,* 1154–1166.

Doukas, D. J., & Gorenflo, D. W. (1993). Analyzing the values history: An evaluation of patient medical values and advance directives. *Journal of Clinical Ethics, 4* (1), 41–45.

Dresser, R. (2001). Advance directives in dementia research: promoting autonomy and protecting subjects. *IRB Ethics and Human Research, 23* (1), 1–15.

Folstein, M. F., Folstein, S. E., & McHugh, P. R. (1975). "Mini-mental state": A practical method for grading the cognitive state of patients for the clinician. *Journal of Psychiatric Research. 12* (3), 189–198.

Fox, N. C., Crum, W. R., Scahill, R. I., Stevens, J. M., Janssen, J. C., & Rossor, M. N. (2001). Imaging of onset and progression of Alzheimer's disease with voxel-compression mapping of serial magnetic resonance images. *Lancet, 358,* 201–205.

Geldmacher, D. S., & Whitehouse, P. J. (1997). Differential diagnosis of Alzheimer's disease. *Neurology, 48* (Suppl. 6) S2–S9.

Grand, A., Grand-Filaire, A., Bocquet, H., & Clement, S. (1999). Caregiver stress: A failed negotiation? A qualitative study in southwest France. *International Journal of Age and Human Development, 49* (3), 179–195.

Gray, V. K. (1983). Providing support for home care. In M. Smyer & M. Gatz. (Eds.), *Mental health and aging* (pp. 197–214). Beverly Hills, CA: Sage Publications.

Gray-Davidson, F. (1999). *The Alzheimer's sourcebook for caregivers: A practical guide for getting through the day.* Los Angeles: Lowell House.

Ham, R. J. (1997). After the diagnosis: Supporting Alzheimer's patients and their families. *Post Graduate Medicine, 101* (6), 57–70.

Lambert, P., Gibson, J. M., & Nathanson, P. (1990). The values history: An innovation in surrogate medical decision-making. *Law, Medicine and Health Care, 18* (3), 202–212.

Lawton, M. P. (1994). Quality of life and Alzheimer's disease. *Alzheimer's Disease and Associated Disorders, 8* (Suppl. 3), 138–150.

Lipkin, L. V., & Faule, K. J. (1987). Dementia: Educating the caregiver. *Journal of Gerontology, 13,* 23.

Mace, N. L., & Rabins, P. V. (1999). *The 36-hour day: A family guide for persons with Alzheimer disease, related dementing illnesses, and memory loss in later life.* Baltimore: Johns Hopkins University Press.

Mayeux, R., Saunders, A. M., Shea, S., Mirra, S., Evans, D., Roses A. D., et al. (1998). Utility of the Apoplipoprotein E Genotype in the diagnosis of Alzheimer's Disease. *New England Journal of Medicine, 338* (8), 506–511. Erratum appears in *New England Journal of Medicine,, 338* (18) (1998), 1325.

Meyers, B. S. (1997). Telling patients they have Alzheimer's disease. *British Medical Journal, 314* (7077), 321–322.

Post, S. G. (1997). Physician-assisted suicide in Alzheimer's disease. *Journal of the American Geriatrics Society, 45,* 647–651.

Post, S. G. (2000). *The moral challenge of Alzheimer disease* (2nd ed.). Baltimore: Johns Hopkins University Press.

Post, S. G., & Whitehouse, P. J. (1995). Fairhill guidelines on ethics of care of people with Alzheimer's disease: A clinical summary. *Journal of the American Geriatrics Society. 43,* 1423–1429.

Post, S. G., Whitehouse, P. J., Binstock, R. H., Bird, T. D., Eckert, S. K., Farrer, L.A., et al. (1997). The clinical introduction of genetic testing for Alzheimer's disease: An ethical perspective. *Journal of the American Medical Association, 277* (10), 832–836.

Reilly, R. B., Teasdale, T. A., & McCullough, L. B. (1994). Projecting patients' preferences from living wills: An invalid strategy for management of dementia with life threatening illness. *Journal of the American Geriatrics Society. 42,* 997–1003.

Ross, J. W., Glaser, J. W., Rasinski-Gregory, D., Gibson, J. M., and Bayley, C. (1993). Appendix 11.1. Values History Form. *Health Care Ethics Committees: The Next Generation.* Chicago: American Hospital Association Publishing.

Teitel, R. (2001). *The handholder's handbook: A guide for caregivers of people with Alzheimer's and other dementias.* New Brunswick, NJ: Rutgers University Press.

Volicer, L. (2001). Management of severe Alzheimer's disease and end-of-life issues. *Clinics in Geriatric Medicine, 17* (2), 377–391.

Wilen, S. B., Harman, S. M., & Alexander-Israel, D. (1997). Home care and the Alzheimer's disease patient: An educational imperative. *Caring, 16* (1), 44–46, 48–49.

Yale, R. (1999). Support groups and other services for individuals with early-stage Alzheimer's disease. *Generations, 23* (3), 57–61.

Zarit, S. H., & Zarit, J. M. (1982). Families under stress: Interventions for caregivers of senile dementia patients. *Psychotherapy: Theory, Research, and Practice, 19* (4), 461–471.

CHAPTER SEVENTEEN

Changing Patterns of Protection and Care for Incapacitated Adults

Perspectives from a European Society in Transition

Eugenijus Gefenas, M.D., Ph.D.

The idea of developing a European-American dialogue on palliative care for persons with Alzheimer disease (AD) presupposes two more or less homogeneous groups of discussion partners bringing different perspectives on the issue. The problem is, however, that the European counterpart of this dialogue is no longer a homogeneous one. Even though European integration is supposed to be based on common European values and perspectives (which are often presented as being in opposition to American ones), the process of European unification has revealed striking differences between European states themselves, especially those called transition societies and those regarded as welfare states. A discussion sensitive to sociocultural differences should take this situation into account.

What are the main principles and features of the changing attitudes toward incapacitated persons taking place in modern society? How should these changes be evaluated from the perspective of Central and East European (CEE) countries? Should caring for such adults be regarded as a priority area in the context of a social and health care of post-Communist societies, also called transition societies? These are the central topics dealt with in this chapter.

The chapter starts with an overview of legal reform in the field of the protection of fundamental rights of incapacitated persons as reflected in a recently adopted European Recommendation on Principles Concerning the Legal Protection of Incapable Adults (Council of Europe, 1999). Even though legal regulations are not the only factor influencing the model of care existing in the society, the analysis of the existing legislative framework concerning one of the most vulnerable groups of the population highlights ethical principles prevalent in a particular society. It also helps us to predict the tendencies of future developments in different countries and sociocultural contexts.

Changing Attitudes toward Incapable Persons

In 1999, the attempt to facilitate the process of reform in the member states of the Council of Europe resulted in adoption of the Recommendation on the Principles Concerning the Legal Protection of Incapable Adults. In general, the recommendation has been based on the recognition that existing freedoms and capacities of people suffering from different types of mental disorders (including AD) should be preserved as much as possible. This general principle has also been applied in the field of health care interventions.

The adoption of the recommendation was possible because the notion of protection of incapable persons has significantly changed in many democratic welfare societies in the last few decades. The most important feature of these changes has been the strengthening of respect for decision making by the affected persons themselves. That is why the legal reform dealing with the protection and care of incapable persons could also be regarded as a manifestation of a broader ethical development. This development is based on the increasing role of two fundamental ethical principles: human dignity and respect for personal autonomy.

Even though the principles and values constituting the ideological background of the recommendation could be regarded as self-evident and firmly established in Western countries with a stronger tradition of protecting human rights, they are not really implemented or sometimes even recognized in the context of European societies in transition. From this point of view, the recommendation is a most important document for the European transition societies as it helps to define the main features of reform badly needed in CEE countries.

❧ Traditional and Alternative Types of Legal Framework

According to a survey on the issues concerning incapacitated adults conducted in the process of drafting the European Recommendation, the present member states of the Council of Europe have wide disparities in legislative systems of protecting incapable adults (Council of Europe, 1998). Two opposite models within the variety of the existing systems can be distinguished:

1. The traditional system is characterized mainly by a deprivation of all, or almost all active, legal capacity to make decisions, coupled with the appointment of a guardian who represents the person concerned in almost all matters. This type of system denies any meaningful participation of the incapacitated person into his or her own care-related decision making.

2. An alternative system is based on protection and assistance, rather than on deprivation of legal capacity. This type of legal system consistently is based on the ethical principles of human dignity and respect for personal autonomy. It usually employs a flexible formal measure, which is modified to suit a particular case.

The movement from the first toward the second type of legal system marks a significant historical development in the attitudes toward incapacitated persons.

❧ Basic Trends and Principles of the Reform

Basic trends in the new approach to legal protection are explicated as fundamental principles of the recommendation; among the most important are

1. Respect for the wishes and feelings of the person. This is especially important because it takes into account that the decision-making capacity of the person is getting increasingly compromised by the disease. This principle allows the caregiver to refer to previously expressed wishes and the life story of the person.

2. Prominence given to the interests and welfare of the person. This is stressed because it should be the paramount consideration in the implementation of a measure of protection or care, and it is important to counteract the tendency to use the assets of the person to benefit other parties.

3. Subsidiarity, or minimum necessary intervention. The idea behind the

principle is that of deciding whether the measure of protection or care is necessary. Preference should be for any less formal arrangements that might be used rather than formal ones, and for any assistance that might be provided by family members or public authorities.

4. Proportionality. This closely related principle stresses that the measure of protection should be proportional to the degree of capacity of the person concerned and tailored to the individual circumstances of the case. This principle is especially important as it replaces the traditional attitude of depriving the person of almost all legal capacity.

To summarize, the above principles are aimed at respect for persons with incapacitating conditions such as AD and maximum preservation of their remaining mental capacity. This goal is achieved by (1) honoring any residual capacity of the person and involving that person in the process of decision making; (2) respecting arrangements made by the affected person; and (3) distinguishing various forms and degrees of incapacity, which helps to replace a total deprivation of legal agency.

The legislative reform introducing an alternative type of care and protection for people with various degrees of impaired mental capacities has already been started, and even completed, in many West and North European countries, Canada, and the United States. At the same time, however, the traditional type of system is still prevalent in many CEE countries (Council of Europe, 1998).

Protection of Incapacitated Adults in CEE

It is extremely difficult to implement a system of care and protection of incapacitated adults tailored to the values and life story of the person concerned if the legal background is a traditional one and does not correspond to the basic principles of an alternative type of system. Lithuania can be regarded as a typical example of a CEE country with a traditional type of legal framework. In Lithuanian legislation, there are only two types of protective measures for adults. A less restrictive measure is called *rupyba,* which literally means "taking care of" and might be translated as a partial guardianship. This measure is used only in two circumstances:

1. For those dependent on the use of alcohol and drugs
2. For those who are mentally capable, but who due to their somatic health problems are unable to exercise their rights and everyday activities

In a partial guardianship, a person acts jointly with the selected guardian (e.g., in a case of alcohol or drug abuse, the freedoms of the person concerned are limited to small personal spending). However, according to Lithuanian law, this measure could not be extended to protect a person suffering from dementia.

The second measure—the more restrictive—is *globa,* which might be translated as "guardianship." This measure might be applied to a person who, according to Lithuanian law, is unable to understand and control his or her actions due to mental illness or mental retardation (Civil Code of the Republic of Lithuania, 2000, art. 3.277). The person is declared to be legally incapable by a court, with the consequent appointment of a guardian who has power over all spheres of personal welfare and financial affairs of the incapable person. No legal time limit is envisaged for the measure of guardianship, and there is no regular review of the case.

Very few adults with AD and other dementias have this kind of protective measure. The most usual motive in applications for guardianship is an attempt by family members to take care of the property of the person concerned. The existing legislation does not protect incapacitated adults because it does not explicate any specific aspect of protection or care centered on the interests and integrity of such persons themselves. The protection of their interests mainly depends on the goodwill of those around them, usually relatives.

In a number of CEE countries, resistance and/or delay in introducing an alternative system of legal protection means that the culture or ideology of personal autonomy is still weak and not practically implemented in systems of caring for incapable adults.

☙ Different Meanings of Personal Autonomy and Care

The shift from the traditional paternalism toward a culture of respect for personal autonomy in the field of caring for incapable adults is a complicated process. On the one hand, as has been shown above, the reform of protection and care for incapacitated adults has been explicitly based on the principle of respect for personal autonomy. On the other hand, the principle of autonomy has itself been criticized as providing insufficient background for bioethics, especially in the care of persons with impaired mental capacities. In particular, the criticism has been directed toward a minimalist account of bioethics based on a libertarian interpretation of personal autonomy (Pellegrino & Thomasma, 1988).

To understand the role of personal autonomy in the process of establishing a system of care and protection for incapacitated persons, we therefore need to analyze the concept of autonomy in more detail. To put it in a very tentative way, at least two different meanings or dimensions of personal autonomy might be distinguished. These two meanings could also be used to understand a historical shift from a traditional-paternalistic to autonomy-oriented health care ethics in the CEE region.

The first interpretation is based on the libertarian-minimalist account of personal autonomy as noninterference with the decision making of a person (Engelhardt, 2000). In the context of caring for persons with AD, for example, a minimalist account of personal autonomy would favor a decision based on the living will of the person. This interpretation of personal autonomy has been criticized as reducing the relationship between health care provider and patient to a simple contract between provider of services and consumer (Gefenas, 1998). Taken in isolation, such a model, of course, distorts and neglects very important aspects of health care; namely, the patient's vulnerability and the caring character of the doctor-patient relationship.

The second concept of autonomy emphasizes the authenticity of a decision-making process (Miller, 1987; Welie, 1998). This is a much broader and richer interpretation of autonomy, sometimes also conceptualized as a separate and distinct principle, as seen in ten Have's chapter in this book. Without going into the complex analysis of the interrelationship between the concepts of autonomy and authenticity here, I will nevertheless distinguish two aspects of authenticity that are especially important in dealing with incapable persons. First of all, autonomy as authenticity is implemented as decision making in the context of the values and life story of the person (Collopy, 1988). This is especially the case when people close to the patient and having an intimate knowledge of his or her character make choices that are congruent with the patient's personality as it developed in the past.

Another important feature of authenticity is that it captures and emphasizes an emotional component of decision making. It helps us to elucidate not only rational and conscious choice but also a deeper, unconscious motivation of persons with impaired capacities. This kind of motivation is becoming increasingly important as long as cognitive abilities of a person are decreasing. Illhardt's chapter 12 gives examples and interesting interpretations of a sensitive communication with persons who have AD. For example, the reluctance of the AD patient to stop playing with his wife's jewelry box while she was talking to a third person might be interpreted as the patient's attempt to express a protest, as if he would say: "Be aware that I, too, am here." Sensitivity to the actual feelings and emotions of the patient helps to develop a relationship free of coercion—one that is more respectful toward the patient.

The concept of autonomy as authenticity is much more complex and difficult to implement than libertarian or minimalist approaches. However, at the same time this interpretation of autonomy is more relevant for the protection of vulnerable populations and opens new perspectives in caring for persons with AD.

A health care provider is assigned different roles within the different conceptions of autonomy. According to the libertarian-minimalist account of personal autonomy as noninterference with the decision making of a person, the health care provider might predominantly be seen as a potential intruder into the life story of a patient. In contrast, the second interpretation of autonomy emphasizing authenticity of decision making assigns to those dealing with a vulnerable patient the role of a facilitator of patient's preferences and values (which sometimes have to be reconstructed from the life story of the patient). This is, of course, a much more demanding role for the health care provider. However, it is at the same time a much more plausible one if we wish to implement an alternative model of protection and care for incapacitated persons.

❧ Personal Autonomy and Development of Bioethics in the Transition Society

Even in this very tentative sketch of different interpretations of personal autonomy, we can make some preliminary observations about the prospects of caring for incapacitated adults in the CEE countries. It could plausibly be argued that the CEE countries are still coping with the first dimension of the shift from traditional paternalism to personal autonomy; namely, the attempt to implement a principle of informed consent into the relationship between health care provider and patient. This shift is first of all based on a minimalist-libertarian concept of personal autonomy.

There have already been some achievements in this process, at both the national and European level. For example, the principle of informed consent has already been introduced into the legal systems of many post-Communist countries (not to mention West Europe) as it is also implemented into international documents such as the Council of Europe Convention on Human Rights and Biomedicine (Council of Europe, 1997). Legalizing the principle of informed consent could be regarded as a fundamental presupposition to implementing a minimalist account of autonomy. This is a very important step toward reforming the relationship between the health care provider and patient in the context of a transition society. Think, for example, about fields such as biomedical research or organ transplantation, where the principle of informed consent is a most important safeguard against the abuse of potential research subjects and organ donors and their families. It should be stressed, however, that a minimalist account of personal autonomy is not actually implemented in the care of persons with impaired mental capacities. Such practices as writing down living wills do not exist in many CEE countries.

The second and more complicated step will be to develop a provider-patient relationship that is sensitive to what has been described with respect to autonomy as authenticity of a person's values, motivation, and life story. This is a crucial dimension of any attempt to develop relevant caring attitudes toward incapable people. As the survey of European legislation shows, West and North European countries have already adopted the legislation conducive to the account of personal autonomy as authenticity. These countries are now trying to implement this perspective into their practice. Unfortunately, the CEE countries have not even started to implement the alternative legal system, not to speak of a culture of provider-patient relationships.

This situation should be taken into account very seriously when thinking about the role that autonomy plays in developing a sensitive care system for incapacitated adults. It is understandable why many Western bioethicists are critical of a minimalist interpretation of personal autonomy and stress its limitations, especially in a field such as caring for incapacitated persons. They represent the perspective of the society, which takes it as granted that a libertarian account of autonomy has already been implemented into the health care practice and that the principle of informed consent is not only legalized but also followed in everyday practice.

On the other hand, the CEE countries have recently started a process of very rapid health care reform. In this context, implementation of a libertarian interpretation of personal autonomy in the form of making informed consent a legal rule followed in everyday practice is of paramount importance. Replacing traditional paternalism could be seen not only as a safeguard against patient abuse but also as a necessary presupposition to developing a broader understanding of the respect for persons, as it is stressed by those who emphasize the importance of authenticity of decision making.

❦ The Sociocultural Context of the Changing Attitudes

In addition to the absence of legislation conducive to a respect for the autonomy of persons with decreasing mental capacities, this group of people is in a very unfortunate position in the post-Communist society due to several other circumstances.

The main reason why these societies are still in the initial state of integrating respect for personal autonomy into decision making related to health care is that during the few decades of totalitarian regime the values and principles of a free and democratic society were heavily suppressed in this part of Europe. In particular, respect for personal autonomy was regarded as secondary to the "best interests of the society," and every act of self-determination was severely punished. In such a way, paternalistic attitudes have been strongly enforced by the authoritarian character of Soviet society.

Secondly, for political reasons, people suffering from mental disorders were hidden from society and usually kept in institutions, where almost all of their civil rights were taken away. The purpose of such a practice was not to spoil the utopian vision of the successful development of the Soviet system. Both of these features have resulted in a very serious social marginalization of people with impaired capacities. Unfortunately, these features are still playing a negative role in reforming the system of caring for such people.

Thirdly, the current economic situation makes it very difficult to argue for priority in allocating resources to develop a legal and institutional framework and train professionals with skills to care for persons with decreasing mental capacities. In the majority of CEE countries, the annual per-person expenditure for health care amounts to approximately 10 percent of the resources allotted for the same purpose in West or North Europe (e.g., annual per capita expenditure on health care is about US$250 in Lithuania, compared with about US$1,700 in Sweden and almost US$4,000 in the United States). In such a situation, reversing the lack of very basic material essentials is a more important task than an attempt to change a pattern of care that is not sensitive enough with regard to respect for personal autonomy. Such a situation limits the current discourse on personal autonomy to what was described as its libertarian-minimalist interpretation enforced by new legislation on patients' rights legalizing the principle of informed consent. But it will be a very long and hard struggle to implement a shift in attitude in the area of protecting those whose decision-making capacity needs sensitive and active support.

Finally, demographic data on the prevalence of AD in Lithuania (probably other CEE countries as well) do not prove that this is the most prevalent type of dementia. For example, there are 4,956 diagnosed dementia cases in the Lithuanian population of 3.7 million. Only 381 of these, or fewer than 10 percent, are categorized as Alzheimer cases, which is far less than the number reported in West Europe, where AD accounts for about 60 percent of all dementia cases. The reasons behind such a significant difference would have to be explored; however, at the moment, the group of people suffering from this particular disorder would not be regarded as having a special priority status on the basis of their prevalence in Lithuanian society.

It seems that those dealing with the protection and care of incapacitated persons in Lithuania and other transition societies find themselves in a very different situation compared with those in West European countries or North America. First of all, in transition societies access to social and health care is very dependent on the ability to pay. With very limited resources allotted to social and health care within the transition society, very often the quality of care available to persons with impaired capacities depends on their (or their relatives') out-of-pocket payments. Despite equitable access to health care being regarded as a priority in official health policy documents, there is in fact a libertarian type of health care (Ministry of Health of the Republic of Lithuania, 1997). Paradoxically, this is a consequence of the decades spent in a society that declared the principles of equality and solidarity to be the most important ones in all spheres of public life. It seems that the European transition societies resemble the American situation. A popular distinction between European bioethics as egalitarian and American bioethics as libertarian is not strictly applicable to European transition societies (Wulff, 1999).

Another popular distinction between American and European bioethics is supposed to be related to the claim that Europeans reject the historical importance of autonomy in bioethics (Marshall, 1998). It should be stressed again that from the perspective of the CEE countries, respect for personal autonomy is to be regarded as a fundamental principle. Both of its components—autonomy as noninterference with the decision making of the patient and autonomy as fostering authenticity of decisions—are needed to establish a relevant system of care, bearing in mind the need to replace strong paternalistic attitudes in a short period of reform.

Finally, I would like to stress that the legal reform concerning incapacitated persons in the United States appears to be based on the same principles as those of West and North European legal reform. This kind of reform is still to be implemented in the CEE countries, which have retained a traditional system of dealing with incapacitated persons.

In summary, Europe is not a homogeneous region of states fostering a single set of values and principles. The process of European integration has forced its member states to apply the same legal and institutional standards to evaluate and compare different areas of social life. It has created a basis for harmonizing legislative and institutional frameworks between different European regions. However, at the same time it has clearly highlighted the demographic and socioeconomic differences between the states. We have to take these circumstances into consideration if we wish to achieve a realistic dialogue between Europeans and Americans on pressing bioethical issues.

REFERENCES

Civil Code of the Republic of Lithuania. (2000) art. 3.277.

Collopy, B. J. (1988). Autonomy in long term care: Some crucial distinctions. *Gerontologist, 28,* 10–17.

Council of Europe. (1997). Convention for the Protection of Human Rights and Dignity of the Human Being with regard to the Application of Biology and Medicine: Convention on Human Rights and Biomedicine. Oviedo, Spain, April 4, European Treaty Series No. 164.

Council of Europe. (1998). *Explanatory report to the recommendation on principles concerning the legal protection of incapable adults.*

Council of Europe. (1999). *European recommendation on principles concerning the legal protection of incapable adults.* Recommendation no. R (99) of the Committee of Ministers, adopted February 23. Strasbourg, Council of Europe Publishing.

Engelhardt, H. T., Jr. (2000). The cardinal principle of contemporary bioethics. In P. Kemp, J. Rendtorff, & N. M. Johansen (Eds.), *Bioethics and biolaw* (pp. 35–46). Copenhagen: Rhodos International Science and Art Publishers.

Gefenas, E. (1998). A contract or an encounter. In M. Evans (Ed.), *Advances in bioethics, Vol. 4, Critical reflection on medical ethics* (pp. 307–321). London: JAI Press.

Marshall, P. A., Thomasma, D. C., & Bergsma, J. (1998). Intercultural reasoning: The challenge for intercultural bioethics. In J. F. Monagle & D. C. Thomasma (Eds.), *Health care ethics* (pp. 584–593). Gaithersburg, MD: Aspen.

Miller, B. L. (1987). Types of autonomy and their significance. In B. A. Brody & H. T. Engelhart (Eds.), *Bioethics: Readings and cases* (pp. 105–109). New York: Prentice Hall.

Ministry of Health of the Republic of Lithuania. (1997). Lithuanian Health Programme, 1997–2010 (pp. 31–34). Vilnius, Lithuania.

Pellegrino, E. D., & Thomasma, D. S. (1988). *For the patient's good: The restoration of beneficence in health care.* New York: Oxford University Press.

Welie, J. V. M. (1998). *In the face of suffering.* Omaha, NE: Creighton University Press.

Wulff, H. R. (1998). Contemporary trends in health care ethics. In H.A.M.J. ten Have & H.-M. Sass (Eds.), *Consensus formation in health care ethics* (pp. 63–72). Dordrecht, Netherlands: Kluwer Academic Publishers.

CHAPTER EIGHTEEN

Social Marginalization of Persons with Disability

Justice Considerations for Alzheimer Disease

Ruth B. Purtilo, Ph.D.

The trends that point to an increasing number of persons with Alzheimer disease (AD) worldwide and the perceptions of escalating financial and other burdens occasioned by this increase have prompted growing discussion by governments, private insurers, and national and international organizations about how best to allocate resources to address the new challenges. From the ethicist's point of view, answers to these challenges best are derived from the biddings of justice and, more fundamentally, should be based on a clear understanding of the situation of all those affected by the allocation decisions. Thus, this chapter lays out some basic areas of consideration that should be taken into account when allocation policies are forged.

It will not surprise readers that persons with AD and their families do not fall easily into one health care or social services policy niche. AD is one of those confoundingly complex, long-lasting, progressively debilitating medical-social conditions that renders it at high risk of falling through the policy slats. In both the United States and Europe, interventions are piecemealed together through various medical and social service sources, changing sometimes abruptly as new manifestations of the disease appear. The overall spectrum of care almost always is, at best, fragmented.

Of the several common health care allocation categories, the members of our international dialogue concluded that AD is least often viewed as an "acute care" problem, though acute symptoms do occur. In the United States, in Western Europe, and in Central and Eastern Europe it is viewed variously as a chronic disease, a long-term care challenge, or a terminal illness. But most frequently it is treated, over time, as an impairment that has become a disability. When do impairments reach the point of disability? According to the medical model, the disability ensues when the impairments are deemed to merit medical intervention. Presumably, the proffering of health care (and other social service) benefits are judged according to the level of impairment. In short, this approach focuses on the "broken person" approach (Silvers, 1998). Susan Wendell's (1996) term *the unhealthy disabled* aptly fits the societal perception of AD, though such a category does not appear in policy-making arenas. Thus, a just basis for allocation policy cannot be determined without an exploration and understanding of the effects of this social perception of persons with AD.

Any person judged to have a disability—more importantly, a mental disability—is perceived to present a special challenge involving special burdens on society. Mental disability is a more stigmatizing attribute than physical disability (Nussbaum, 2001). In fact, the label of mental disability is an occasion for social disregard and disrespect toward members of society who otherwise might continue to have a voice in policy matters (Daniels, 1988). This lack of regard (i.e., having an identity deemed worthy of others' attention) and respect (i.e., having an identity deemed worthy of others' caring and having one's contributions considered worthwhile) goes beyond the psychological damage imposed on persons with impairments by virtue of important personal and social identity props being withheld or withdrawn. There are also damaging social effects on such persons because society does not deem them deserving of resources that are being allocated.

What can be done to help assure that persons with AD and their caregivers do not become unduly marginalized? An apt starting point for assessment is John Rawls's (1971) conception of justice since it takes seriously the role of regard and respect and how they are key in a social contract approach to allocations that treat everyone fairly.

✎ Justice Allocations through Rawls's Social Contract Approach

Rawls's social contract approach has become an extremely influential foundation for disability and health policy within the United States and elsewhere. Some have found his approach useful on the basis of his "circumstances of justice," which include (1) a situation of moderate scarcity; (2) the presence of a cherished but scarce resource, and especially (3) the requirement that any arrangement for the distribution of resources among legitimate claimants must meet the requirement of benefiting the least well off. His approach does not preclude that dramatic disparities in resource allocation toward the most advantaged and least well off may occur, but his maximin principle requires that the least advantaged group not be left out of the equation altogether.

Rawls uses a hypothetical model for choosing among the various basic goods that a society has to distribute. He proposes that under a "veil of ignorance" about the place in society each planner will have, each will choose a societal arrangement that would protect him or her in the unfortunate luck-of-the-draw that would land that person in a situation among the least well off members of society. The goal of societal arrangements that result is to foster and support self-respect and self-regard for everyone. At the same time, the practical reason these are supported is that only in such a situation can persons come to the negotiating table as fully developed moral agents capable of understanding and defending the societal arrangements that will serve everyone best overall.

Rawls's hypothetical exercise has its basis in real life—psychological considerations that are relevant to the situation of persons with AD—especially in regards to the damage that is done when regard and respect are withdrawn. Mainstream members of society enjoy social affirmations that support the formation of a strong self-identity, have ready access to institutional mechanisms designed to address their basic needs, and can *expect* society's willingness to acknowledge their contributions. One can sum it up by saying that mainstream members come to expect *regard* and *respect*. Many ethicists, theologians, and philosophers assert that individuals possess a basic, inherent human dignity from which regard and respect should be understood and that will override any compromises of the person's moral status on the basis of specific attributes that he or she may have or lack. At the same time, allocation decisions seldom are made on the basis of inherent dignity. Society's interpretation of the person's worthiness drives allocation decisions.

Persons with AD often are robbed of this regard and respect. One must marvel that a U.S. president or a mother who has raised several children or run a publishing company can, through this disease, become a member of a group that is not prized. The terrible truth is that they have acquired attributes that others do not want to acknowledge and cannot identify with. They also lack the characteristics required for society to accept their contributions as meaningful. In other words, they are not viewed as worthy of society's attention and do not have a role worthy of others' support and admiration (Abel, 2000).

Persons with AD may *themselves* come to consider that they are unworthy of regard and respect. Drawing on the work of developmental and moral psychologists, Rawls reminds us of the close association between the regard/respect one receives from others and *self*-regard/respect. Put another way, self-regard and self-respect grow as a result of positive feedback from society's assurances that the person "is somebody!" The connection is important because strong self-regard and self-respect positions a person psychologically to lay claim to resources needed to survive and thrive. This is especially the case in societies where individual self-determination, say-so, autonomy is prized. When self-regard and self-respect are dealt a blow by society's negative treatment, the person may internalize the experience as shame, and his own confidence in his value suffers. Moreover, the shame takes on a moral dimension: "In such a society we are liable to *moral* shame when we lack characteristics that our own identity depends on for a feeling of worth and fulfillment and which society encourages us to realize" (Rawls, 1971, pp. 332–333). Under such duress, he says, we eventually can come to doubt whether we are even worthy of our moral standing as human persons because we lack key characteristics society requires for a person to legitimately lay claim on human resources:

> What makes the situation more difficult for a person who cannot measure up is that some actions and traits are joined in a special way to shame, since they are peculiarly indicative of the failure to achieve self-command.... In moral shame, we focus on our infringement of what we have come to believe are the just claims of others and the injury we have done to them and on their probable (deserved) resentment or indignation towards us (p. 334).

In short, Rawls's description highlights how an individual's self-identity and his feelings of social belongingness work together to create a self-perception of moral worthiness. He also shows how "defects" become occasions for moral shame and, working together with society's disapproval, marginalize the person from the decision maker's attention when basic goods are being allocated. In *The Moral Challenge of Alzheimer Disease,* Stephen Post draws out this point: "There are many rival theories of what justice is, but we know that it is unjust when persons in great need are ignored, and this is the current state of affairs with regard to persons with dementia and their loved ones. . . . Maybe because we write off people with dementia as 'dead,' as 'useless' or as 'non persons,' we do not think of them as *deserving* distributional fairness" (Post, 2000, pp. 136–137). In short, one area that requires much more attention as foundations for a just allocation of resources for persons with AD are laid is a thorough examination of how societal blows amounting to disregard and disrespect leave them at high risk of becoming neglected victims of injustice. In the words of psychologist Sabat, society has a tendency to *position* such persons so that the lens through which they are viewed narrows the actual range of characteristics and capabilities they have (Sabat, 2001).

❧ Just Allocation through Protection of Vulnerable Populations

As the above discussion highlights, the strengths of Rawls's conception of justice are that regard and respect are taken seriously as both psychological and social-political forces and the fact that some persons, in less advantaged situations than others in society, must not be ignored. Still, this social contract approach has been the subject of criticism. It is not within the purpose of this chapter to critique Rawls's conception thoroughly, but two aspects of it do deserve further consideration. The first, discussed here, springs from his assumption that by identifying and attending to less-advantaged or *vulnerable* groups, policymakers will be counseled in the direction of justice.

It goes without saying that vulnerability can be attributed to persons with AD. We have shown that they fall prey to the same negative judgments often made of any group whose mental functions are compromised by illness, injury, or disease. In a now classic work, Diana Crane (1975) showed that patients judged to have serious *mental* disabilities (in contrast to acute problems or physical impairments) consistently fared least well when physicians were asked about their quality of life and the extent to which the physician's interventions were merited. A measure of the vulnerability that many patients experience in the health care system as a mental impairment runs its course is their own increasing awareness of being devalued by the larger society, usually because they are in a *group* of people diagnosed with AD. The devaluation often takes the form of (and is described by others as) a "downhill course" into necessarily deeper dependence, not only on health professionals whom they fear increasingly devalue them but also on virtually everyone with whom they are in relationships.

For example, in his account of Murray Wasserman, a man experiencing the progression of AD, James Buchanan recounts how Murray's awareness of his heightening dependence finally altered his basic identity as a person: "In his more lucid moments—and they became fewer and fewer—Murray knew that he was a fallen angel, a wounded animal which could not survive except as a scavenger feeding from its host" (1989, p. 41). Where did this conclusion spring from? It is not surprising that as a member of U.S. society, this man was aware of the link between self-sufficiency and his qualification to demand moral regard and respect. He was now a member of a group that was, at best, a drain on society. This assumption is deeply embedded in Western social consciousness (Jaworska, 1999). In short, Rawls's approach does not take this type of devaluation of such groups into account fully enough.

A second criticism of Rawls's approach is his focus on a social contract mechanism of societal consensus. Eva Feder Kittay (2001) raises the important concern that the social contract approach entails an assumption of autonomy of individuals coming together to agree on what is best for all. In Rawls's conception, the person with self-regard and self-respect will be "fully functioning"; that is, will be a "self-originator," able to speak up for what he or she needs from society. It is difficult to see how this condition can be met by someone whose vulnerability is in the form of a severe cognitive impairment and, on that basis, is unable to speak for herself. What is missing from this approach, Kittay contends, is a fundamental fact of human existence; namely, that vulnerability, as a lived experience, never stands alone. It is intrinsically tied to the companion notion of dependence. Rawls does allude to dependency concerns—any individual can become dependent—but he treats it as a concern only because of the potential equal vulnerability of everyone. Policies from such a stance can gloss over the lived reality—emphasized in many chapters of this book—that the vulnerability of AD involves a specific relationship of care receiver / caregiver (often a family member, other times combined with or solely a professional). Turning the focus from solely vulnerability to the reality of dependency requires society to deal with the allocation challenge as one of sustaining a necessary set of relationships. A corrective to Rawls's approach would result "if dependency is recognized as one of the circumstances of justice. This would take into account that the dependent is a fully functioning person in a period of dependency" (Kittay, 2001, p. 84). As it stands, his approach is not concerned with the justice or injustice about how dependency needs are met for any of the parties in the relationship, except that his maximin principle requires that the group shown to be the "worst off" cannot be dropped from consideration altogether when societal goods are being distributed.

As these criticisms point out, the strengths of Rawls's approach also have some cause for concern embedded in them. The social devaluation of vulnerability and the link of vulnerability to dependency relationships warrant further examination in regards to the situation of persons with AD. The goal of a just allocation is to promulgate policies in which dependency needs are addressed in a manner that is equitable to everyone. But this task requires that attention then be given to societal dynamics that currently act as barriers to this laudable goal.

❧ Dependency, Relationships, and Just Allocation

In economically developed countries, *dis*ability often has been equated with an *in*ability to contribute to the well-being of society, and the contribution usually is judged on the value it has to the economy. Adults who cannot do this are judged not only to be "dependent" but, more fundamentally, to have a serious shortcoming or "defect" (Jette, 1994). Mental disability brings fully into focus the devalued characteristic of adult extreme dependency on others, creating a situation of disdain or even suspicion (Silvers, 1998). Mainstream society's hesitance to reckon positively with individuals in it who exhibit perceived shortcomings or "defects" takes several deleterious forms. Among the most serious are two companion assumptions; namely, that persons with impairments cannot meet reasonable expectations placed on other people, and, in contrast, that their family caregivers must assume a level of responsibility for caregiving that goes beyond reasonable expectations. While one could argue that the family relationship is being viewed as a unit of consideration in such a position, these distortions of the role of each in contributing to the larger society does not support a healthy foundation for the individuals concerned, for their relationship, or for the larger society. In short, the attempt to base a just allocation on such distortions will lead to further harm. The distortion is so important that the next two sections examine each in turn.

❧ Low Expectations of What Persons with AD Can Contribute

As noted above, one of the most important ways that adults gain a recognized place in society is through their contributions to that society's well-being. A central feature of adulthood is the satisfaction and self-fulfillment that accompanies assuming one's share of the responsibilities (Reeves, 1999). But society places decreased expectations on persons judged to have disabilities—often a self-fulfilling prophecy (Marienelli, 1999). Disability results in lower societal expectations of persons because those around them assume a disabled person's "suffering" prohibits him or her from handling the challenges imposed by the condition (Spelman, 1997). Spelman does not judge this assumption sympathetically; rather, he argues that mainstream society's insistence on directing its attention to the *suffering* of disability—whether or not the person with the condition actually experiences suffering—reinforces the idea of a disabled person's inferiority. This societal disservice robs disabled persons of their ability to participate meaningfully in the various communities to which they belong and upon which they depend (Reeves, 1999). It is not difficult to imagine that persons with AD would be negatively affected by this assumption, which of course impoverishes the larger community as well.

Society's unwillingness to include in the labor pool and deep social fabric highly qualified but disabled persons is appropriately interpreted as discrimination akin to racism, homophobia, and ageism. For example, Koppelman (1996) shows that in the United States, unemployment patterns among disabled people follow patterns of people of color, not those whose skills have become obsolete. The irrationality of this unwillingness has caused some people with impairments to opt for minority- or social- rather than medical-based models of disability (Silvers, 1996). We return to his line of thinking later in this chapter: but first a look at the caregiver's situation.

❧ Unreasonably High Expectations on Family Caregivers

When faced with a loved one who shows the debilitating effects of Alzheimer disease, most family caregivers initially rise to the occasion with remarkable courage, good spiritedness, and, if all else fails, resignation. They often enjoy the admiration ("regard") of others on the basis of having assumed this new identity. Even people who previously were not seen as noteworthy may become objects of approbation, judged as being a stalwart defense against the incursions of the loved one's disease and troublesome symptoms. As Post highlights, "once care is in place, the issues that emerge in the natural course of the disease can be addressed in an informed manner. *Informal family caregivers are vital in the culture and practice of care*" (Post, 2000, p. 20; italics added).

An all-too-often devastating long-term effect is that attention to other vitally important aspects of the caregiver's identity becomes almost immediately *dis*regarded, with social *dis*respect leading to marginalization quickly ensuing. Neglect over time replaces the initial attention afforded "heroic" caregivers to the point that their own basic needs are ignored and their contributions unappreciated. The family caregiver for AD joins other caregivers of persons with disabilities as a group doomed to a downward spiral into increasing isolation and, for some, eventually ineffective caregiving (Levine, 1999).

Study after study reveals that the everyday, lived reality of most family caregivers is governed by society's belief that the family member must now accept a role characterized by his or her *unbounded obligation* toward the affected loved one by virtue of their wedding vows, commitment as a parent, spouse/partner, son or daughter, or even as "only living relative" (Williams, 2001). It is simply expected by society. This social attitude, which persists today, is deeply embedded in social roles and expectations worldwide, especially for women caregivers (Abel, 2000). Caregivers who complain or, more unthinkable, abandon their station are deemed morally reprehensible at best and unworthy to be considered a "person" at worst (Kittay, 2001). A case in point is a U.S. woman who, a few years ago in her home state of Oregon, drove her demented father to the steps of a hospital where she knew he would be cared for and left him there, much as desperate mothers over the ages have left infants in doorways. The ensuing press coverage demonized her, overwhelming her attempts to explain her desperation and failure by all other means to call attention to her and her father's life-threatening symptoms. Albeit an extreme example, her story strikingly illustrates that her desperation evoked a societal response that served to further compromise her ability to make reasonable claims on society's resources.

In Martha Nussbaum's recent review entitled "Disabilities: Who Cares?" she notes that a common theme is how disability is altering family life in the United States (2001). She cites the U.S. Department of Labor Women's Resources Division statistics that in an estimated one out of four households (22.4 million people) home care is being provided by family members for persons over fifty years of age. Caregiving in the home traditionally has fallen to women, and in the great majority of cases it still does. At the same time, data show that an increasing number of men also are changing their work and social roles dramatically to become family caregivers.

A high incidence of stress-related disorders among family caregivers is extremely disquieting, as is a rising incidence of serious caregiver physical injury from lifting, violence perpetrated by the person with AD, and poor judgment stemming from exhaustion. Yet these conditions are barely on the screen of consideration by policymakers. Worse still, if family caregivers' quality of life is compromised because safety and comfort are barely attended to, their autonomy is more neglected except in the form of temporary "respite" mechanisms sometimes provided through government or other sources. While important, the more fundamental social regard and respect for the implications of the caregiver's and dependent's changing relationship largely are ignored.

The family also often bears a disproportionately greater financial burden than before as a result of the caregiver's necessity of quitting work, cutting back hours, or scaling down a level of responsibility in the workplace. Almost no policies are in place to assist the caregiver in reentering the workplace once institutionalization or death of the loved one occurs or to retrain caregivers for salary-bearing jobs that can be carried out within the constraints of caregiving demands (Mahowald, Levinson, & Cassel, 1996). For this reason, some have advocated that such caregiving responsibilities be treated economically as care *work,* and remunerated accordingly (Jacques, 1993). The lack of support for this position at present, and opposition based on the assumption that "natural bonds" of family should override all other considerations, probably is a reflection of society's belief in the caregiver's unbounded obligation.

Family caregiving under these conditions is taking its toll economically, not only in economically developed nations but also in developing ones (United Nations Development Programme, 1999). Resistance to change leads to the conclusion reached in the United Nations report that this unpaid work, a major source of disadvantagement to women (and increasingly so in the new global economy) arises from a social dynamic akin to racism against the predominantly female population of family caregivers, further exacerbating their social marginalization.

The conclusions from this examination of the two major parties in the dependency relationship is not difficult to reach: society's unreasonably high expectations on caregivers, combined with disproportionately low expectations placed on persons with disabling conditions, create an unhealthy environment for both parties by socially (and often physically) marginalizing them from sources of social and financial support. Kittay observes correctly, however, that "we cannot eliminate dependency work, nor would we want to" (Kittay, 2001, p. 95). In fact, she reflects an observation that dominated the U.S.–European dialogue from which this book took root: such realities of human life move us more to seek social alliances than the idea of remaining independent and invulnerable from all others. In short, a just allocation must focus on the relationship of caregiver and care receiver, taking into account the *contributions and needs* of each in the dependency relationship. An allocation approach based on vulnerability considerations of the person with AD alone does not accomplish this end.

✢ Just Allocation: Goods, Services, and Social Structures

The above sections show some of the strengths and challenges encountered in trying to find an approach to a just allocation of resources that take the situation of persons with AD into account. The preceding section discussed some of those within the appropriate context of the relationships that should be honored. In this final section, one additional tension is addressed; namely, the question of whether a just allocation ever is possible if the focus remains on individuals or groups in vulnerable or dependent situations in society, or whether, instead, the entire focus must be shifted away from individuals or groups with a given set of characteristics.

One insight into where such an analysis should start is offered in Daniel Brock's critique of approaches based on vulnerability (2002). He observes that bioethicists fail to address the claims of vulnerable populations adequately because (with the goal of influencing practice and policy) they have focused attention on health care resource prioritization. In short, he says, this focus has been too fully on health care, to the exclusion of those health issues not entirely under social control. These approaches to solving problems of vulnerable populations are "resourcist" (i.e., focused on the distribution of goods and services) rather than "welfarist" (i.e., focused on health as a component of overall well-being). Faced with realities such as he points out, many have suggested that in order for justice to be served, it becomes necessary to shift the emphasis away from limited individuals to limited social structures. As Silvers, Wasserman, and Mahowald (1998, pp. 1–11) note, traditionally disabled persons have had to live with social practices that treat an impairment as a "limiting case," a practice that "cannot help but marginalize individuals."

Elizabeth Anderson (1999) takes up this line of reasoning in her notion of "democratic equality," contrasting it with what she calls "luck equality." Theories of luck equality deal with the concept of "the unfortunate," the vulnerable. Two people or groups become equal by the equal amount of some distributable good they are able to enjoy. By contrast, democratic equality places the emphasis on the development of society's structures that allow two people to be equal. In such development, *each* accepts the obligations to justify their own positions by principles acceptable to the other, and mutual consultation, reciprocation, and recognition are taken for granted.

Concerned with some of the same problems anticipated by Anderson, Silvers advocates for a social model of disability to replace the medical model. The medical model, it may be recalled, emphasizes that goods and services may become appropriate according to an impaired person's need in comparison with another's:

> The medical model assumes that disabilities are, fundamentally, deficits of natural assets rather than of social assets. . . . [In contrast,] the social model of disability transforms the notion of "handicapping condition" from a state of a minority of people, which disadvantages them in society, to a state of society, which disadvantages a minority of people. The social model traces the source of this minority's disadvantage to

a hostile environment and treats the dysfunction attendant on (certain kinds of) impairment as artificial and remediable, not natural and immutable. It transfigures individuals with disabilities from patients into persons with rights, which, when acknowledged, should eliminate the social disadvantages that are attendant upon their being a minority. Their environment is inimical to them because, in respect to almost all social venues and institutions, people with disabilities are neither numerous nor noticeable (Silvers, 1998, pp. 74–75).

Positive signs of social respect for persons with disability, expressed through laws designed to destroy structural barriers, have appeared. For example, the U.S. Americans with Disabilities Act of 1990 (ADA), based on thinking consistent with the social model, provides a measure of legal nourishment for the social environment through its attempt to cover discrimination against persons with disabilities in employment situations and access to public services or public accommodation. The act also was designed to provide protection from retaliation or coercion for exercising ADA-described rights. Still, how such protections and encouragement apply to persons with serious cognitive and other symptoms associated with AD is unclear, except insofar as the act places responsibility on society to eliminate structural barriers to social participation. Some commentators also worry that the act's "separate but equal" position may create a new social-legal landscape wherein new discrimination and other forms of disregard and disrespect could take root (Gostin & Looney, 1995).

Although European nations appear to have made more strides in creating social enablers that work for all, the consensus in the U.S.–European dialogue was that, in this regard, worldwide, much more needs to be done.

❧ A Just Allocation in Global Perspective

This chapter focuses on several challenges that face ethicists and policymakers in their quest for a just allocation of societal resources in the face of an increasing incidence of AD worldwide. Although this can provide only a starting point—a brief survey of key concerns in current approaches—it should be a springboard for others who will take analyses deeper. One serious shortcoming of the present analysis is the assumption of a moderate degree of scarcity of resources that can be brought to bear on the challenges described in this chapter. In our United States–European dialogue that became the foundation for this book, the Central and Eastern European colleagues reminded the others that their countries (and the majority of the world) experience a dire scarcity of resources for even the most basic human needs. Any allocation policy ultimately must be cast in global perspective. Such acknowledgement supports further exploration of a social model of disability and a welfarist orientation over those that stretch goods and services as their primary goal.

REFERENCES

Abel, E. K. (2000). *Hearts of wisdom: American women caring for kin, 1850–1940.* Cambridge: Harvard University Press.

Anderson, E. (1999). What is the point of equality? *Ethics, 109,* 287–337.

Brock, D. W. (2002). Health resource allocation for vulnerable populations. In M. Doris, C. Clancy & L. R. Churchill (Eds.), *Ethical dimensions of health policy* (pp. 283–310). New York: Oxford University Press.

Buchanan, J. H. (1989). *Patient encounters: The experience of disease.* Charlottesville: University Press of Virginia.

Crane, D. (1975). *The sanctity of social life: Physicians' treatment of critically ill patients.* New York: Russell Sage.

Daniels, N. (1988). *Am I my parents' keeper?* New York: Oxford University Press.

Gostin, L., & Looney, B. L. (1995). Disability: Legal issues. In W. T. Reich (Ed.), *Encyclopedia of bioethics* (Rev. ed.) (pp. 622–625). New York: Simon & Schuster Macmillan.

Jacques, R. (1993). Untheorized dimensions of caring work: Caring as a structural practice and caring as a way of seeing. *Nursing Administration Quarterly, 17* (2) 1–10.

Jaworska, A. (1999). Respecting the margins of agency: Alzheimer's patients and the capacity to value. *Philosophy and Public Affairs, 28* (2) 105–138.

Jette, A. (1994). Physical disablement: Concepts for physical therapy research and practice. *Physical Therapy, 74,* 381.

Kittay, E. F. (2001). *Loves labor: Essays on women, equality, and dependency.* New York: Routledge.

Koppleman, A. (1996). *Anti-discrimination law and social equality.* New Haven, CT: Yale University Press. [Cited in a footnote in A. Silvers, D. Wasserman, & M. Mahowald, (Eds.), *Disability, difference, discrimination* (p. 175). Lanham, MD: Rowman & Littlefield.]

Levine, C. (1999). The loneliness of the long-term care giver. *New England Journal of Medicine, 340,* (15), 87–88.

Mahowald, M., Levinson, D., & Cassel, C. (1996). The new genetics and women. *Milbank Quarterly, 74,* (2), 268–270.

Marienelli, R. P., & Dell Orto, A. E. (Eds.). (1999). *The psychological and social impact of disability* (3rd ed.). New York: Springer.

Nussbaum, M. (2001). Disabled lives: Who cares? *New York Review of Books,* January 11, 34–37.

Post, S. (2000). *The moral challenge of Alzheimer disease: Ethical issues from diagnosis to dying* (2nd ed.). Baltimore: Johns Hopkins University Press.

Rawls, J. (1971). *A theory of justice.* Cambridge: Harvard University Press.

Reeves, P. M. (1999). An update on adult developmental theory: New ways of thinking about the life course. *New Directions of Adult and Continuing Education, 84* (winter), 19–28.

Sabat, S. R. (2001). *The experience of Alzheimer's disease: Life through a tangled veil.* Malden, MA: Blackwell.

Silvers, A. (1996). "Defective" agents: Equality, difference, and the tyranny of the normal. In R. Manning & R. Trujillo (Eds.), *Social justice in a diverse society* (pp. 54–175). Menlo Park, CA: Mayfield.

Silvers, A. (1998). Formal justice. In A. Silvers, D. Wasserman, & M. B. Mahowald (Eds.), *Disability, difference, discrimination* (pp. 13–147). Lanham, MD: Rowman & Littlefield.

Silvers, A., Wasserman, D., & Mahowald, M. B. (Eds.). (1998). *Disability, difference, discrimination.* Lanham, MD: Rowman & Littlefield.

Spelman, E. (1997). *Fruits of sorrow: Framing our attention to suffering.* Boston, MA: Beacon Press.

United Nations Development Programme. (1999). Human Development Report 1999 (pp. 77–83). New York: Oxford University Press.

U.S. Congress. (1990). Americans with Disabilities Act, U.S. Public Law 10.

Wendell, S. (2001). Unhealthy disabled: Treating chronic illnesses as disabilities. *Hypatia, 16,* 17–33.

Willams, J. (2001). *Unbending gender: Why family and work conflict and what to do about it.* New York: Oxford University Press.

Commentary on Part V

*A Clinician's Commentary from a Post-Soviet Society
on Organizational Issues of Care for Alzheimer Disease*

Givi Javashvili, M.D., Ph.D.

In this part of the book (part V), my collaborators have addressed organizational issues of care for persons with Alzheimer disease (AD) raising ethical aspects of care. They emphasize correctly that the goal is to actually change the lives of people with AD. But for these changes to occur, a variety of organizational issues must be given attention, including development of an appropriate legal framework, adaptation of public health policy, elaboration of professional standards, revision of training curricula for doctors and nurses, and implementation of a system of quality control, to name some.

Writing as the only other contributor to this volume who represents Central and East European (CEE) countries, I want to draw attention to the contribution by Eugenius Gefenas. I will also comment briefly on others. Gefenas (chapter 17) emphasizes social, cultural, and other differences between CEE countries and the rest of Europe (developed European states) and shows how these differences eventually led to the formation of different legal frameworks for dealing with the problem of autonomy of incapacitated persons (including persons with AD). These differences are highlighted in today's era of integration when the legal frameworks of member states of the Council of Europe (COE) must be made compatible with the binding legal texts (i.e., conventions or recommendations) of the COE. He explores existing distinctions between legal systems in relation to the protection of incapacitated persons (the traditional type of system versus an alternative type of system) and comments on existing realities in CEE countries, attributing the delay in introducing an alternative system to cultural and ideological peculiarities of the CEE countries. Certainly, the ideology of totalitarian states in Central and Eastern Europe supported the sacrifice of individualism and personal autonomy for the "best interest of the society," and these states very often succeeded in implementing that ideology in practice. This was true in the health care setting as well, and health care professionals usually did not acknowledge the principle of patient autonomy. However, it is inaccurate to say that the culture of the entire CEE society was geared to disregard completely the principle of personal independence during the years of the authoritarian regime, particularly in those states that became part of the Communist group only after World War II. It is worth noting that the ideology and resulting legislation in the latter countries did not necessarily fully reflect the culture and true attitudes of the larger society. This assumption may be supported by Gefenas's observation about Lithuania that "very few adults with AD and other dementias have this kind of protective measure. The most usual motive in applications for guardianship is an attempt by family members to take care of the property of the person concerned." The cultural specificity of different populations in the post-totalitarian era has deep roots and warrants further research and analyses.

Another notable subject dealt with in Gefenas's chapter is the different meanings of autonomy in the context of care for incompetent persons and the tendencies in CEE countries to implement a libertarian concept of personal autonomy. Certainly, modern democratic societies should avoid establishing an oversimplified concept of informed consent, which sometimes becomes the only legal prerequisite for medical interventions and may be used by health care professionals mostly to protect themselves from liability. This is particularly relevant when it comes to decision making about the care of incompetent persons, including those with AD. A strict, rigid model of informed consent may leave unacknowledged real values of the person. However, I absolutely agree with the author in saying that legalizing and implementing informed consent in CEE countries is a very important movement toward enforcing the role of patients, particularly in areas where there is a high risk of abuse (e.g., biomedical research, human organ transplantation). Legalization of autonomy understood as authenticity may be the next step for these countries. Such legalization would be very difficult to introduce in a top-down manner. It must come from the public's belief that it is in their best interest that individual autonomy be legalized.

Also of interest in Gefenas's chapter is his characterization of CEE health care systems as libertarian, resembling the U.S. model. However, the author appropriately points out that the situation in transition societies (where individuals are expected to take responsibility for their own health, and access to health care services depends on the ability to pay) basically is triggered by extremely limited resources. Consequently, in transition societies the abovementioned state of affairs is *caused* by a scarcity of resources, not solely by cultural norms, as in the United States.

In chapter 18, Purtilo examines the societal roots of disregard and disrespect toward persons with AD, a situation that eventually leads to difficulties in assuring that appropriate resources will be allocated for palliative care of Alzheimer patients. She speaks from a U.S. and West European framework of thought, drawing on the well-known philosopher John Rawls. She notes that one of the fundamental determinatives causing persons with AD (and their families) to suffer from social marginalization is the tendency to put a price on a person's worth and consequently to assess whether he or she deserves regard and respect. Due to this kind of approach, people with dementia, including persons with AD, "often are robbed of regard and respect." This societal attitude often is mirrored in the perceptions of people with dementia, who come to "consider that they are unworthy of regard and respect." The ensuing state of affairs concerning allocation of resources is the tendency for persons with disability to be marginalized "from the decision maker's attention when [society's] basic goods are being allocated." The situation could apply every bit as much to transitional societies such as the CEE countries, but as Gefenas emphasizes (and Purtilo notes at the end of her chapter) the problem must be viewed also in the context of a situation where there are not sufficient resources for even the most fundamental types of health care. One might expect on that basis alone that the patient with AD would become an even lower priority when there are so many other competing needs.

Taking this reality into consideration, I want to comment on advance directives, which we are very interested in implementing: does an advance directive (which is supposed to be one tool to preserve a patient's autonomy) adequately reflect the values of "disabled" persons? I think it is quite possible that decisions about future care, particularly about end-of-life care, made by "disabled" people are considerably affected by the combination of societal attitudes toward the "disabled" and the lack of resources available to them. There is a possibility that the significant financial burden on their families may lead them to decide to refuse life-sustaining (or even life-saving) or expensive treatment; or they may prefer isolation, just to be hidden from the eyes of others. Accordingly, under existing societal circumstances, the true value of short, succinct advance directives made by competent persons with AD may be under question. A more appropriate approach may be the explication of the true values of patients (e.g., through completion of a Values History Form as advised by Scheirton in chapter 16). However, changing society's attitude to make judgments "on the basis of inherent dignity" has to remain the ultimate goal.

Scheirton's chapter, outlining a comprehensive guide to educational strategies to be implemented while caring for patients with AD, and Furlong's promises of the hospice approach as a means for ensuring effective palliative care for patients with AD (chapter 15) describe ideals that should be promoted whenever possible. They aim at a type of care for comforting patients and ensuring a higher quality of life in contrast to just prolonging life by means that could make patients suffer more and also may undermine their dignity.

In short, the U.S. authors seem optimistic about the possible elimination of existing barriers in palliative care, particularly for patients with AD. However, such a solution to the dilemmas may be an outcome that is feasible only in highly developed countries, like the United States, while others still have to cope with hard decisions related to resource allocation. (To mention a similar situation: renal dialysis in the United States became widely available and therefore there was no need to "select patients" for this type of treatment—as the "Seattle Committee" was doing in the United States in the 1960s.) A global approach in research and assessment of ethical aspects of resource allocation regarding AD therefore will remain vital for many years.

In spite of these caveats, as a clinician I want to add my voice to Furlong's final, enthusiastic Yes! in favor of a palliative model of care aimed at preserving the quality of life, autonomy, and dignity of patients with Alzheimer disease.

Part VI / Research Underpinnings for an Ethical Model of Palliative Care

CHAPTER NINETEEN

Biomedical Research in Alzheimer Disease

Patricio F. Reyes, M.D.

Until three and a half decades ago, there was little biomedical research in aging—not in aging in general, nor in Alzheimer disease (AD) in particular. This was largely because for many years societal efforts and resources were geared toward the young. Aging and medical conditions that affect older patients were viewed with fatalism by the lay and scientific communities. Advanced medical care coupled with increased longevity inevitably led to heightened awareness and research interest in age-related issues. As a consequence, dementing conditions clinically characterized by progressive deterioration of cognition, behavior, and activities of daily living became a major focus of medical and scientific investigations.

Several systemic and primary neurologic entities can cause dementia, but in the Western world AD is the most common etiology among middle-aged and elderly persons. AD affects between 5 percent and 10 percent of the population above sixty-five years of age (Ernest & Hay, 1994). Recent studies and the incidence and prevalence of AD increase with advancing age have indicated that at least 4 million Americans and 50 percent of nursing home patients in the United States suffer from the disorder (Hebert et al., 1995). The annual cost for AD has been estimated to be $110 billion, and since the fastest growing segment of our population is the elderly, the number of affected patients is expected to rise steeply during the next several decades (Ernest & Hay, 1994; Hebert et al., 1995). If we take into account loss of income from caregivers, who frequently suffer from depression and other medical conditions, the total cost of caring for AD patients could easily escalate.

The early symptoms of AD are often difficult to appreciate because they are nonspecific, intermittent, and insidious; its clinical course usually evolving over a period of six to ten years. It affects all ethnic groups, but its incidence and age of onset may be modified by certain risk factors such as the frequency of the APOE-4 gene (Terry & Katzman, 1983). Although its etiology remains elusive, advancing age, genetic background, head trauma, and gender are considered other risk factors (Desai & Grossberg, 1999). Future investigations designed to offer a better understanding of the disease, develop more reliable diagnostic techniques, and provide safer and more effective treatment will have to be pursued in order to meet the challenges of prevention, early detection, and definitive therapy.

In general, memory loss for recent events is the clinical hallmark of AD. However, careful neurobehavioral assessment frequently reveals concomitant impairment of language functions, comprehension, judgment, orientation, calculation, and attention span. Behavioral symptoms, including depression, anxiety, delusions, hallucinations, insomnia, wandering, and violent behavior, are not uncommon manifestations that could precede decline of intellectual functions (Jost & Grossberg, 1996). Difficulty carrying out daily activities at home or at work may herald or coexist with cognitive and behavioral manifestations. As the disease progresses, patients will require more supervision and caregiving, either at home or in chronic care facilities. There is insidious loss of general body functions, and death usually occurs several years later from pneumonia, sepsis, or trauma.

Current epidemiological and clinical data have generated unprecedented enthusiasm in investigating factors that influence normal aging and AD. This was a major departure from the old notion that dementia and AD were untreatable normal consequences of aging. For the past three decades, neuroscientists, physicians, and other health care providers have independently or collaboratively produced an exponential amount of new and interesting data that have considerably enhanced our understanding, diagnosis, and treatment of AD.

Advances in biomedical research may be divided into (1) diagnostic; (2) therapeutic; and (3) preventive categories. These are essential because successful management of a disease requires accurate diagnosis as well as safe and effective treatment and preventive measures.

Diagnosis of AD was significantly advanced by the introduction of validated clinical instruments for assessing (a) cognition: the Mini-Mental State Examination (MMSE), the Alzheimer disease assessment scale (ADAS), and the clinical dementia rating scale (CDR); (b) behavior: the neuropsychiatric inventory (NPI); and (c) activities of daily living: the progressive deterioration scale (PDS) and the global deterioration scale (GDS). These measures allow clinicians to verify presence, severity, and stage of disease and provide appropriate and timely recommendations to families and caregivers. Similar measures were recently utilized to identify seemingly "normal" individuals with mild cognitive impairment (MCI), many of whom represent the early stages of AD (Petersen et al., 1999).

Other diagnostic tools consist of neuro-imaging techniques such as computerized tomography (CT), magnetic resonance imaging (MRI), single photon emission computerized tomography (SPECT), and positron emission tomography (PET) scans. CT and MRI offer structural and anatomical views of the brain and cranium. Although there are no specific lesions associated with Alzheimer disease, CT and MRI are useful in excluding other conditions (e.g., strokes, tumors, and infections) that can mimic AD symptomatology. Functional MRI enables the simultaneous investigation of brain function and structure, whereas SPECT offers valuable information on cerebral blood flow changes that may differentiate strokes from AD. PET is presently a research tool that measures metabolism in certain parts of the brain. In some clinically diagnosed AD patients and asymptomatic cases with APOE-4 gene, PET has shown hypometabolism in posterior parietal and temporal regions (Ojemann et al., 1997). Results of longitudinal studies will determine whether PET could be a reliable method for diagnosing AD.

Another important component of the diagnostic workup for AD includes tests that utilize serum, cerebrospinal fluid, and brain tissue. These are critical in order to exclude systemic and other neurological disorders that can mimic the symptoms of AD. In spite of a comprehensive workup, AD is solely established by neuropathologic examination of postmortem brain tissue. Diagnosis is confirmed by the presence of large numbers of neuritic plaques (NPs) and neurofibrillary tangles (NFTs). Synaptic changes and neuronal loss are important observations but are not required for neuropathologic diagnosis (Wright, Geula, & Mesulam, 1993).

AD treatment was purely symptomatic until cholinergic and other neuro-transmitter deficits were discovered in the brains of affected patients. Among the various neurochemical abnormalities, the level of cholinergic deficiency corre-lated best with severity of dementia in AD (Coyle, Price, & DeLong, 1983; Perry et al., 1998; Schegg et al., 1992). Cholinergic neurons in the nucleus basalis of Meynert are lost, in addition to there being diminished activity of choline-acetyltransferase (ChAT), the synthesizing enzyme for acetylcholine (ACh), and reduced levels of neocortical ACh, a neurotransmitter vital for maintaining memory related processes (Geula, 1998; Younkin et al., 1986). Clinical trials uti-lizing acetylcholinesterase inhibitors have produced modest response and de-layed symptom progression in AD patients with mild to moderate dementia (Anand, Messina, & Hartman, 2000; Nordberg & Svensson, 1998; Polinsky, 1998; S. L. Rogers & Friedhoff, 1998; Schneider, Anand, & Farlow, 1998). Neuroprotec-tive agents such as vitamin E, estrogen (for postmenopausal and surgically ster-ilized women), and nonsteroidal anti-inflammatory drugs are prescribed to reduce neuronal degeneration (Desai & Grossberg, 1999; Gibbs & Aggarwal, 1998; J. Rogers, 1995). Furthermore, the public is inundated with herbs, food sup-plements, and other forms of medicinals that are advertised as "safe and effec-tive" treatment for memory loss, depression, anxiety, and other forms of cognitive and behavioral deficits without the benefit of controlled clinical inves-tigations. We have to verify the purity, beneficial effects, and complications of herbs before they can be endorsed for therapeutic purposes. To date, there is no cure for AD, and none of the pharmacological agents approved for its treatment can reverse or stop the progression of the disease.

Molecular biology and genetics have produced some of the most exciting knowledge on aging and AD. Studies on Down syndrome and familial AD cases have yielded invaluable information that will influence our therapeutic ap-proach. Initial experiments were largely driven by the concept that beta amyloid, the protein core observed in NPs, is central to the etiopathogenesis of AD. For the past several years investigations have focused on beta amyloid's biochemical, ultrastructural, molecular, functional, and toxic properties. Similarly, NFTs are now known to be mainly made up of hyperphosphorylated protein called tau. Future research in these areas could provide clues as to the evolution of AD and lead to formulation of novel pharmacologic compounds that might avert disease development and/or progression. Successful development of such drugs could offer preventive as well as definitive therapies. Genetic studies have confirmed mutations of chromosomes 1, 14, and 21 in early onset familial AD and identified certain secretases, the enzymes that are thought to cleave the beta amyloid protein from its parent molecule, the amyloid precursor protein (Cruts & Broeckhoven, 1998). Drugs that can block the action of such secretases may prevent the NP formation. Moreover, a transgenic mouse model for AD has been developed, and APOE-4 gene is now considered to be a risk factor because its presence significantly raises disease susceptibility (Saunders, 2001).

Most recently, biomedical scientists found a class of stem cells, called pluripotent due to their potential to develop into different cell types in the body (Svendsen & Smith, 1999). These cells are found in embryos and fetal tissue. In the few years since this discovery, evidence has emerged that these stem cells are, indeed, capable of becoming almost all of the specialized cells of the body and may have the potential to generate replacement cells for a broad array of tissues and organs. Thus, this class of human stem cell holds the promise of being able to repair or replace cells or tissues that are damaged or destroyed by many devastating and currently untreatable diseases that are usually associated with serious disabilities and fatal outcome. New data have emerged that stem cells from adults can be found in bone marrow, cornea, retina, and the brain. Adult and embryonic stem cells have different properties. The latter are currently preferred for experimental purposes.

The potential role of stem-cell research in clinical practice has generated significant controversy after investigators have shown that differentiated cells obtained from both adult and embryonic stem cells can repair or replace damaged cells and tissues. Researchers are pursuing two fundamental strategies to explore this discovery. One is, by starting with undifferentiated neural cells, to grow differentiated cells in a laboratory dish that are suitable for implantation into a patient. The other repair strategy relies on finding growth hormones and other "trophic factors" that can stimulate a patient's own stem cells and endogenous repair mechanisms to allow the body to cope with damage from disease or injury. Efforts to develop stem-cell based therapies for Parkinson's disease provide a good example of research aimed at rebuilding the central nervous system. Historically, one of the first attempts at using cell transplantation in humans was tried in Parkinson's disease cases (Allen et al., 1989). Although dramatic improvement in Parkinson's patients was initially reported after transplanting dopamine-producing cells from the patients' own adrenal glands to the affected area of their brains, subsequent studies showed limited, short-lived, and inconsistent improvement of patients' symptoms. Similarly, previous human transplantation studies on Parkinson's disease using fetal brain tissue removed from an elective abortus demonstrated encouraging but inconsistent benefit to patients. Although not all patients improved, some patients who received fetal tissue transplants had a clear reduction in the severity of their symptoms. Furthermore, autopsies done on these few patients revealed a robust survival and differentiation of the grafted neurons. Most investigators remain optimistic that cell-transplantation will be effective in treating Parkinson's disease. At present, there has been no therapeutic trial utilizing stem-cell transplantation for AD.

Potential adverse events may accompany stem-cell use in medicine. If embryonic stem cells are injected into a mouse with a compromised immune system, a benign tumor called a "teratoma" can develop. For this reason, scientists do not anticipate that undifferentiated embryonic stem cells will be used for therapeutic applications. These cells will need to be differentiated or otherwise modified before they can be used clinically. Current challenges are to direct the differentiation of embryonic stem cells into specialized cell populations and to control their development or proliferation once placed in the patient. With the exception of the clinical application of hematopoietic (blood making) stem cells, adult stem cells are not ready to be utilized for therapy. In order to use adult stem cells safely in tissues other than the tissue from which they were isolated, researchers will need purified populations of adult stem cells. In addition, modifications to the cells, to the immune system, or both will be a major requirement for their potential application in instances of tissue rejection after stem-cell transplantation.

The development of stem-cell technology (SCT) has offered hope to many patients and families who suffer from incurable diseases such as cancer, brain and spinal cord trauma, AD, Parkinson's disease, heart failure, and several genetic and degenerative disorders that cause irreversible organ damage. It also raises important ethical, legal, and economic concerns that have polarized segments of our society. Therefore, it is imperative that we approach such a subject with sufficient background knowledge, utmost objectivity, and minimal emotionalism.

It is clear that SCT could become a viable form of treatment for particular diseases, and stem cells may be derived from embryonic, fetal, and adult tissues. In general, materials from elective abortions are preferred and utilized for research studies. As technology evolves, it is conceivable that adult tissues could provide the needed number of cells for clinical application. If SCT becomes a treatment option, the need for aborted fetuses and embryonic tissues would increase exponentially. This could lead to a disproportionate rise in the number of abortions, as well as private ventures designed to generate revenues from products of abortion. Second, significant scientific concerns like tumor-growth complications, long-term survival of cells, effects of environment on cell integrity and lifespan, and other factors that influence successful stem-cell treatment must be addressed before we can recommend SCT for therapeutic purposes. Moreover, we have to determine the overall cost for the type, extent, and duration of benefits we intend to achieve and the potential adverse events that may accompany SCT. More importantly, introduction of SCT as a therapeutic tool must take into account our legal system, economic resources, and ethical, moral, and spiritual values.

A preventive approach for AD is in its infancy due to our limited insight into the pathogenesis of AD. However, we now know that certain risk factors could increase the chance for developing the disease. These include advancing age, APOE-4 gene, female gender, and head trauma (Desai & Grossberg, 1999; Terry & Katzman, 1983). Investigations of neurobiologic phenomena involved in normal aging and AD have to be pursued to obtain relevant information on cell death, degeneration, and regeneration. Paradoxically, increased knowledge on cell death, due to necrosis and apoptosis, and regeneration is crucial in order to prevent cell degeneration and promote quality of life in later years. It is important to emphasize that unlike chromosome mutations that almost always lead to Alzheimer disease, APOE-4 gene is a susceptibility gene that simply augments the risk for the disorder. Estrogen is believed to have neuroprotective properties in postmenopausal women, and nonsteroidal anti-inflammatory drugs (NSAIDs) have been advocated to reduce neuronal damage due to inflammation. Vitamin E, a known antioxidant, is prescribed to lessen the deleterious effects of free radicals in the brain parenchyma (Desai & Grossberg, 1999; Gibbs & Aggarwal, 1998; J. Rogers, 1995). Head trauma can predispose patients to AD (Reyes et al., 1989), months or years after the injury. It is hoped that in the future we could reduce our exposure to or counteract the ill effects of risk factors and/or neutralize the influence of genetic abnormalities. These possibilities have given rise to heightened enthusiasm and expectation that AD could potentially be arrested, if not be prevented.

The availability of new diagnostic tests and therapies for AD has considerably influenced our medical approach and management of AD and other previously untreatable neurodegenerative disorders. It has given patients and families hope for safer and more effective treatment options. These same developments, however, have generated interesting and challenging medical and philosophical issues. Who should undergo and pay for more sophisticated and comprehensive neurobehavioral assessment? When do we start and terminate treatment? Who should have genetic testing and access to the results of genetic testing? Lastly, as we develop more sophisticated scientific techniques such as SCT, we also need to establish strict guidelines for their use in medical practice. Otherwise, we can potentially destroy the humanity we are attempting to save.

REFERENCES

Allen, G. S., Burns R. S., Tulipan N. B., & Parker, R. A. (1989). Adrenal medullary transplantation to the caudate nucleus in Parkinson's disease: Initial clinical results in eighteen patients. *Archives of Neurology, 46, 487–491.*

Anand, R., Messina, J., & Hartman, R. (2000). Dose-response effect of rivastigmine in the treatment of Alzheimer's disease. *International Journal of Geriatric Psychopharmacology, 2, 68–72.*

Coyle, J. T., Price, K. L., & DeLong, M. R. (1983). Alzheimer's disease: A disorder of cortical cholinergic innervation. *Science, 219, 1184–1190.*

Cruts, M., & Broeckhoven C. (1998). Molecular genetics of Alzheimer's disease. *Annals of Medicine, 30, 560–565.*

Desai, A., & Grossberg, G. (1999). Risk factors and protective factors for Alzheimer's disease. *Clinical Geriatrics, 7* (11), 43–52.

Earnest, R. L., & Hay, J. W. (1994). The U.S. economic and social costs of Alzheimer's disease revisited. *American Journal of Public Health, 84, 1261–1264.*

Geula, C. (1998). Abnormalities of neural circuitry in Alzheimer's disease: Hippocampus and cortical cholinergic innervation. *Neurology, 51, S18–S29.*

Gibbs, R. B., & Aggarwal, P. (1998). Estrogen and basal forebrain cholinergic neurons: Implications for brain aging and Alzheimer's disease-related cognitive decline. *Hormone and Behavior, 34, 98–111.*

Hebert, L. E., Scherr, P. A., Beckett, L. A., Albert, M. S., Pilgrim, D. M., Chown, M. J., Funkenstein, H. H., Evans, D. A. (1995). Age-specific incidence of Alzheimer's disease in a community population. *Journal of the American Medical Association, 273,* 1354–1359.

Jost, B. C., & Grossberg, G. T. (1996). The evolution of psychiatric symptoms in

Alzheimer's disease: A natural history study. *Journal of the American Geriatrics Society, 44* (9), 1078–1081.

Nordberg, A., & Svensson, A. (1998). Cholinesterase inhibitors in the treatment of Alzheimer's disease. *Drug Safety, 19,* 465–480.

Ojemann, J. G., Buckner R. L., Corbetta M., & Raichle, M. E. (1997). Imaging studies of memory and attention. *Neurosurgery Clinics of North America, 8,* 307–319.

Perry, E. K., Perry, R. H., Blessed, G., & Tomlinson, B. E. (1998). Changes in brain cholinesterases in senile dementia of Alzheimer type. *Neuropathology and Applied Neurobiology, 4,* 273–277.

Petersen, R. C., Smith, G. E., Waring, S. C., Ivnik, R. J., Tangalos, E. G., & Kokmen, E. (1999). Mild cognitive impairment: Clinical characterization and outcome. *Archives of Neurology, 56,* 303–308.

Polinsky, R. J. (1998). Clinical pharmacology of rivastigmine: A new-generation acetyl-cholinesterase inhibitor for the treatment of Alzheimer's disease. *Clinical Therapeutics, 20,* 634–647.

Reyes, P. F., Booth, K., Sacchetti, T., & Carner, E. (1998). Dementia among retired elderly boxers [Abstract] (April 13–19). Chicago: American Academy of Neurology.

Rogers, J. (1995). Inflammation as a pathogenic mechanism in Alzheimer's disease. *Ärztliche Forschung, 45,* 439–442.

Rogers, S. L., & Friedhoff, L. T. (1998). Long-term efficacy and safety of donepezil in the treatment of Alzheimer's disease: An interim analysis of the result of a U.S. multicentre open label extension study. *European Neuropsychopharmacology, 8,* 67–75.

Saunders, A. M. (2000). Apolipoprotein E and Alzheimer's disease: An update on genetic and functional analyses. *Journal of Neuropathology and Experimental Neurology, 59,* 751–758.

Schegg, K. M., Harrington, L. S., Nielsen, S., Zwieg, R. M., & Peacock, J. H. (1992). Soluble and membrane-bound forms of brain acetycholinesterase in Alzheimer's disease. *Neurobiology of Aging, 13,* 697–704.

Schneider, L. S., Anand, R., & Farlow, M. R. (1998). Systematic review of the efficacy of rivastigmine for patients with Alzheimer's disease. *International Journal of Geriatric Psychopharmacology, 1,* S26–S34.

Svendsen, C. N., & Smith, A. G. (1999). New prospects for human stem-cell therapy in the nervous system. *Trends in Neurosciences, 22,* 357–364.

Terry, R. D., & Katzman, R. (1983). Senile dementia of the Alzheimer type. *Annals of Neurology, 14,* 497–506.

Wright, C. I., Geula, C., & Mesulam, M. M. (1993). Neuroglial cholinesterases in the normal brain and in Alzheimer's disease: Relationship to plaques, tangles, and pattern of selective vulnerability. *Annals of Neurology, 34,* 373–384.

Younkin, S. G., Goodridge, B., Katz, J., Lockett, G., Nafziger, D., Usiak, M. F., & Younkin, L. H. (1986). Molecular form of acetylcholinesterase in Alzheimer's disease. *Federation Proceedings, 45,* 2982–2989.

CHAPTER TWENTY

Conducting Research in the Alzheimer Disease Population

Balancing Individual, Group, Family, and Societal Interests

Søren Holm, M.D., Ph.D., Dr.Med.Sci.

Research into the best ways of providing palliative care for persons with Alzheimer disease (AD) and other dementias is of paramount importance. The number of people with dementia is projected to rise rapidly in most countries (Fratiglioni, DeRonchi, & Aguero Torres, 2000). Although treatments are being developed and marketed, most of them are not targeting the underlying disease process and are able only to temporarily ameliorate the symptoms of the condition.

Most patients with dementia will therefore progress to a state of moderate to severe dementia before they die, and many will need specialized palliative care. Such care should be evidence-based and not driven only by the different theoretical commitments of practitioners in the field.

I address some of the major research challenges in regards to dementia. When I talk about dementia, it is always dementia caused by AD. I believe the general line of argument put forward is valid for a range of other dementias, but the specific symptoms of the different kinds of dementia vary and therefore the palliative approach may also vary according to specific circumstances.

❧ The Traditional Problem: Research without Consent

The traditional research ethics problem discussed in connection with dementia research is the problem of research involving persons who are incapable of giving valid informed consent. This problem has been extensively analyzed, and at the regulatory level of research ethics a close to complete consensus has developed on the requirements that have to be fulfilled for such research to be deemed ethically acceptable. These requirements are

1. Consent must be sought from the person's representative (proxy)
2. If the person is able to assent or dissent, although unable to consent, the person's assent must be obtained
3. The research must either be directly beneficial to the person or it must be beneficial to the patient group to which the person belongs, and it must be impossible to perform the research in a group of patients who can consent
4. The risk to the person must be minimal in those circumstances where there is no direct benefit

This consensus is expressed in paragraphs 24–26 of the most recent revision of the Helsinki Declaration from the World Medical Association:

24. For a research subject who is legally incompetent, physically or mentally incapable of giving consent or is a legally incompetent minor, the investigator must obtain informed consent from the legally authorized representative in accordance with applicable law. These groups should not be included in research unless the research is necessary to promote the health of the population represented and this research cannot instead be performed on legally competent persons.

25. When a subject deemed legally incompetent, such as a minor child, is able to give assent to decisions about participation in research, the investigator must obtain that assent in addition to the consent of the legally authorized representative.

26. Research on individuals from whom it is not possible to obtain consent, including proxy or advance consent, should be done only if the physical/mental condition that prevents obtaining informed consent is a necessary characteristic of the research population. The specific reasons for involving research subjects with a

condition that renders them unable to give informed consent should be stated in the experimental protocol for consideration and approval of the review committee. The protocol should state that consent to remain in the research should be obtained as soon as possible from the individual or a legally authorized surrogate. (World Medical Association, 2000)

Very similar provisions can be found in the Council of Europe's Convention for the Protection of Human Rights and Dignity of the Human Being with regard to the Application of Biology and Medicine:

Article 17—Protection of persons not able to consent to research

1. Research on a person without the capacity to consent as stipulated in Article 5 may be undertaken only if all the following conditions are met:

i. the conditions laid down in Article 16, sub-paragraphs i to iv, are fulfilled;

ii. the results of the research have the potential to produce real and direct benefit to his or her health;

iii. research of comparable effectiveness cannot be carried out on individuals capable of giving consent;

iv. the necessary authorization provided for under Article 6 has been given specifically and in writing; and

v. the person concerned does not object.

2. Exceptionally and under the protective conditions prescribed by law, where the research does not have the potential to produce results that directly benefits the health of the person concerned, such research may be authorized subject to the conditions laid down in paragraph 1, subparagraphs i, iii, iv and v above, and to the following additional conditions:

i. the research has the aim of contributing, through significant improvement in the scientific understanding of the individual's condition, disease or disorder, to the ultimate attainment of results capable of conferring benefit to the person concerned or to other persons in the same age category or afflicted with the same disease or disorder or having the same condition;

ii. the research entails only minimal risk and minimal burden for the individual concerned. (Council of Europe, 1997)

The consensus is quite clear that persons who can give informed consent to become a research participant is the paradigm case and that research on persons incapable of giving consent is an aberrant case that, if it is allowed at all, must be accommodated within the consent paradigm.

This accommodation is achieved by seeking a "consent equivalent" and by restricting the types of research that persons can participate in if they are incapable of consenting. The restriction on types of research in this latter case can be justified in three partially different ways:

The first is based on the historical fact that vulnerable groups have often been used in ethically problematic research and that if incompetent people could be used as research participants in ordinary projects there is a risk that they would become an easy source of research material.

The second focuses on the intersection of interests between the person with a specific condition and the group of sufferers with that condition. The argument is that even if a person does not realize a personal benefit from the research, he is benefited indirectly through the benefits accruing to the group. However, this justification is problematic in many cases. One situation where the argument is of doubtful validity is where the membership of the group in question is temporary and where most persons who are part of the research will no longer be members of the group when the benefits materialize. This could be the case where, for instance, a condition is rapidly progressive, or where research projects are very drawn out in time. Another such situation is where the benefits are of a kind that can be enjoyed only by people who are not yet members of the group. This could be the case if, for instance, the knowledge sought in a project is exclusively knowledge about how to prevent the occurrence of the condition.

The third possible justification is the pragmatic one that unless we allow some kinds of research without consent into conditions where all sufferers are incompetent, very little progress will be made in the treatment of such conditions (the "golden ghetto" argument), but such research should be limited to those projects that cannot be performed in any other way in order to minimize the infringements caused by research without consent.

❧ Less-traditional Research Ethics Problems

Even if we accept the traditional consensus outlined above, this does not exhaust the research ethics problems raised by dementia research. Two problems that are not solved by the traditional consensus are (1) what topics should be researched; and (2) what kind of research should be conducted.

The Council of Europe's position on restricting research to "research [that] has the aim of contributing, through significant improvement in the scientific understanding of the individual's condition, disease or disorder, to the ultimate attainment of results capable of conferring benefit to the person concerned or to other persons in the same age category or afflicted with the same disease or disorder or having the same condition" provides very little constraint with regard to what research can be performed within the dementia field. All kinds of research topics, ranging from basic science to institutional design, can fall within this categorization. Similarly its restriction to "research [that] entails only minimal risk and minimal burden for the individual concerned" provides only limited constraints on the research methods that can be used.

Both choice of research topics—and, perhaps more importantly, what research topics should receive priority and funding—and choice of research methods are ethically charged. Different groups of stakeholders in the research process have different interests with regard to these issues, and it requires further analysis to decide whether these interests are in conflict and subsequently whether such conflicts can be resolved.

❧ Identifying the Interests

A necessary first step in the analysis is to identify the various stakeholders. Dementia is a problem not only for the affected person but also impinges on family and other informal caregivers, formal caregivers, commercial providers of goods and services, and society as a whole. Each of these groups can be seen as a stakeholder group, but it is important to remember that there may be differing interests even within such a group.

The interests of persons with early or moderate AD may differ from the interests of those in later stages, and the interests of family members actually caring for persons with dementia may differ from the interests of those who do not.

For the moment, I will allow myself to bracket that problem in order to identify the main potential conflicts of interests between the different stakeholder groups.

Persons with Moderate or Severe Alzheimer Disease

For persons who are presently suffering from moderate or severe Alzheimer disease, it is unlikely that any current research into the disease process or pharmacological means of alleviating symptoms will be able to produce results that can be introduced into clinical practice within their lifetime or before their condition progresses so far that they are outside the range of any possible treatment. As a group, these persons are therefore unlikely to benefit from research into these areas. Future members of the group will probably benefit, but we have no a priori reasons to believe that the interests of present patients are connected with the interests of future patients in any strong sense (see above).

Given the genetic component in Alzheimer's dementia, it could be argued that this group nevertheless does have a direct interest in preventive and curative research, not because they themselves will benefit but because their children and other relatives will benefit. This argument may be valid for the small group of patients with early onset dementia where there is a strong genetic component, but it is of questionable strength when it comes to the much larger group of elderly people with dementia. The interest of this group of persons with respect to research topics will primarily be various kinds of palliative interventions aimed at improving their quality of life during the further progression of their disease.

With regard to research methods, the interests of this group will be to have the research performed in a way that causes the minimal amount of distress or confusion and thereby interferes as little as possible with their daily life. The cognitive impairments of persons with moderate to severe dementia entails that they are less likely to be able to understand the meaning of interventions that interfere with their body or disrupt their daily routines and that they are therefore much more likely to be distressed by such interventions than normal, adult, competent persons.

Informal Caregivers and Family Members

The interests of informal caregivers and other family members may not coincide with the interests of the persons with dementia themselves. As O'Brien, Pinch, Purtilo, and other contributors to this book have highlighted, caring for a person with dementia is time-consuming, emotionally draining, and may involve considerable expense. The informal caregivers may therefore have an interest in any kind of intervention that can reduce the strain of caring for their relatives with dementia.

Professional Caregivers

The interests of professional caregivers are, on the one hand, their professional interest in providing high-quality treatment and care and, on the other hand, their interest in a work environment that is not too stressful and demanding.

Commercial Interests

A number of industries have economic interests connected to the treatment and care of persons with dementia. These include the pharmaceutical industry, the nursing home and home-services industry, and the producers of various aids used in caring for those with dementia. All of these industries are working in competitive markets with a substantial degree of state involvement and control. This creates a two-pronged pressure to produce competitively priced products with a documented effectiveness and quality.

Most of the products marketed by these different industries are not "sold" directly to persons with dementia, but "sold" to caregivers or to society. The commercial interests may therefore be more aligned to the interests of these other groups than to the interests of persons with dementia.

In a recent overview of the ethical concerns in drug clinical trials in dementia, the authors point to the need for research on the psychosocial, familial, environmental, cultural, and community aspects of dementia to keep pace with the "scientific" (*sic*) and clinical developments in antidementia drug research (Issa, 2000). Haddad addresses some of these problems in chapter 21.

Society

Society itself has a strong interest in research that can either decrease the economic impact of dementia or decrease the suffering caused by dementia. These two interests are potentially in conflict.

Society also has a long-term interest in prevention and/or cure of dementia since that would presumably be the most effective way of reducing costs. Furthermore, society has an interest in the proper conduct of research in general, an interest that is pursued through the requirement for research ethics committee approval and other forms of regulation of biomedical research.

✿ Two Examples of Potential Conflict

All of the interests of the different stakeholder groups outlined above are legitimate. These interests can come into conflict in many different ways, and while it is outside the scope of this chapter to try to describe and analyze all these potential conflicts, illustrative examples can be given. The following case highlights some of the conflicts that are important in the research situation and that center on the choice of research topic.

A pharmaceutical company is developing a drug that decreases the tendency to wander that characterizes many persons with moderate dementia (Algase, 1999). The drug is superior to common sedatives and neuroleptics since it does not cause general drowsiness or long-term side effects like tardive dyskinesias and does not seem to increase the number of falls (with the attendant risk of femoral and other fractures). The drug does, however, lead to some reduction in social interaction. Two large-scale controlled trials are being planned in order to gain conclusive evidence concerning clinical effectiveness and cost/benefit in the nursing home and home care population respectively.

In this example, the drug targets a behavior or symptom that, while it is a major problem for carers, does not normally decrease the quality of life of most persons with dementia. The behavior is a problem that also creates costs in the nursing home sector because of the staff resources necessary to control wandering, unless it is controlled by (the inappropriate) use of sedatives or neuroleptics.

Another example of potential conflict of interests focusing on choice of research methods occurs in research projects where two goals are pursued simultaneously, the first being to study the effectiveness of a given intervention and the second being to study its mode of action. If the study of the mode of action of the intervention involves invasive or distressing research procedures, it may well be, on the one had, in the interest of the persons with dementia to have the effectiveness studied and, on the other hand, against their interests to have the mode of action studied. However, the study of the mode of action is clearly in the interests of the developers of the treatment.

☙ Resolving Conflicts of Interest within the Current Research Ethics Paradigm

In the current research ethics paradigm as it is laid down in international declarations and conventions and in national regulations of biomedical research, there are three (or in some cases, four) actors involved in the chain of decisions leading to the participation or nonparticipation of a specific incompetent person with dementia in a specific research project. These actors are the research ethics committee that evaluates the project; the institution (e.g., a nursing home) that decides whether or not to participate in the project (this is especially relevant for institutionalized persons with dementia); the proxy decision maker who gives or withholds consent; and the person with dementia who gives or withholds assent (except in cases of very severe dementia, where not even assent or dissent may be possible).

None of these actors—except, in certain circumstances, the institutions—are proactive initiators or designers of research. Each acts in a reactive mode, responding to individual research projects that have been designed by others. They are therefore able only in an indirect way to promote their own research interests or the interests of the persons with dementia. Even this indirect way of promoting interests is circumscribed in the case of research ethics committees since in general they are unable to disallow research projects with legitimate purposes within the scope of the regulations, and, as seen above, the regulations may allow research that is not clearly in the interest of the persons with dementia. Given the multiplicity of interests, it is also unlikely that the other actors (e.g., the institutions and the proxies) will always consistently make decisions based only on the interests of the persons with dementia.

We thus can see that the current research ethics paradigm cannot ensure that the right research topics and the right research methodologies are chosen. It has been argued above that, for many people with dementia, their main needs are palliative, and that seems to indicate that a substantial part of the research in this field should be directed toward palliative interventions. In the future, we therefore need to consider some mechanism other than research ethics committees for ensuring that research in the context of moderate to severe dementia is directed toward palliative interventions that are in the interest of those with this condition. In the interim, it is important that members of research ethics committees considering proposals for dementia research are knowledgeable about the specific features of this condition. At least, then, oversight of research methodologies will be knowledgeably performed.

REFERENCES

Algase, D. L. (1999). Wandering: A dementia-compromised behavior. *Journal of Gerontological Nursing, 25,* 10–16.

Council of Europe. (1997). Convention for the protection of human rights and dignity of the human being with regard to the application of biology and medicine: Convention on human rights and biomedicine. Oviedo, Spain, April 4, 1997. European Treaty Series No. 164.

Fratiglioni, L., De Ronchi, D., & Aguero Torres, H. (1999). Worldwide prevalence and incidence of dementia. *Drugs and Aging, 15,* 365–375.

Issa, A. M., & Keyserlingk, E. W. (2000). Current and future clinical trials for Alzheimer's disease: Evolving ethical concerns. *Progress in Neuro-Psychopharmacology & Biological Psychiatry, 24,* 1229–1247.

Neal, M., & Briggs, M. (2000). Validation therapy for dementia, *Cochrane Database Systematic Review, 2,* CD001394.

World Medical Association. (2000). *World Medical Association Declaration of Helsinki: Ethical principles for medical research involving human subjects.* Adopted by the 18th WMA General Assembly, Helsinki, Finland, June 1964, and amended by the 29th WMA General Assembly, Tokyo, Japan, October 1975; 35th WMA General Assembly, Venice, Italy, October 1983; 41st WMA General Assembly, Hong Kong, September 1989; 48th WMA General Assembly, Somerset West, Republic of South Africa, October 1996, and the 52nd WMA General Assembly, Edinburgh, Scotland, October 2000.

CHAPTER TWENTY-ONE

Drugs and Dementia

Pharmacotherapy and Decision Making
by Primary Caregivers

Amy M. Haddad, R.N., Ph.D.

The overall aim of this chapter is to review the literature regarding the experiences of primary caregivers (i.e., family members who care for a person with Alzheimer disease) and decisions about drug therapy. Specifically, the purpose is to describe the experience of acetylcholinesterase inhibitor (AChEI) therapy of primary caregivers of persons with Alzheimer disease (AD), outline the inherent ethical issues that are part of drug therapy decisions, and suggest areas for future, empirical research.

Since there is no cure, the primary goals when treating patients with probable AD are enhancing independence and functional abilities and maintaining quality of life for patients and caregivers. Presently, there is only one group of drugs on the market that hold potential for amelioration of the symptoms of AD (i.e., acetylcholinesterase inhibitors, or AChEIs). So far, in the United States four AChEI drugs have been approved by the Food and Drug Administration for use in AD (i.e., tacrine, donepezil, rivastigmine, and galantamine). Of these, the last three have some advantages in that they can be given once daily and produce fewer side effects. All of these drugs have demonstrated some beneficial effects, albeit modest and unsustainable. At their best, these drugs could be classified as an intermediate type of antidementia drug. Intermediate drugs both improve decreased cognitive functioning and slow the rate of progression of dementia to some extent (Hirai, 2000). A drug that would completely arrest the progression of dementia is the ultimate goal, but the ideal drug is not yet available. It is unlikely that one class of drug will ever provide a cure for diseases as complex as AD, and patients and families must settle for drugs that work for some patients with varying degrees of benefit but that will not appreciably change the trajectory of the disease (Moghul & Wilkinson, 2001).

Little empirical evidence exists to understand the varied experiences that patients and caregivers have with drug therapy decisions and AD. The unique nature of the disease, its impact on patients and families, the limited treatment options, and the action of AChEIs combine to produce numerous questions about decision making and drug therapy. For example: How do these primary caregivers identify and weigh the benefits and burdens of pharmacotherapy in AD? What do they expect will happen? Does hope play a role in drug decisions and AD? What factors impinge on decisions about drug therapy (e.g., caregiver factors such as age, education, work status, relationship to the patient, the care setting; factors in the patient, such as quality of life, drug side effects, severity of dementia, functional abilities, age; and cost of medication)? How do primary caregivers monitor the effectiveness of AChEI therapy when no specific marker exists? What sorts of ethical problems are involved in decisions about drug therapy?

To provide partial answers to these questions, a review of the literature in three major areas follows: (1) decision making and AChEI therapy; (2) factors influencing primary caregivers' decisions; and (3) ethical issues and pharmacotherapy. However, before exploring the literature, some background information on AChEI therapy is necessary.

Acetylcholinesterase Inhibitors

Pharmacotherapy may benefit some patients with AD. During the last two decades, biomedical research on the neurobiology of AD has led to a profusion of pharmacological treatments. The most established and investigated of these are the cholinergic drug treatments (Davies & Maloney, 1976). The discovery of severe cholinergic cell loss in the basal forebrain has been the rationale behind a group of drugs designed to potentiate central cholinergic function (Bartus et al., 1982). Four AChEI drugs are currently approved by the FDA for treating AD: tacrine (Cognex®), donepezil (Aricept®), rivastigmine (Exelon®), and galantamine hydrobromide (Reminyl®). All four drugs increase the effective amount of acetylcholine available at the cholinergic receptor by binding at post-synaptic cholinergic receptors. "This prevents hydrolysis and increases the availability of acetylcholine, which is thought to prevent or slow memory loss" (Hanson & Galvez-Jimenez, 2000, p. 443). The overall possible action of these drugs is that of maintaining nerve signals. However, they are a chemically diverse group of drugs, which vary in mechanism of action and specificity for brain acetylcholinesterase.

It should be emphasized that the effectiveness of all four drugs declines as the disease progresses and fewer cholinergic neurons remain functionally intact. The most common effects are on cognition and function (Morris et al., 1998). AChEIs probably have no effect on the underlying pathological process that occurs in AD. A summary of reported pharmacological effects are (1) amelioration of the disease in the form of slowing or sometimes temporarily or partially reversing cognitive decline; (2) delay in nursing home placement; (3) improvement of behavioral disturbances such as anxiety, apathy, hallucinations, and motor restlessness; and (4) the patient's increased ability to perform activities of daily living such as dressing or being able to feed oneself (Daly, 1999). Long-term studies for periods longer than a year (up to 4.5 years) suggest that in the presence of the drug, benefit differences can be maintained in a number of patients (Giacobini, 2000).

A certain percentage of patients do not respond to AChEIs. A small percentage of patients with AD actually do worse on AChEIs, in that they become more agitated or depressed or have side effects severe enough to warrant discontinuation of the drug. In clinical trials, compared with those in the group taking placebo, two to three times as many people taking active treatment experienced adverse events sufficient to lead to withdrawal from the study (Wilcock, 2000). Depending on when AChEIs therapy is discontinued, there is a decline to the nontreatment level of cognition. Because of this, families may believe that discontinuing the drug causes the patient's condition to worsen, when in fact interruption of drug treatment allows the disease to progress to the same level as those who did not receive drug treatment. Given the modest benefit that these drugs provide and family concerns regarding "causing" a decline in their loved one's cognitive abilities, there is very little incentive to discontinue the drugs. AChEIs could thus be thought of as a pharmaceutical manufacturer's dream in that they will be prescribed for the remainder of the patient's life (Garber, 2001).

❧ Decision Making and AChEIs

Even though the benefits from AChEIs therapy may be modest, drugs that hold the promise of stabilizing or retarding the cognitive decline of AD are ardently desired on the part of patients, caregivers, and health professionals. Furthermore, "the current emphasis on medications not only reflects advances in neuroscience and pharmaceutical marketing, but also results from a reliance on technology that has expanded to the point where patients [and caregivers] and physicians think nothing is being done if a pill is not prescribed" (Filley, Chapman, & Dubovsky, 1996, p. 204). Thus, we have a situation in which there is no cure for a disease with a devastating pathology, desperate need for relief from the symptoms of the disease, overburdened family caregivers, and a society with a predilection for drug use. Some have suggested that AChEI therapy is really just a way to help patients and particularly family members cope with this devastating diagnosis: "Acetylcholinesterase inhibitors might be compared with treating the symptoms of a growing brain tumor with aspirin. While aspirin can in fact help with some symptoms, the underlying tumor is unaffected and remains terminal. The inhibitors do not affect the underlying progression of neuronal loss in AD, but they may have a preventive capacity that will help society navigate the AD crisis" (Post, 1999, p. 106).

At the advent of AChEI therapy, numerous questions were raised about the appropriate use of a drug that appeared to reverse some of the cognitive decline associated with AD, but did not alter the ultimate outcome of the disease. For example, there were concerns about whether there would be pressure from family caregivers to take the medication even if there were unpleasant side effects, since the patient's behavior would be more acceptable. Furthermore, there were questions about whether or not it was right to restore memory to people when one result might be their increased awareness of decline (both previous and eventual decline) in cognitive ability.

Anecdotal accounts of unexpected negative effects from the drugs began to appear in the literature. These negative effects cannot really, in the true clinical sense, be called side effects in the way that nausea, vomiting, anorexia, or diarrhea are; rather, families found themselves weighing the positive aspects, such as improved memory and the ability of the patient to perform basic activities of daily living such as dressing and eating, against the negative effects of agitation or depression. The decision is more difficult than it appears. Primary caregivers spend considerable time, up to three hours a day on average, handling difficult and often inappropriate behavioral symptoms such as wandering or delusions, which add to levels of caregiver stress (Teri, 1997). Thus, any assistance in minimizing such behaviors is highly desirable. Furthermore, it is sometimes difficult to tell if the drugs are working or not, yet there is a reluctance on the part of primary caregivers to discontinue the drug because of fears about "plummeting" or causing the patient to "crash" to a lower level of functioning. The following cases illustrate some of the more subtle problems associated with decisions about these drugs.

Case 1. At age fifty-seven, Mr. A was diagnosed with probable AD. At age sixty-two, he began taking one of the AChEIs, first as part of an experimental study, then on open-label treatment for three years. During this time, his rate of deterioration appeared to slow, and he remained physically robust. He could no longer participate in any meaningful social or occupational activities, but because he could still carry out basic self-care, the family could not bring themselves to consider placement outside the home. The emotional drain on the family in providing continuous supervision and protection from injury was profound, as was the effect of interacting constantly with someone who was not the same person as before and could not reciprocate in any significant way. As the problems with interacting with the patient gradually progressed, he became more irritable and resistant to directives from the family. However, the family continued to hope that the medication might one day reverse his deterioration. (Filley, Chapman, & Dubovsky, 1996, p. 203)

Case 2. Mrs. D, aged fifty-eight, has AD at a severe stage. AChEI therapy was prescribed to improve cognition. After three months of therapy, the daughter, the primary caregiver, reports that "the therapy made a substantial improvement in memory and intelligence. She understands all the things I show her, but now that she is aware of her physical state says that she is nothing." The daughter confirms that the patient is frequently depressed, but that attention, cooperativeness, and autonomy in basic activities is considerably improved. (Bianchetti & Trabucchi, 1999, p. 913)

Case 3. Ms. W. describes the case of her mother-in-law, Ms. J., who had previously been well-adjusted to the routine in her nursing home. She was in a relatively benign state emotionally and seemed to be enjoying the art and music programs, in which she participated actively. After beginning Aricept®, however, Ms. J. regained insight into her situation. For example, she remembered that she did not want to be in a nursing home and insisted that she be allowed to leave. She also refused to participate in the support programs because the participants are "too slow for me." Ms. J. appeared to be a well-adjusted AD patient (i.e., she was no longer anxious about her losses and reasonably happy while living more or less in the pure present). After this successful early period in the nursing home, however, she is now noncompliant and resentful of the circumstances. This is disruptive for Ms. J., her family, and the nursing home. If she is allowed to leave, she will soon again reach the level of incapacitation that justified her initial nursing home placement. (Post & Whitehouse, 1998, p. 785)

Case 4. If Mr. L. had sought out diagnosis and treatment when his symptoms first appeared, his story might have turned out differently. As it was, by the time his wife forced him to see his family physician, Mr. L. had many of the symptoms of mild-moderate AD. The family physician was not completely sure what was wrong with Mr. L., but he did recommend nursing home placement to try to assist the exhausted Mrs. L. Several years later, the first AChEI, tacrine, became available. Although he had been managed with psychotropic drugs in the nursing home when he was agitated, no other drugs had been available to treat what the family physician now suspected was AD. By this time, Mr. L. was in the moderate to severe stage of the disease. Tacrine was approved for use in the early stages of AD, but the family physician reasoned, "What could it hurt to try it." Mrs. L. was in favor of trying anything if her husband would only recognize her again. She was somewhat concerned about the cost of the medication, but if it worked then it would be worth it. After a month of drug therapy, there was no appreciable change in Mr. L., and only mild side effects. However, when Mrs. L. asked about discontinuing the drug, her physician said, "I'm afraid that might do serious harm." So the drug was continued until Mr. L. died from a respiratory infection.

These cases highlight the kinds of decisions that family members face when initiating or discontinuing AChEI therapy. Some of the problems are the same as those encountered with other types of drug therapy (i.e., off-label usage and misinformation about the efficacy of the drug in question). However, there are really no other diseases or classes of drugs like AD and AChEI therapy. Antipsychotic drugs do change the mental state of psychotic patients, but, unlike AD, mental illness due to schizophrenia is more like a chronic disease than a terminal one. In addition, if antipsychotics are taken routinely, the patient can be stabilized as long as the drugs continue. Even with complete compliance, patients who take an AChEI drug will continue to decline, but at a slower rate. With AChEI therapy, patients (when they are able) and primary caregivers are asked to make difficult, if not impossible, trade-offs. "Thus temporary improvements of some months duration [or years] may or may not enhance quality of life for patients or caregivers" (Post & Whitehouse, 1998, p. 784).

❧ Factors Influencing Primary Caregivers' Decisions

Another aspect of AD sets it apart from other categories of diseases and other types of drug therapy. Individuals with probable AD suffer a gradual and inexorable decline over a prolonged period of time, much of which is spent in the community, where typically they are cared for by family members (Wimblad & Wimo, 1999). As cognitive impairment progresses, family members assume important decision-making roles to a greater degree than in other chronic conditions (Forbes, Bern-Klug, & Gessert, 2000). Although it is possible, and ethically required, that a person in the early stages of the disease be involved in decision making about treatment, AChEIs are prescribed off-label at all points along the continuum of the disease. So even if a person with probable AD was involved in the initial decision involving drug therapy, there will come a time when he or she will have to rely on a surrogate decision maker to make choices about continuing or discontinuing drug therapy. Furthermore, drug therapy for persons with AD is not just for the patient, as the cases illustrate. As several other chapters in this book have illustrated, it is difficult to disentangle the well-being of the person with AD from that of the primary caregiver or caregivers.

Compared with the amount we know about the mechanism of action and pharmacology of AChEIs (and it is extensive), very little is known about surrogates' perception of, understanding of, and experience with decisions about these drugs. Most of the caregiver research in AD has focused on issues such as caregiver burden and the many forms it takes (Cohen et al., 1990; Parks & Pilisuk, 1991; Teri, 1997). Most of the clinical trials with AD patients have focused on outcome measures concerned solely with the patient (Rogers et al., 1998; Wilkinson, 2001). However, more and more studies have shifted the focus to the affect of AChEIs on caregiver burden (Fillit, Gutterman, & Brooks, 2000; Gauthier, 1999). In the study by Fillit and colleagues, the caregivers of patients taking donepezil reported significantly lower levels of subjective distress or difficulty with respect to their caregiving activities compared with individuals who cared for patients not taking this drug (2000, p. 397). Gauthier and colleagues in a poster presentation noted overall improvement in caregiver burden with donepezil treatment over a four-month period (Gauthier, 1999). Since caregiver burden is one of the principal predictors of institutionalization among elderly patients with dementia, the impact of AChEI therapy on caregiver burden, usually evidenced in fatigue, depression, or illness, is particularly important.

The primary caregiver plays a key role in the decision to start drug therapy, monitor its effectiveness, and decide whether or not to continue. Unlike professional knowledge, caregiver knowledge has its roots in the experience of an illness (Helman, 1994; Williams & Popay, 1994). Thus, a failure to acknowledge primary caregivers' understanding of their role in decision making about these medications is an important oversight.

Finally, in addition to mitigating some of the burden of caregiving, there may be a more compelling reason to decide to use AChEI therapy. This reason was alluded to in the quote previous cited from Post: "they may have a preventive capacity that will help society navigate the AD crisis." AChEI therapy may be more than preventive; it may be a source of hope to primary caregivers. Both clinicians and researchers have described hope as contributing to the quality of life and affecting the course of the disease/disorder (Farran, Herth, & Popovich, 1995). In his book *The Psychology of Hope*, Stotland (1969) stresses the importance of hope to humankind and says that humans try to cling to, restore, and protect hope when it becomes threatened. It is possible that AChEI therapy, with its modest benefits and in spite of its troubling negative effects, may give primary caregivers something to cling to even with a hopeless diagnosis like AD.

Although no studies were found in the literature dealing with hope and AD, there are some possible corollaries between AD and recurrent cancer in that both present a fairly dire prognosis. Ballard et al. (1997) noted that patients with recurrent cancer drew hope from faith and that the hope of these patients was different than that of newly diagnosed cancer patients. Other factors have been shown to influence hope in cancer patients such as marital status, length of illness, income level, job responsibilities, and being active in one's own care (Herth, 1992). Do primary caregivers of patients with AD view hope in the same way as patients with cancer or are there differences?

A concept that is similar to hope is expectation. What do primary caregivers of patients with AD expect will happen in the course of the disease and how will the drugs have an impact on this? In a panel discussion regarding slowing the progression of AD at the time the first AChEIs were introduced, Whitehouse, one of the panelists, raised the issue of family expectations and the possible impact that this could have on decision making, "It might be interesting to ask those families what their expectations were for slowing progression of the disease. One wants to make sure that in the spirit of informed consent they actually have a sense of what you are trying to do and what that might mean. Slowing the progression of the disease is a magic term. It is a very linguistically powerful concept. I think that we have to dissect what we mean" (General discussion, 1997, p. S37). Expectations are shaped by many things, including personal experience with AD, media representation of persons with AD, and information provided by health professionals and support organizations such as the Alzheimer's Association.

Once again, there is a paucity of research about the expectations of primary caregivers and the impact these expectations might have on decision making. However, a recent survey study conducted by the Alzheimer's Association in the United States indirectly addressed the expectations of family members. The survey found large gaps between what caregivers, on the one hand, and physicians, on the other, say they discussed on treatment and caregiving issues when family members were first diagnosed with AD:

> Fifty seven percent of caregivers said they wanted information about what to expect as the disease progressed, only 38 percent said they received such information. But 83 percent of physicians said they do provide information on the progression of the disease to caregivers. Forty-six percent of caregivers said they wanted information about medications and what to expect from them, 41 percent of caregivers said they actually received information, but 91 percent of physicians said they talked to caregivers about the issue (Alzheimer's Association, 2001).

The differences between what physicians believe they discuss and what families hear is its own problem, but what is an important finding from this survey is that families wanted to know what to expect. Unbundling what *expect* means to these families and how it differs from or is an adjunct to hope remains unexplored.

❧ Ethical Issues

Many of the ethical problems that pharmacotherapy and the treatment of AD raise can be easily accommodated by well-established principles of ethics such as doing good and avoiding harm. "Clearly one has a duty to do good to patients in the widest possible sense: not just improve their scores on cognitive tests (although that in itself can be counted as a good), but also improve things more globally. The good of others needs balancing in the equation, but not at the cost of doing harm" (Hughes, 2000, p. 539). But how is good defined? Do AChEIs provide enough good to outweigh the negative effects of the drugs?

The strongest argument in favor of using AChEIs, unless there are severe side effects, is the effect it has on cognitive and functional abilities, thus decreasing the amount of time in long-term care institutions and thus lowering the costs of care overall. However, the burden for care is shifted to the family. Is this shift in the setting of care worth it? In a study by Small, Donohue, & Brooks (1998), a comparison was made between patients (N=376) receiving donepezil for AD versus nontreatment (matched for basic demographics and severity of disease). In the treatment group, direct medical costs were calculated to include physician visits, emergency department use, hospital stays, drug costs, institutionalization, and support services such as nursing visits. The only significant difference in resource use between the two groups occurred in the rate of institutionalization— lower in the treatment group. There was no significant difference in total direct medical costs between the two groups.

Additionally, slowing the progression of the disease does not always mean that the quality of life is enhanced for the patient. "An antidementia drug may keep a patient out of a nursing home for a period of time and possibly save money, but this may not benefit him or her emotionally or cognitively" (Post et al., 1997, p. 27). Thus, we keep returning to the central ethical issue involved in decisions about AChEIs therapy, the balancing of the goods and harms between patients and families.

To further complicate the issue, families may be willing to preserve whatever level there is to preserve, or may even push for it, often far further than the patient would have wanted or health professionals would deem appropriate. The prolongation of morbidity in AD would need strong ethical justification, given the helpless position of the patient.

Another ethical issue concerns the harms that result for the patient when he or she has to live through decline and loss more than once. If AChEIs are used appropriately—that is, for the early stages of AD—then patients and their caregivers need not live through the difficult stages of AD twice. However, physicians retain the right to prescribe off-label, and so the odds are high that patients in the advanced stages of AD will receive the drugs and that they and their families will have to readjust to losses and cognitive decline. Some have argued that readjustment and even some depression are a small price to pay to slow the progression of AD: "We believe that because the patient lives through the same decline twice or regains awareness of the disease should not be reasons to limit the use of new antidementia drugs; rather we should increase our attention to patient quality of life and needs so that all strategies to reduce discomfort are explored" (Bianchetti & Trabucchi, 1999, p. 913). How primary caregivers decide to balance potential goods and harms in the area of drug therapy and AD remains to be explored.

✿ Suggestions for Future Research

An exploration of primary caregivers' experience with drug decisions should be undertaken as an initial attempt to broaden understanding of this phenomenon. Why focus on primary caregivers? Because they are the ones who deal with the outcomes of drug therapy and the ones most intimately connected to the person with AD. Their viewpoints regarding these drugs and the impact the drugs have on their lives are significant for the formulation of meaningful interventions and teaching strategies.

Information from primary caregivers will help us to understand the experience of drug therapy designed to slow down the cognitive decline in AD. A quantitative/qualitative design would be most appropriate for the complex phenomenon of drug therapy decisions. With a proper understanding of the experience of caregivers and drug therapy, we can formulate hypotheses for health care interventions, for patients and for family members, to assist them in the struggle with AD and in turn promote their well-being.

REFERENCES

Alzheimer's Association. (2001). Caregiver/physician survey. www.alz.org/intranet/insite/abtassoc/awareness/release/relintro.htm (accessed March 2001).

Ballard, A., Green, T., McCaa, A., & Logsdon, M. C. (1997). A comparison of the level of hope in patients with newly diagnosed and recurrent cancer. *Oncology Nursing Forum, 24* (5), 899–904.

Bartus, R. D., Dean, R. L., III, Beer, B., & Lippa, A. S. (1982). The cholinergic hypothesis of geriatric memory dysfunction. *Science, 217,* 408–417.

Bianchetti, A., & Trabucchi, A. (1999). Ethical problems in the use of antidementia drugs. *Journal of the American Geriatrics Society, 47* (7), 913.

Cohen, D., Luchins, D., Eisdorfer, C., Paveza, G., Ashford, J. W., Gorlick, P., et al. (1990). Caring for relatives with Alzheimer's disease: The mental health risks to spouses, adult children, and other family caregivers. *Behavior, Health and Aging, 1,* 171–182.

Daly, M. P. (1999). Diagnosis and management of Alzheimer disease. *Journal of the American Board of Family Practice, 12* (5), 375–385.

Davies, P., & Maloney, A. J. F. (1976). Selective loss of central cholinergic neurons in Alzheimer's disease (letter). *Lancet, 2,* 1403.

Farran, C. J., Herth, K. A., & Popovich, J. M. (1995). *Hope and hopelessness: Critical clinical constructs.* Thousand Oaks, CA: Sage.

Filley, C. M., Chapman, M. M., & Dubovsky, S. L. (1996). Ethical concerns in the palliative drug treatment of Alzheimer's disease. *Journal of Neuropsychiatry, 8* (2), 202–205.

Fillit, H. M., Gutterman, E. M., & Brooks, R. L. (2000). Impact of donepezil on caregiving burden for patients with Alzheimer's disease. *International Psychogeriatrics, 12* (3), 389–401.

Forbes, S., Bern-Klug, M., & Gessert, C. (2000). End-of-life decision making for nursing home residents with dementia. *Image, 32* (3), 251–258.

Garber, K. (2001). An end to Alzheimer's? *Technology Review* (March), 70–77.

Gauthier, S. (1999). Managing expectations in the long-term treatment of Alzheimer's disease. *Gerontology, 45* (Suppl. 1), 33–38.

General discussion. (1997). Panel presentation. *Alzheimer Disease and Associated Disorders, 11* (Suppl. 5), S37–S39.

Giacobin, E. (2000). Cholinesterase inhibitor therapy stabilizes symptoms of *Alzheimer disease. Alzheimer Disease and Associated Disorders, 14* (Suppl. 1), S3–S9.

Hanson, M. R., & Galvez-Jimenez, N. (2000). Effective treatment of Alzheimer disease and its complications. *Cleveland Clinic Journal of Medicine, 67* (6), 441–448.

Helman, C. G. (1994). *Culture, health, and illness* (3rd ed.). Oxford, UK: Butterworth-Heinemann.

Herth, K. (1992). Abbreviated instrument to measure hope: Development and psychometric evaluation. *Journal of Advanced Nursing, 17,* 1251–1259.

Hirai, S. (2000). Alzheimer disease: Current therapy and future therapeutic strategies. *Alzheimer Disease and Associated Disorders, 14* (Suppl. 1), S11–S17.

Hughes, J. (2000). Ethics and the anti-dementia drugs. *International Journal of Geriatric Psychiatry, 15,* 538–543.

Moghul, S., & Wilkinson, D. (2001). Use of acetylcholinesterase inhibitors in Alzheimer's disease. *Expert Review of Neurotherapeutics, 1* (1), 61–69.

Morris, J. C., Cyrus, P. A., Orazem, J., Mas, J., Bieber, F., Ruzicka, B. B., et al. (1998). Metrifonate benefits cognitive, behavioral, and global function in patients with Alzheimer's disease. *Neurology, 50,* 1222–1230.

Parks, S. H., & Pilisuk, M. (1991). Caregiver burden: Gender and the psychological costs of caregiving. *American Journal of Orthopsychiatry, 61,* 501–509.

Post, S. G. (1999). Future scenarios for the prevention and delay of Alzheimer disease onset in high-risk groups: An ethical perspective. *American Journal of Preventive Medicine, 16* (2), 105–110.

Post, S. G., Beerman, B., Brodaty, H., Gaines, A. W., Gauthier, S. G., Geldmacher, D. S., et al. (1997). Ethical issues in dementia drug development: Position paper from the international working group on harmonization of dementia drug guidelines. *Alzheimer Disease and Associated Disorders, 11* (Suppl. 3), 26–28

Post, S. G., & Whitehouse, P. J. (1998). Emerging antidementia drugs: A preliminary view. *Journal of the American Geriatrics Society, 46* (6), 784.

Rogers, S. L., Farlow, M. R., Doody, R. S., Mohs, R., Friedhoff, L. T., & Donepezil Study Group. (1998). A 24-week, double-blind, placebo-controlled trial of donepezil in patients with Alzheimer's disease. *Neurology, 50,* 136–145.

Small, G. W., Donohue, J. A., & Brooks, R. L. (1998). An economic evaluation of donepezil in the treatment of Alzheimer's disease. *Clinical Therapeutics, 20* (4), 838–850.

Teri, L. (1997). Behavior and caregiver burden: Behavioral problems in patients with Alzheimer's disease and its association with caregiver distress. *Alzheimer's Disease and Associated Disorders, 11* (Suppl. 4), S35–S38.

Wilcock, G. K. (2000). Treatment for Alzheimer's disease. *International Journal of Geriatric Psychiatry, 15,* 562–565.

Wilkinson, D. (2001). Drugs for the treatment of Alzheimer's disease. *International Journal for Clinical Practice, 56* (2), 129–134.

Williams, G., & Popay, J. (1994). Lay knowledge and the privilege of experience. In J. Gabe, D. Kelleher, & G. Williams (Eds.), *Challenging medicine* (pp. 118–139). London: Routledge.

Winblad, B., & Wimo, A. (1999). Assessing the societal impact of acetylcholinesterase inhibitor therapies. *Alzheimer's Disease and Related Disorders, 13* (Suppl. 2), S9–S19.

The Declaration of Berg en Dal on Ethical Principles Guiding Palliative Care of Persons with Alzheimer's Disease

Preamble

Alzheimer's Disease presents a mounting challenge to caregivers and society at large. Palliative care is a promising interdisciplinary answer to this challenge. The following ethical principles are intended specifically to guide the provision of palliative care for persons with Alzheimer's Disease, while acknowledging that general ethical principles in health care apply equally.

1. Principle of Respect for Dignity

Persons with Alzheimer's Disease have human dignity irrespective of their capacities. In preserving the dignity of these persons with Alzheimer's Disease, we also acknowledge our own dignity. The dignity of persons with Alzheimer's Disease demands that we not exclusively mourn their losses, but also acknowledge and encourage their present abilities, while respecting their past and fostering their future opportunities.

2. Principle of Well Being

The well being of persons with Alzheimer's Disease must be thoroughly considered when planning and providing care.

3. Principle of Participation
Irrespective of their capacities, persons with Alzheimer's Disease should be enabled to participate as much as possible in their own care.

4. Principle of Equal Consideration
Structures of care must provide that the dignity and well being of caregivers of persons with Alzheimer's Disease are considered equally with the dignity and well being of the persons receiving this care.

5. Principle of Non-Abandonment
Persons with Alzheimer's Disease and their caregivers should be adequately supported and never abandoned.

6. Principle of Moderation
Care for persons with Alzheimer's Disease should be provided in the least intrusive and least restrictive yet adequate manner.

7. Principle of Proportionality
Care for persons with Alzheimer's Disease should be offered at the level of organizational complexity that is proportionate to the needs and concerns of the persons with Alzheimer's Disease and their caregivers.

Commentary on the Declaration
Jos V. M. Welie, M.MedS., J.D., Ph.D., and Bert Gordijn, Ph.D.

Palliative care is a major focus of treatment for the more than 12 million sufferers from Alzheimer disease worldwide. This condition is characterized by dramatic alterations in cognition, behavior and everyday activities of living. In recent years, a number of scholars have examined the ethical aspects surrounding the treatment of persons with Alzheimer disease as well as biomedical research of the disease itself and potential remedies (Berg, Karlinsky, & Lowy, 1991; Post, 1995; Nordenram, 1997; Post & Whitehouse, 1998). Notwithstanding significant diagnostic and therapeutical advances, most persons with Alzheimer disease still face an extended period of ever increasing debilitation in the final years of their lives. Yet clinicians, ethicists, and policymakers have only begun to examine the ethical concerns that arise in providing comfort care measures when the patient's downward course persists for a decade or more and takes its toll on patients, families, and society (Luchins & Hanrahan, 1993; Rhymes & McCullough, 1994; Bonnel, 1996; Filley, Chapman, & Dubovsky, 1996; Simard, 1999; Volicer, 2001).

In response to this void, an international and multidisciplinary research project was organized by the directors of the Center for Health Policy and Ethics at Creighton University Medical Center, Omaha, Nebraska, and the Department of Ethics, Philosophy, and History of Medicine at the University Medical Centre Nijmegen, the Netherlands. In the fall of 2001 and with the financial support of the Greenwall Foundation, New York, the participating scholars, representing eight countries and a variety of disciplines (including medicine, nursing, dentistry, pharmacy, bioethics, philosophy, theology, law, policy, and education) convened in the Dutch town of Berg en Dal (near the city of Nijmegen). One of the objectives of this working conference was to draft a declaration of ethical principles that can guide the provision of palliative care for persons with Alzheimer disease.

Scope of the Declaration

As is true of the research project overall, the Declaration of Berg en Dal specifically focuses on the provision of palliative care. It is not designed to cover all ethical principles that should guide care of persons with Alzheimer disease. In that regard, it differs from and is intended to complement existing declarations such as the 1994 Fairhill Guidelines, the legal rights of patients document developed by Alzheimer Europe, and similar ethical guidelines developed by the American Alzheimer's Association (Post & Whitehouse, 1994; Alzheimer Europe www.alzheimer-europe.org; Alzheimer's Association, 1988; Alzheimer's Association, 1997). The Preamble therefore concludes with the sentence that "general ethical principles in health care apply equally."

The Method Employed

The Declaration of Berg en Dal was developed in two steps. Initially, the twenty-two participants each drafted three ethical guidelines based on their own research and submitted them prior to the conference. Since each participant focused on a different aspect of palliative care for persons with Alzheimer disease, the net result was a long list of very diverse guidelines. During the working conference, the group forged out of this diversity a single, comprehensive document that would be acceptable to all. In order to achieve this goal, the authors of this commentary developed a fast-track decision-making tree.

During the first session, the conference participants determined that the Declaration of Berg en Dal should clarify morally important considerations and offer professional and lay caregivers a framework of basic ethical principles. Although it should focus on the care of persons with Alzheimer disease, consideration should be given as well to those giving care. Given the desire to guide the actual provision of care, the conference participants deemed it important to strive for succinctness. By outlining a concise set of primary ethical principles, foregoing more detailed instructions, the Declaration of Berg en Dal would also be germane to culturally, religiously, or politically diverse contexts. At the same time, the wording should leave no doubt that the document was intended to be normative, rather than descriptive.

In the second session, the conference participants divided into small groups, each of which selected the five most important guidelines, combining several draft guidelines where appropriate. In the third session, the draft document was scrutinized for clarity and comprehensiveness. After eliminating one paragraph about which consensus could not be attained, the remaining text of the Declaration of Berg en Dal was underwritten by all conference participants.

REFERENCES

Alzheimer's Association. (1997). *Ethical issues in dementia research.* Adopted by the Alzheimer's Association (U.S.A.) National Board of Directors, May 1997. Available online at www.alz.org/aboutus/overview/statements.htm#ethical

Alzheimer's Association. (1988). *Treatment of patients with advanced dementia.* Adopted by the Alzheimer's Association (U.S.A.) National Board of Directors, May 1988. Available on-line at www.alz.org/aboutus/overview/statements.htm#eatment

Alzheimer Europe: *Legal Rights.* (n.d.) Available on-line at www.alzheimer-europe.org

Berg, J. M., Karlinsky, H., Lowy, F. H. (1991). *Alzheimer's disease research: Ethical and legal issues.* Toronto: Carswell.

Bonnel, W. B. (1996). Not gone and not forgotten: A spouse's experience of late-stage Alzheimer's disease. *Journal of Psychosocial Nursing Mental Health Services, 34* (8), 23–27.

Filley, C. M., Chapman, M. M., & Dubovsky, S. L. (1996). Ethical concerns in the use of palliative drug treatment for Alzheimer's disease. *Journal of Neuropsychiatry and Clinical Neurosciences, 8* (2), 202–205.

Luchins, D. J., & Hanrahan, P. (1993). What is appropriate health care for end-stage dementia? *Journal of the American Geriatrics Society, 41* (1), 25–30.

Nordenram, G. (1997). *Dental care of patients with dementia: Clinical and ethical considerations.* Stockholm: Karolinska Institute.

Post, S. G. (1995). *The moral challenge of Alzheimer disease.* Baltimore: Johns Hopkins University Press.

Post, S. G., & Whitehouse, P. J. (1994). *Fairhill guidelines on ethics of the care of people with Alzheimer's disease: A clinical summary.* Available on-line at gitt.cwru.edu/ap_ethics.html

Post, S. G., & Whitehouse, P. J. (Eds.). (1998). *Genetic testing for Alzheimer disease: Ethical and clinical issues.* Baltimore: Johns Hopkins University Press.

Rhymes J. A., & McCullough L. B. (1994). Nonaggressive management of the illnesses of severely demented patients: An ethical justification. *Journal of the American Geriatrics Society, 42* (6), 686–687.

Simard, J. (1999). Making a positive difference in the lives of nursing home residents with Alzheimer disease: The lifestyle approach. *Alzheimer Disease and Associated Disorders, 13* (Suppl. 1), S67–S72.

Volicer, L. (2001). Management of severe Alzheimer's disease and end-of-life issues. *Clinics in Geriatric Medicine, 17* (2), 377–391.

Note: This document was prepared on behalf of the members of the European–U.S. Dialogue on Ethical Foundations of Palliative Care for Alzheimer's Disease during their working meeting in Berg en Dal, Netherlands, in September 2001. The membership consisted of the contributors to this volume and the volume's coeditors.

Framework for an Educational Module for Health Professionals

Richard L. O'Brien, M.D., and
Wim J. M. Dekkers, M.D., Ph.D.

Members of the European–U.S. Dialogue on Ethical Foundations of Palliative Care for Alzheimer's Disease, funded by the Greenwall Foundation, New York, met in Berg en Dal, Netherlands, for a working conference in the fall of 2001. One of the products they generated is a framework for a teaching and learning module to educate and sensitize professional caregivers. Recognizing their crucial role in the care of persons with Alzheimer disease (AD), the purpose is to assist health professions educators to adapt this framework to the specific needs of their students, either those enrolled in health professions schools or practicing health professionals seeking continuing education. It is readily adaptable to interdisciplinary courses to facilitate team building in the care of persons with Alzheimer disease. Though specifically designed for health care professionals, it may also be adapted to the education of others involved in AD (e.g., health care administrators, bioethicists and philosophers, health policymakers, attorneys).

The framework is designed for structuring curricula that may be offered as short or extended courses designed for learners at varying levels of educational attainment. It is not a syllabus or an accumulation of teaching materials. Emphases, depth and breadth of presentations, material covered and specific pedagogical modalities will depend on the needs and abilities of educators and learners. Course content and structure also will vary depending on the time and budget available, the professional disciplines, level of knowledge and learning goals of participants, specific cultural patterns, and other relevant factors. References to useful resources should be easily found in this book or by a literature search.

Goal

Those who complete the course will understand the most important ethical aspects of palliative care for persons with AD, their families, and caregivers.

Objectives

Those who complete the course will be able to

- Describe AD and its different phases in general terms: genetics, pathology, behavioral patterns, prognosis, and treatment
- Describe the burden of AD on primary caregivers and the rewards of caregiving
- Describe the range of palliative care modalities relevant for patients with AD
- Analyze moral problems in the care of patients and their families
- Reflect on their technical and ethical performances on behalf of persons with AD
- Reflect on their moral sensibility and attitude as they apply to selected cases
- Reflect on relevant societal norms and values including solidarity and distributive justice
- Collaborate in care for persons with AD and caregivers
- Compare and contrast traditional bioethical principles with the principles of caring described in the Declaration of Berg en Dal on Ethical Principles Guiding Palliative Care of Persons with Alzheimer's Disease
- Interpret and apply the principles of the Declaration of Berg en Dal

Content

I. *Introduction: Palliative care*

At the present time, the care of patients with AD is necessarily palliative. Given the current state of knowledge and the modes of treatment, the only possible therapeutic goals are relief of symptoms, a comforting environment, and relief of the stress of AD on patients and caregivers. We adopted the definition of palliative care of the World Health Organization (*Cancer Pain Relief and Palliative Care,* Report of a WHO Expert Committee, Technical Report Series, No. 804, 1990; also available at www.who.int/dsa/justpub/cpl.htm; accessed January 2003).

WHO definition of palliative care

Palliative care is the active total care of patients whose disease is not responsive to curative treatment. Control of pain, of other symptoms, and of psychological, social and spiritual problems is paramount. The goal of palliative care is achievement of the best possible quality of life for patients and their families. Many aspects of palliative care also are applicable earlier in the course of the illness, in conjunction with . . . [other] treatment. Palliative care

- affirms life and regards dying as a normal process;
- neither hastens nor postpones death;
- provides relief from pain and other distressing symptoms;
- integrates the psychological and spiritual aspects of patient care;
- offers a support system to help patients live as actively as possible until death;
- offers a support system to help the family cope during the patient's illness and in their own bereavement.

[Specific disease treatments] have a place in palliative care, provided that the symptomatic benefits of treatment clearly outweigh the disadvantages. Investigative procedures are kept to a minimum. (www.who.int/cancer/palliative/definition/eu)

II.   Understanding AD

- The nature of the disease—pathology and pathophysiology
- Symptoms and complications—Variability
- Cognitive impairment and retained functions
- Progression and outcomes
- Available therapies
- Current research directions—Hope for the future
- Patients' experiences of AD
- Family and professional caregivers' experiences of AD

- Vulnerability, fragility, suffering, finiteness
- Language sensitivity in the daily care for persons with AD

III.   Needs of patients, family, and caregivers

- Intellectual, emotional, and physical comfort
- Independence and expressions of autonomy
- Safe and comfortable environment
- Socialization and social support
- Religious and spiritual support
- Meaningful life
- Well informed and trained caregivers (for patients and caregivers)
- Respite care (for caregivers)

IV.   Family and societal responsibilities

- Distributive justice
  legitimate claims of AD sufferers and caregivers on society
- Solidarity
- Research
  genetics, prevention, diagnosis, treatment, pathogenesis
  economics and sociology
  theological/philosophical reflection

V.   The person of the caregiver

- Moral sensibility and attitude of caregivers
- How health care professional caregivers view their contribution to the welfare of patients
- The idea of a good life and good death
- Palliative care as part of a good life
- Does palliative care contribute to the welfare of caregivers?
- Virtue ethics; Important personal (moral) qualities (virtues)
- Accounting for one's actions
- Narrative ethics

VI.   Principles of caring

- Respect for dignity
- Preservation of well-being

- Participation
- Equal consideration of caregivers and patients
- Nonabandonment
- Moderation
- Proportionality

VII.   *Ethical competencies for health professionals (these all derive from the Declaration of Berg en Dal; see appendix A)*

- Understand each individual patient's condition
- Understand each patient's and caregiver's specific needs
- Identify each patient's potential and assist the patient develop it
- Inform patients of the nature of the condition and what to expect
- Assist patients and caregivers prepare for disease progression and outcome
- Encourage patients, when they are competent, to plan for future contingencies
- Monitor each patient's progress and adjust the environment and circumstance to accommodate it
- Provide appropriate relief of physical and emotional symptoms
- Respect patients for their present selves and retained abilities
- Honor autonomy even when patients seem no longer able to make rational decisions
- Impose no inessential interventions that patients indicate they do not want
- Keep any restraints on a patient's activities to the minimum necessary to assure safety
- Attend to prevention of complications
- Enable surrogate decision makers to have all information relative to any decision they are asked to make
- Provide appropriate patient care for all health needs, but interventions that prolong dying, that do not add quality life, are not justified
- Attend to bereavement (prior to death)
- Assure appropriate spiritual care in all settings
- Assure cultural/ethnic sensitivity in treatment planning
- Monitor and address the well-being of caregivers (respite)
- Support and advocate on behalf of persons with AD and caregivers resources for care and research

- As possible and appropriate educate policymakers and the public about the nature of AD and the needs of patients and caregivers

Note: This document was prepared on behalf of the members of the European–U.S. Dialogue on Ethical Foundations of Palliative Care for Alzheimer's Disease during their working meeting in Berg en Dal, Netherlands, in September 2001. The membership consisted of the contributors to this volume and the volume's coeditors.

Index